BETWEEN DOCTORS AND PATIENTS

BETWEEN DOCTORS AND PATIENTS

The Changing Balance of Power

LILIAN R. FURST

UNIVERSITY PRESS OF VIRGINIA
Charlottesville and London

The University Press of Virginia
©1998 by the Rector and Visitors of the University of Virginia
All rights reserved
Printed in the United States of America

First published 1998

∞ The paper used in this publication meets the minimum requirements of the
American National Standard for Information Sciences—Permanence of Paper
for Printed Library Materials, ANSI Z 39.48-1984.

Library of Congress Cataloging-in-Publication Data

Furst, Lilian R.
    Between doctors and patients : the changing balance of power /
Lilian R. Furst.
        p.   cm.
    Includes bibliographical references and index.
    ISBN 0-8139-1755-7 (alk. paper)
    1. Physician and patient. 2. Physician and patient in literature. 3. Power (So-
cial sciences) I. Title.
R727.3.F89 1998
610.69'6.dc21   97-17695
                                                 CIP

CONTENTS

FOREWORD

$-\cdot-\cdot-\cdot-\cdot-\cdot-\cdot-\cdot-\cdot-\cdot-\cdot-\cdot-\cdot-\cdot-\cdot-$

POWER COMES EASILY TO DOCTORS, slipping into their lives as readily as they acquire the special language in medical school, as rapidly as they learn the proper placement of a stethoscope round their necks, as effortlessly as they don a white costume. During my twenty-nine years as a practicing surgeon I never yielded any of my power. I never shared my language or listened to the patient's language or asked a proper question: What does it feel like to have heart disease and to await surgery and suffer? I allowed no negotiation and no true communication. To do so would be to get involved, to drop my surgical mask, to feel the patient's pain, to yield power.

I first learned of the disparity of this power between doctor and patient when a friend repaired my not so simple inguinal hernia; my inclination was to be treated like any other patient, as I would treat any other patient. When I was awoken at three in the morning by the nurse to check my dressing and at six by my doctor, I quickly discovered that I did not enjoy being treated like any other patient. At six on the morning of one's discharge, who can conjure questions and what surgeon will take the time to listen?

My patients were cheated. They deserved more than my expertise in the operating room; they needed understanding, participation, and comfort. Simply put, psychologically and physiologically, patients do better when they are energetically engaged in their own care, when they share power. In retaining all the power in our relationships, I cheated not only my patients but also myself: I could have done better.

To be able to convey to me, twenty-nine years a clinical surgeon, what I have not understood about the practice of medicine might have been an impossible task for an academic embedded in a humanities department, even one so formidable as to hold an endowed chair in comparative literature at the University of North Carolina at Chapel Hill. Yet Lilian Furst manages this task very well indeed, with an exemplary clarity in her capacity to think and explain, grounded in a vast knowledge of literature and a profound appreciation of the practice of medicine, past as well as present.

To trace the origins and ramifications of the power relationships between doctor and patient, she interweaves the discourse of novels, documents, and essays from the nineteenth century to the present. She shows how the development of medicine as a science and the introduction of technical devices, starting with the stethoscope, have altered the balance of power between doctor and patient. She documents how changes in hospitals and laboratories have impinged on the connection between physician and patient. She writes of the effect of the arrival of students at the bedside and the advent of women into medical practice. She carries us into the current dilemmas of managed care, third parties, and health care providers, all insisting on intruding with their own power, always impacting, sometimes disrupting the doctor-patient relationship. And especially intriguing is the discussion of how vital language can be in the transaction of power between doctor and patient. We doctors can learn much here of medical history, of literature, and of the courtesy of power that our patients need from us. Most of all we can learn about ourselves.

LAWRENCE I ZAROFF, M.D.

PREFACE

— · — · — · — · — · — · — · — · — · — · — · — · — · — · — · — · — · —

Eᴛɪǫᴜᴇᴛᴛᴇ ᴀɴᴅ ᴘᴏᴡᴇʀ ᴀʀᴇ ᴛᴡᴏ concepts that seem to be contradictory, even mutually exclusive. Etiquette is the performance of a socially ordained ritual, a body of usages, forms, manners, and ceremonies prescribed by convention to regulate the behavior of individuals toward one another in a social or professional context. Power, by contrast, is more of an instinctual drive, the impulse to exert and impose one's will upon others. The conciliatory courtesies of etiquette are subverted and overruled by the controlling domination central to power.

But these two conflicting concepts do converge in the special code between doctor and patient. The etiquette governing communication in the professional consultation is at once stringent and delicate. The physician is empowered by virtue of knowledge, while the patient is submissive because of need. So the situation permits the probing of most intimate personal details by a person whom the patient may well never previously have seen (say, in a hospital), yet it predicates, too, a certain measure of consideration for the patient's privacy. Power may be exercised, but it has to be done with tact and respect.

Most of us have already had the experience of being patients, and almost all of us will before we finally die. We tend to accept the ruling etiquette between doctor and patient because we have been conditioned to it, and also because we can hardly envisage an alternative. Yet alternatives are even now being introduced through the expansion of managed health care, which undercuts the doctor's power through scrutiny, and possibly emendation of his or her decisions and recommendations by a fiscally potent extraneous agency. This rapidly growing new system, insofar as it modifies the directness of the doctor-patient interaction, forces us to reconsider the traditional etiquette of power. What is more, once we begin to ruminate and to investigate the issue from a historical perspective, we discover, perhaps to our surprise, that doctors' present ascendancy has by no means always been the norm any more than has their high social standing (and income). Before about the mid–eighteenth century, surgeons, as their association with barbers denotes, were regarded more as skilled tradesmen than as learned professionals. The beginnings of their rise to their present-day authority originated, without doubt, in the momentous scientific advances of the mid- to later nineteenth century such as germ theory, asepsis, and the introduction of various specifically effective remedies. Medicine's increasing capacity to cure, mitigate, and prevent the ravages of many diseases led to the elevation of physicians to a commanding position.

The development of modern medicine into a learned and prestigious profession has been amply chronicled, especially in recent years through the establishment of medical history as a distinctive field of scholarship. However, as I shall argue later, the patient is conspicuously missing from these accounts. Although an actively cooperative rapport between physician and patient is recognized as a positive factor in the healing process, relatively little attention has so far been paid to the historical evolution of this aspect.

One possible reason for this lacuna has been obliquely put forward by the medical historian John Harley Warner, who laments the "methodological difficulties inherent in determining what nineteenth-century physicians actually did at the bedside."[1] I propose that at least a partial solution to this difficulty can be found in literary works, rich documents for a humanistically oriented sociocultural history of medicine. The many vividly portrayed encounters between doctors and patients offer revealing insight into the etiquette of power and its changes over the past century and a half. Medical history can therefore be complemented by the analysis of literary works. Their testimony not only supplements the underlying data, endowing the skeleton of dates and statistics that provide the outline of medical history with substance—flesh, as it were. It also gives access to another kind of information, about the fabric of human relationships, and certainly about the position and role of medicine and physicians within particular cultures. Medical history concentrates on recording the advent of various diagnostic tools and therapeutic interventions, how they were discovered and when they were brought into use; however, my essay, in mapping cultural history in and through literature, is concerned mainly with the ways in which the predominant styles and beliefs of medical practice have affected the doctor-patient alliance.

Apart from these intellectual roots, this book also has personal ones. I am a frustrated physician. Both my parents graduated from medical school in Vienna and were passionately committed to their work. Since many of their friends were physicians too, I grew up on medical talk, which always fascinated me. The magazines that came into our house in my adolescence were the *Lancet,* the *British Medical Journal,* and the *British Dental Journal* (my father practiced dentistry, which had been a specialized branch of medicine in Austria). It never occurred to me that I would choose any profession other than medicine. So it was a shock to discover that my abilities lay in languages, not sciences. Eventually I found my appropriate niche in comparative literature, a happy choice for me. But my early interest in medicine never faded totally and was immediately rekindled in 1987 when I met Peter W. Graham, then associate editor of *Literature and Medicine,* who opened up this whole new field to me.

Also, as a result of my peripatetic life I have myself experienced quite disparate types of medical culture. Partly from memory but more from hearsay, I know of the conduct of practice in prewar Central Europe. In England after the war I witnessed the institution of the National Health Service and the transition from attendance by a family doctor to the prevalence of group practice and a multitiered organization in which socialized and private medicine coexisted uneasily. On coming to the United States I was exposed to yet another system, in which, to my considerable surprise, even patients with chicken pox went to the doctor's office. In recent years my rather bizarre medical history has provided me with more firsthand knowledge than I would have wished to have. This is not, however, a personal book except insofar as my experiences have raised my consciousness of the complexities of the etiquette between doctor and patient and have made me ponder and investigate the topic.

An earlier version of parts of chapter 3 appeared as "Struggling for Medical Reform in Middlemarch," *Nineteenth-Century Literature,* December 1993, 341–61.

The translation of citations is mine, and the italics or emphases are the authors'. Sources are given briefly in endnotes, keyed to a full bibliography at the end.

It is a pleasure to express my thanks for the significant support I have received in this endeavor. The National Endowment for the Humanities awarded me a fellowship during 1994–95 that enabled me to write a first draft. The Stanford Humanities Center in the summers of 1991 through 1996 granted me the visiting-scholar status that gave me access to the Green Humanities and Social Sciences Library and the Lane Medical Library. In a number of long conversations at crucial junctures, Peter W. Graham encouraged me by his enthusiasm and helped me with his valuable suggestions. Equally important to me were my good friends Stephen and Madeline Levine, who let me indulge in "shoptalk" and try out my ideas at several relaxed brunches at their house. My colleagues in the University of North Carolina's psychoanalytic theory seminar James L. Peacock III and William J. Peck brainstormed one afternoon over coffee to produce a starter reading list. My research assistants, Véronique Machelidon, Ian Wilson, Melissa Moorehead, and Kristin Daly, successively provided willing legs. I am much indebted to Jürgen Buchenau as well as to Susan Groag Bell and Edith Gelles for discussion of historians' methodologies. Jürgen Buchenau was also most generous in sharing with me his computer expertise. My former student Ester Zago read an early version of the first two-thirds of the manuscript and let me have the benefit of her astute judgment and honest criticism. Mark G. Perlroth, M.D., of Stanford Medical Center, kindly gave me valuable bibliographical information. Last but by no means least, Stephen M. Ford, M.D., of Duke Medical Center, has sustained and supported me through his interest and his humane as well as professional caring.

BETWEEN DOCTORS AND PATIENTS

1.

"THE DOCTOR KNOWS BEST"

Knowledge itself is power.—FRANCIS BACON

THE DOCTOR KNOWS BEST" is a watchword that not only acknowledges and endorses the physician's entitlement to power but also implies the etiquette between doctor and patient that buttresses and validates that power.

In the late twentieth century, convention endows the physician with extensive powers while relegating the patient to relative powerlessness. This imbalance is to some extent the natural outcome of the predicament or crisis that instigates the encounter. Patients are likely to be disturbed, probably anxious, about symptoms that, at best, are disrupting their lives through discomfort or pain or, at worst, may prove a potential threat to their very existence. They are ready to adopt "the sick role,"[1] submitting perforce to the physician's superior judgment and advice. The physician is thus empowered by both the patient's need and the recognition of his or her ability to meet that need through his or her specialized expertise. In this situation, etiquette therefore sanctions the asking of multiple questions with the expectation of frank answers, the intrusion of physical examination, often supplemented by a plethora of diagnostic tests, the prescription of medications, and the recommendation of what are euphemistically called "procedures." All these steps may be distressing to patients: they may have to avow self-destructive habits (smoking, lack of exercise, overindulgence) or submit to a loss of dignity, to unpleasantly invasive investigations, to nasty side effects of drugs, or to frightening surgery. But on the whole patients tend to comply in hopes of regaining health, or at least of attaining alleviation. This desire provides a strong motivation for the willing investiture of power in the doctor.

However, etiquette grants certain powers to patients too. They in turn have the right to pose questions so as to elicit explanation of the possible meanings of their symptoms, to seek a second (and a third) opinion in a complex or murky syndrome, and, as a last resort, to refuse the proposed treatment. Ultimately, certainly theoretically, they own their bodies and may dispose of them as they sees fit. But in practice the urge to live is so intense in most patients as to make them willing and even glad to defer to the doctor's competence in making decisions, based on his or her accumulated knowledge and experience.

The extent of the doctor's power as a therapeutic tool was analyzed by the Hungaro-British psychiatrist Michael Balint in his book *The Doctor, the Patient, and His Illness,* which was a landmark when it appeared in 1957 and has since become a classic. Balint ascribes to the physician a quasisacerdotal mystique, asserting that the doctor's mere presence as a concerned listener has an effect so potent as to warrant description as "the drug 'doctor'" (1). Although the influence to which Balint refers is clearly psychological, its impact extends equally to physical pathologies. Many patients, notably Norman Cousins, have confirmed this with the observation that the doctor's arrival in the sickroom ushers in an atmosphere of hope that devolves from the patient's implicit trust in the doctor's healing powers. Such confidence is encouraged by the medical profession as likely to be conducive to a good outcome; at the same time, it intensifies the patient's dependence on the doctor, whose power is thereby further heightened.

The balance of power in the medical field is nowadays further complicated by the jurisdiction of insurance or managed care companies. This recent development has introduced a new and very troubling perspective to the entire issue of doctors' and patients' powers. Economic motives are widely suspected of ousting the patient's well-being as the overriding factor. The denial of certain courses of action prescribed by physicians amounts to a reduction of their authority, a constraint on their autonomy through the intervention of a third party. Choosing the most appropriate therapeutic option is no longer solely a matter of counsel and trust between doctor and patient; both may now have to bow to an outsider unfamiliar with the circumstances of the particular case and making rulings according to standardized criteria. The changes currently under way prompt retrospective reconsideration of the balance of power between doctor and patient. For it is a constantly evolving tradition that over the past two centuries has undergone a transformation so fundamental as to amount to an almost complete reversal.

The difference between doctors' present enormous prestige and their formerly much more precarious position becomes fully apparent in Daniel Webster Cathell's *Book On the Physician Himself,* which was published in Philadelphia in 1881, had run to eleven editions by 1902, and continued to be reissued until 1922. Cathell, who was born in Maryland in 1839 and graduated from the Long Island Hospital Medical College in 1865, wrote only this one work. A respected practitioner in Baltimore and an active member of the profession, he lists on the title page of the second edition (1822) the many professional offices he has held. The *Book On the Physician Himself,* which bears the subtitle "Things That Concern His Reputation and Success," is a conduct book, a manual of tact and a recipe for success directed at aspiring doctors. To gain a foothold in the profession was difficult at that time of severe overproduction of doctors in the United States. The figures cited by Cathell for the comparative density of physicians are quite startling: 1:3,500 of the population in Italy; 1:2,500 in Austria; 1:1,814 in France; 1:1,652 in Britain; 1:1,300 in Germany; 1:1,193 in Canada; and 1:600 in the United States (29–30). The orientation of the profession was therefore "*competitive* rather than *cooperative.*"[2]

In setting out guidelines for the newly minted physician on how to attain "reputation and success," Cathell is acutely aware of the need to *woo* patients. He emphasizes impression management, beginning with personal appearance. He thus exhorts the prospective practitioner to eschew "glaring neckties, flashy breastpins, loud, dangling watch-seal, brilliant rings, fancy canes" (19) at one extreme and "appearing in your shirt-sleeves, with unwashed hands, dingy cuffs, egg-spotted or tobacco-stained shirt-bosom, greasy coat, out at elbows; ragged pants, fly-speckled or crumpled hat, and four or five days' beard on the face; rough, creaking, or dirty boots" at the other (80). With the same aim of making a favorable impression he also gets quite carried away in his advice about the appropriate furnishing of the office:

> Exercise care in its arrangement; give it a pleasing exterior; make it look fresh and clean outside, and make it snug, bright and cosy inside, thus showing that the occupant is possessed of good taste and gentility, as well as learning and skill; . . . it is the office of a live, earnest-working, scientific physician, who has a library, takes the journals, and makes use of the various instruments science has devised for him. Take care, however, to avoid running into a quack-

ish display of instruments and tools, and keep from sight such inappropriate or even repulsive objects as catheters, syringes, obstet-
ric forceps, splints, trusses, amputating knives, skeletons, grinning
skulls, jars of amputated extremities, tumors, mannikins, and the
unripe fruit of the uterus. Also, avoid such habits as keeping specula
or human bones on your desk for use as paper weights. It is not
unprofessional, however, to have about you . . . your microscope,
stethoscope, spirit-lamp, test-tubes, re-agents for testing urine, and
other aids to precision in diagnosis; or to hang up your diplomas,
certificates of society memberships, portraits, busts of eminent
professional friends. . . . A neat case of well labelled and well corked
medicines, or a cabinet of minerals, or works of art, are in good
taste; so also are your dictionaries, encyclopaedias, and lexicons for
ready reference; but display no miniature museum of sharks' heads,
stuffed alligators, tortoise shells, impaled butterflies, bugs, miniature ships, mummies, snakes, stuffed birds, lizards, crocodiles, bee-
tles, tape-worms, devil-fish, ostrich-eggs, hornets' nests, or
anything else that will advertise you in any other light than that
of a physician. (5–6)

Cathell's admonitions reveal the extent to which the physician a hundred
years ago was dependent on his patients' favor. His didactic posture is reinforced by such recurrent stylistic devices as direct addresses to an anonymous
"you" and the use of either affirmative, constative constructions or commands.

   Cathell's book has been said to reflect "the exceptional insecurity of
nineteenth-century doctors, their complete dependence on their clients, and
their vulnerability to competition."[3] Competition could be expected from
any one of a range of sectarian practitioners, including homeopaths, Thom-
sonians, Grahamites, not to mention adherents to folk and domestic medicine.
Cathell's generally commonsensical and occasionally (unwittingly) comical
advice is throughout predicated on the explicit and implicit recognition of
the physician's economic subjection to his patients and consequently of the
absolute necessity of keeping in their good graces. This concern leads to an
etiquette whose emphasis is squarely on the ways in which the doctor's behavior can be geared to *pleasing* the patient. "A brusque, tornado-like manner,
or eccentric rudeness is fatal to a physician's success," he warns, advocating

instead a "simple, humane, gentle and dignified manner and a low tone of voice" (45). So as to "preserve a proper degree of dignity and gravity toward patients," vulgar jokes, clownish levity, and undue familiarity are to be avoided, and first names or casual greetings such as "Hallo, Doc!" strongly discouraged (83). Above all, the doctor must take care not to be looked on as "a barbarian or butcher" (85); the desirable image of kindliness can be fostered by remembering the children's names, being polite and courteous, and giving donations to local causes (85–86). Even if patients insist on bizarre or medically worthless remedies such as "saffron-tea, plasters, onions to the feet, etc." (145), Cathell urges prudence in tolerating them so as not to antagonize the patients and risk losing them to more permissive practitioners.

The *Book On the Physician Himself* reflects a power structure in many ways radically different from that of today. It is the doctor rather than the patient who is cast in the subordinate role of supplicant. The financial aspect of the doctor-patient relationship is in the forefront in determining an etiquette that dictates the utmost caution in submitting to patients' whims. Thus Cathell returns again and again to the pressing topic of collecting fees. "It is wise," he affirms near the outset, "to have a small, neat sign, with 'Office Consultations from $1 to $10 cash,' posted in some semi-prominent place in your office" (15). Also, keeping a small case of medicine in the office will "enable you to get fees from patients who can appreciate medicine and advice combined, but who cannot properly value advice alone" (16). The matter of advice without medication is categorically addressed once more later: "You will also occasionally be asked for advice by those about to marry, and by others newly married, who are miserable on account of this or that affliction, defect or fear. . . . Remember in all such cases that your opinions are your capital, and charge your *full fee,* even though you write no prescription" (154).

As the practice becomes better established, tactics may be modified somewhat: charges should be increased, and the "weeding out of worthless [presumably unlucrative] patients" should be undertaken. Cathell emphatically insists that in the final analysis "business is business. You must be clothed and fed, and must support those dependent upon you, just as other people do. Every person naturally and properly looks to whatever occupation he follows for support, therefore let not false delicacy or out-of-place politeness interfere with your business rules in many matters" (245).

A century after its publication the *Book On the Physician Himself* gives a fascinating insight into the etiquette between doctor and patient at that time. The relationship seems quite devious, since the doctor, worried about competition, has to steer a tricky course between protecting his own interests and satisfying his patients. Curiously little reference is made to the power conferred by scientific knowledge, perhaps because it was then less decisive. Cathell assumes that expertise plays a scant role in patients' choice of a physician and that qualified physicians will surely possess the necessary modicum. On the other hand, on the opening page he underscores (literally, by italics) that *"professional tact and business sagacity"* are as vital to attaining "reputation and success" as "it is for a ship to have a rudder" (1). Personal qualities and an understanding of market pressures are here given priority over knowledge. Patients are seen, somewhat reductively, as likely to be impressed above all by appearances and manners, yet they wield considerable power through control of the purse strings. So the doctor faces the difficult task of both winning and keeping the patient *and* asserting his own compromised authority by persuading the patient to follow his medical exhortations. Given this unstable distribution of power, a readiness to negotiate and to make concessions is essential on the doctor's part.

The patient remains a shadowy, voiceless presence in the *Book On the Physician Himself*, a projection by the physician as almost an adversary. In twentieth-century medical histories patients are remarkable for their absence. This hiatus is the more striking in view of the centrality in medical practice of the doctor-patient interaction, which has recently been described as "the irreducible common denominator for most practicing physicians."[4] Yet medical histories have been written as though the patient did not exist. Erwin Akerknecht's *Short History of Medicine* is packed with valuable information about discoveries of disease causality, advances in therapeutics, and the physicians and scientists responsible for the progress made over the centuries but disregards their implications for the recipient, the patient. Richard Shryock's *Development of Modern Medicine* contains two chapters (13 and 16) in which evolving group perceptions of medicine at two discrete periods are discussed, though not the dynamics of the individual rapport. Both Paul de Kruif's *Microbe Hunters* and Sherwin Nuland's *Doctors* give vignettes of the lives and personalities of the researchers whose work they present. Nuland opts for a primarily biographical method, contextualizing the scientific breakthroughs in an account of the personal and medicohistorical circumstances. As a result, in *Mi-*

crobe Hunters as in *Doctors* the physicians and scientists are made to come alive as human beings. However, the impact of their discoveries on patients is no more than a very subsidiary theme.

But the history of medicine is not just the story of diseases, physicians, and therapeutics but also that of patients. Writing about seventeenth-century England, Lucinda Beier comments that "traditional historians, concerned with mapping the advance of medical science, implicitly treated patients as irrelevant, except as the vehicles and beneficiaries of medical discoveries."[5] She argues for increased attention to both sufferers and healers on the grounds that it is impossible to relate illness and medicine to social context without heed of sufferers' feelings, attitudes, and behaviors. Nevertheless, the habitual neglect of the patient persists. For instance, in *Transformations in American Medicine* Lester King reviews the interplay of the intellectual history of medicine with its social history, naming three major relationships: between the physician and the patient, between the physician and nature, and between the physician and the rest of society. Yet even in 1991 the first category is confined to "medical ethics."[6]

This does not mean that the interaction between the doctor and the patient has not been subjected to analysis. In fact, the past twenty years have brought an efflorescence of books and articles devoted to the topic.[7] But they concentrate on the mechanics of the interaction: how to initiate the interview, how to move rapidly toward a diagnosis, how to handle patients' questions, and how to terminate the conversation. As these "how" clauses suggest, they are intended as practical handbooks for the convenience of practitioners; written by and for physicians, they focus on the doctor's behavior toward the patient as the object of scrutiny. No attention is given to the patient's perspective or to such underlying philosophical and psychological issues as the power and trust that bind doctor and patient. The approach to questions of etiquette is not only severely pragmatic and sociological but also firmly based on the automatic assumption of the doctor's preponderance.[8]

The etiquette for the handling of power has a definite linguistic dimension too. Cathell already emphasized the importance of always addressing the patient in a low voice and in decorous language. Since his time the locus of linguistic friction between doctor and patient has shifted away from gentility to the pervasiveness of technical terms as medicine has become increasingly scientific. Doctors need to be able to explain to patients, at least to some extent, what they believe ails them and how they propose to set about treatment. Not merely etiquette but the law itself mandates such explanation for the purposes of informed consent.[9] Nonetheless, it is often hard for doctors to translate complicated pathologies and procedures into a nomenclature comprehensible to patients, free of technical jargon. They have been trained to diagnose and discuss syndromes in a precise terminology in which they can readily communicate with their peers. This discourse unites medical professionals and at the same time alienates the uninitiated so that access to this language becomes a tool of empowerment. Perri Klass recalls how she picked up "endless jargon and abbreviations," as well as "the patterns of speech and the grammatical conventions," during the first three months she worked in a hospital as a medical student. "This special language," she comments, "contributes to a sense of closeness and professional spirit among people who are under a great deal of stress."[10] The converse to that closeness is the exclusion of those unable to understand this parlance, so that in effect a barrier is erected between laypeople and those who have undergone medical training.

Even in the absence of technical vocabulary, however, a discrepancy in the apprehension of ordinary words can create a communicative gap and so destabilize the doctor-patient exchange. The simple terms *illness* and *disease* are good examples. Patients use the former to denote sensations of pain or disturbances of normative function that impel them to invoke medical advice. In response to the patient's complaints, the doctor listens, examines, observes, and tests with the goal of establishing a diagnosis of *disease* as a preliminary to restorative or at least palliative therapy. The semantic divergence between *illness* and *disease* is far more than a linguistic quibble; it indicates the wholly different ways in which patient and doctor relate to the problem that brings them together: patients subjectively and emotionally to a worrisome affliction they cannot handle, doctors objectively and expertly to a clinical entity they want to classify and remediate. In the words of a thoughtful clinician: "The doctor has an agenda of disease; the patient is concerned about his or her life and illness." While the symptoms present a "clinical problem" to the physician, to the patient they may represent a dire threat.[11] So in their initial reaction to the question they confront in common a conspicuous dichotomy of attitude separates patient and doctor. Arguably, it is precisely the doctor's expertise and objectivity that the patient seeks as the most promising means to overcome the affliction. Still, the relationship between patient and doctor is from the outset determined by the intrinsic disparity in their respective stances. Although they share the ultimate aim of restoring good health, the roles they enact and the paths they follow in achieving it are quite heterogeneous, the doctor entitled by knowledge to exercise authority, the patient expected to submit and comply. Tension as well as dependence is innate to the encounter.

What is the appropriate etiquette in this situation? Which behaviors in doctor and patient are most likely to cause or to avert friction? How has the etiquette changed over the past one hundred and fifty years of revolutionary progress in medicine? In what respects has it remained the same? What has been the effect of the rise of the biosciences and of hospitals? To what extent has the balance of power between the two parties shifted? In short, how do patients and doctors come to assume the positions that enable them to work collaboratively with each other or, alternatively, to thwart such cooperation? Many diverse factors come into play here: the assertion of power by the physician and acquiescence in that power by the patient; the tension between the physician's obligation to take charge, perhaps in a seemingly paternalistic manner, and his or her simultaneous need to respect the patient's autonomy; the necessity of establishing and maintaining reciprocal trust; the imperative of tact on both sides and the judgments and decisions this entails; the kind of language and tone expected and used toward each other; and, tangentially, economic interests insofar as they affect professional practice. Even this cursory glance at the issues suggests the conflicting demands constantly shaping and reshaping an etiquette precariously poised between intimacy and impersonality.

A topic as vast as the balance of power is not easily delineated and limited, yet a sharp focus is necessary if vague generalizations are to be avoided. I propose to concentrate on what William Carlos Williams has called "the humdrum, day-in, day-out, everyday work,"[12] the commonplace medical situations faced by almost everyone sooner or later. I do not deal with the highly charged, essentially ethical issues surrounding abortion, organ donation, and continuing life support, many of which have become options only in the past few years. Nor do I cover the psychotherapeutic situation, which has its own pronounced conventions for the interaction between therapist and patient. Child patients are excluded because of the complications of the triangulated situation they create through the intermediacy of their parents. Likewise, pathographies, that is, personal accounts by patients or their survivors of illnesses, are discounted because they form a distinctive genre.[13] Public health issues like the theoretical debates in Henrik Ibsen's *Enemy of the People* are also bypassed since by and large they have no immediate bearing on the rapport between doctor and individual patient, although they may do so in some instances. For example, the controversy in George Eliot's *Middlemarch* over the new hospital sheds light on the way the doctor is perceived by the community of his potential patients.

In exploring continuity and change in the balance of power I dwell on broad international trends in preference to national differences. This is by no means to deny or minimize divergences either between Europe and the United States or within Western Europe. The differences are in fact striking: French leadership in the first half of the nineteenth century through the development of pathological anatomy and the consequent deeper understanding of physiology; German preeminence in the latter half of that century as a result of the basic research conducted in the laboratories of its reorganized universities; the proliferation of sectarian healers in the late-nineteenth-century United States. The persistence in the twentieth century of national idiosyncrasies in styles of medicine is the subject of *Medicine and Culture*, by the medical journalist Lynn Payer, who makes a convincing argument for the priority accorded to the liver in France, to germs in England, and to viruses in the United States. But such cultural quirks are in all probability modulations more in terminology than in therapeutic practice, and, above all, they do not substantially impinge on the basic patterns of conduct between physician and patient.

Nor, indeed, do variations in the timing of advances; what matters are the fundamental shifts in medical methodology. For example, the reliance on the stethoscope as a means of physical examination entails a significant alteration in the bearing of doctor toward patient by creating, paradoxically, at once more penetrating access to the body and a greater distance from it (in comparison with the older practice of listening to the patient's heart and lungs by the placing of the physician's ear directly onto the patient's chest or back). Whether the stethoscope was accepted as a standard instrument as early as the 1820s and 1830s or whether this came about only in the 1840s or even as late as the 1850s (as is reputed of the French provinces) is in the long run of far lesser importance than the nature of the change it wrought. Although cognitive and technological progress occurred at a differing rate from country to country as well as at a different pace at discrete points, the overall trends are parallel across the board. The tables for death rates per 1,000 inhabitants between 1841 and 1926 in England and Wales and·in France illustrate the prevalence of parallelism but not necessarily identity.[14] Thus the particulars of national situations will not be ignored but will be discussed only when they have immediate relevance to the balance of power, as in the case of the admission of women doctors in the final third of the nineteenth century.

Similarly, I refer to "the doctor" and "the patient" as generic categories without specifying differences in their background and personalities that might affect their interaction. Fine research into precisely such differences was carried out in the early 1980s at a family medical center in Charleston, South Carolina, by the sociolinguist Candace West, who examined in *Routine Complications* the permutations attributable to gender, race, and age, that is, how male/female physicians relate to white/black, young/old patients. In the literary texts I analyze here, class and financial standing prove the major factors in defining the balance of power in particular instances. But beyond the differences, there is at each stage in the development of medicine an archetypal paradigm of expected behavior between doctor and patient. Cathell's *Book On the Physician Himself* amply illustrates the cardinal disparity in the basic assumptions between the 1880s and the 1980s. It is these broad lines of evolution that stand in the forefront of this study.

My temporal span extends from about 1830 to the present. Both medico-historical and literary circumstances motivate this choice. There is widespread consensus in siting the beginnings of modern medicine at the end of the eighteenth century. "Modern medicine," Michel Foucault asserts, "has fixed its own date of birth as being in the last years of the eighteenth century."[15] More specifically, Charles Rosenberg points out that "medical therapeutics changed remarkably little in the two millennia preceding 1800; by the end of the century, traditional therapeutics had altered fundamentally."[16] Furthermore, the transformation of medicine in the nineteenth century was as much qualitative as quantitative: "Medicine did not simply become more scientific during the nineteenth century; what was considered science, and what was not, changed."[17] The introduction of the stethoscope, devised by René-Théophile-Hyacinthe Laënnec in 1819, and its gradual adoption as an indispensable tool for physical examination is a major milestone in the development of medicine. The findings of the stethoscope could be confirmed by the prodigious progress in pathological anatomy in the first half of the nineteenth century, which enabled physicians to identify diseases and to describe accurately their manifestations in the body. This startling growth of knowledge forms the foundation for the rise of medical power. The virtual doubling of life expectancy in Western countries from thirty-eight years in 1830 to seventy in 1950 tells the rest of the story: As Michael Crichton stated in 1970, "Far more advances have occurred in medicine in the last hundred years than occurred in the previous two thousand."[18]

The beginnings of modern medicine, in about 1830, are contemporaneous with the prevalence of realism as the dominant literary mode. At the outset the realists liked to envisage themselves as social scientists engaged in a quest for truth parallel to that of their models in the sciences. So Honoré de Balzac proclaimed that "all is true" in his ambitious cycle of novels *La Comédie humaine* (ca. 1830–50; *The Human Comedy*), which sought to give an overview of French society. In the wake of this example, Emile Zola embarked on a similar survey under the title *Les Rougon-Macquart* (1871–93), the name of a large family spread over the spectrum of the social classes and occupations. In tracing its members' lives and fortunes through four generations in both a legitimate and an illegitimate branch Zola claimed to be adopting toward human behaviors an analytical stance imitative of the anatomist's dissecting method. In the preface to the second edition of *Thérèse Raquin* (1867; trans. 1962), written to counter charges of immorality in this lurid tale of adultery and murder, he asserts that in pursuit of his primarily scientific aim he carried out on living creatures "the analytical method that surgeons apply to corpses."[19] He presents his "physiological study" (25) as an expression of "the modern method of universal inquiry which is the tool our age is using so enthusiastically" (26). Whether such a posture as Balzac's and Zola's is fruitful as an artistic theory is, of course, highly debatable.[20] What is important in the present context is the strong impression made on writers by the scientific method and the marked consonance they wanted to establish between the medical and the literary enterprises.

This holds particularly true for realism, whose sustaining conventions, notably its goal of lifelikeness through close adherence to a substratum of factuality, facilitate and justify the connections I want to explore between medical history and literature. During and also beyond the age of realism, writers' fascination with medicine is manifest in sundry ways. Several of the novelists whose works involve medical topics themselves underwent medical training (Arthur Conan Doyle, Somerset Maugham, A. J. Cronin); others came from medical families (Gustave Flaubert, Eugène Sue, Elizabeth Stuart Phelps) or engaged in serious background research (Flaubert again, George Eliot, Zola, Sinclair Lewis). Their own commitment to substantive accuracy validates the intromission of medical history into fiction in the interdisciplinary reading that I am sounding. The coincidence of a new style of medicine with the stethoscope and a new literary style in realism about 1830 not only marks a turning point in both disciplines but is conducive to their rapprochement as well.[21]

This is not to deny that the status of literary texts is still exposed to question by historians who remain suspicious of the contribution fiction can make to an understanding of the past. But the climate of opinion about the reciprocal porosity of history and fiction has been changing over the last quarter of a century, since Hayden White's influential postulate in *Metahistory* (1973) that the construction of "events," however objective in intent, inevitably involves an element of interpretation that allies it narratively with the imaginative processes of fiction. More recently, the new cultural history has moved significantly further in endorsing, indeed welcoming, the appropriation of fiction into historical study. The contributors to the landmark volume *The New Cultural History* (1989), edited by Lynn Hunt, repeatedly insist on the potential for expanding the boundaries of history through the recognition of both "the literary dimension of social experience and the literary structure of historical writing."[22] Language, texts, and narrative structures are underscored as playing an active role in the creation and description of historical reality. Thus the encounter between history and literature is conceived as essentially "dialogic" (128) insofar as the two disciplines complement each other. Nowhere does this hold more true than in the humanistic area of personal relationships that is my topic.

The fruitfulness of the new interdisciplinary approach has already been proven. Medical historians themselves have frequently cited literary texts to support their arguments,[23] though at times without as much attention to such aesthetic factors as perspective, voice, or irony as a literary scholar would wish. Conversely, literary texts can be opened up to a deeper understanding by careful regard to their historical context. For example, it is vital to grasp the implications of Charles Bovary's rank as a "health officer," a level much lower than that of a qualified physician. His incompetence, his hesitations, and ultimately his bungling, as well as his modest social standing, become much more comprehensible once the basic facts of the nineteenth-century French medical hierarchy are grasped.[24] Similarly, the complex conflicts determining Lydgate's reception in *Middlemarch* attain added meaning in light of the medical controversies of that period. To read literary works and medical history in tandem as an interdisciplinary enterprise is a rewarding methodology.

A salient advantage of literary testimony is the instatement of the patient as a central, rounded protagonist whose words and actions are as prominent as those of the physician. By restoring the missing patient, fiction can act as a corrective to the one-sidedness of medical histories. Through its capacity to shift perspective from one figure to another, fictional narrative can give access to the thoughts and motivations of multiple characters in the action. So the factors determining the etiquette of power between doctor and patient can be portrayed with psychological penetration from both angles. The gain is not only in immediacy, plasticity, and vividness but also in the ability to make subtle differentiations in the dynamics of the interaction. The human predicaments, which are the stuff of fiction, flesh out the historical data through lively enactment of the underlying tensions. For instance, the clashes between Lydgate and the other practitioners in Middlemarch are a graphic incarnation of the disputes about germ theory as well as the realignment of the medical hierarchy through the emergence of the general practitioner at that period. *Middlemarch* is medical history translated into personal—and fictional—terms. But just as the novel animates a historical situation, so too the stakes in the struggle between Lydgate and the traditionalists can only become fully comprehensible through an understanding of the medicohistorical context. The reciprocity between history and literature is nowhere more cogently illustrated than in this complex narrative.[25]

Admittedly, though, literature is *not* history and must not be taken to be in a direct equation with it. The demands of the fictional plot may lead to a measure of idealization or vilification that has to be taken carefully into account. Yet precisely such deviations from historical norms can be of special significance insofar as they denote the age's wish (or fear) projections. The contrast between the fate of Lydgate, on the one hand, and those of Mr. Gibson in Elizabeth Gaskell's *Wives and Daughters* (1866) and Dr. Thorne in Trollope's novel (1858) of that name, on the other, is more than a coincidental irony. All three practice in the still semirural English provinces before the middle of the century. Gibson and Thorne fare rather well socially and financially because they meet their patients' modest expectations and mostly show the professional tact that Cathell considered so essential. Lydgate actually practices a far sounder and more advanced style of medicine, having absorbed the most avant-garde notions during his postgraduate studies in Paris. However, despite his initial success with a number of difficult cases, he is ultimately spurned and condemned to failure, partly because his ideas are too startling to be acceptable but even more because he breaches the etiquette of power then prevailing between doctor and patient by arrogating prerogatives not granted at that time to a medical man at his level. He is a striking example of a doctor who knows best at a time when negotiation on a more or less equal basis with paying patients was customary and prudent. In all three novels the requirements of the plot shape the conceptualization of the physician's personality and conduct. Nonetheless, these fictional considerations by no means subvert historicity. Fiction and history are neither synonymous nor incompatible. Indeed, the very problem of how to integrate them is a fertile source of interest in the linkage of medical history to literature.

One of the greatest difficulties is to find an appropriate structure for such a linkage. I adopt a schema from medical history in order to examine how the literary testimony confirms or possibly modifies it. The division of medical history into three distinct phases—*bedside, hospital,* and *laboratory*—was initiated by the doyen of medical historians, Erwin Akerknecht, who used this terminology in both his major works.[26] This outline was subsequently elaborated by the sociologist N. D. Jewson in his seminal 1976 article, "The Disappearance of the Sick-Man from Medical Cosmology, 1770–1870." Jewson distinguishes between the three styles of practice as "ways of knowing (and ignoring)" (226) and as "modes of production of medical knowledge" (228). In noting and explaining the reasons for the disappearance of the sick man from what he calls "medical cosmology" (226) Jewson accepts without demure the banishment of the patient's perspective from consideration.

To retrieve patients from this disappearance is one of the main aims of this study, and that aim can be accomplished by re-placing them within the categories bedside, hospital, and laboratory. This organization has the advantage of capaciousness, so that it can encompass a broad range of medical practice over a long period. As a paradigm it has validity well beyond Jewson's segment,

1770–1870, extending easily into the present. It also has, at least potentially, a high degree of flexibility, although this does not become apparent in Jewson's article because his model remains strongly committed to the idea of succession in a temporal continuum. What Jewson overlooks is the *layering* of the cosmologies; while they become dominant sequentially, they must also be seen as coexisting, overlapping as an imbricated set of continuities. This holds especially true for the first type, bedside, which forms a continuity throughout medical history. Bedside abides as the initial (though not necessarily leading) site of medicine. The resources of laboratory and hospital, invoked for the purpose of diagnosing and treating the patient's disease, are secondary and supplementary to the opening bedside encounter between patient and physician, which is repeated in a series of follow-up "visits" that punctuate the course of the treatment. The persistence of bedside even during the reign of increasingly complex and technological hospital and laboratory medicine is confirmed by the literary testimony, which confutes the tendency in Jewson's article and in much medical history to order the three modes into a discrete sequence.

The relative disinterest in traditional bedside medicine in histories of nineteenth- and twentieth-century practice in favor of the rising areas of hospital and laboratory suggests a reason for the absence of patients in most studies. For it is in the basic bedside situation that the patient is the primary partner in interaction with the physician, in contrast to hospital and laboratory settings, where the orientation is, as Jewson puts it, toward "professional peers" (236). To recognize the continuity of bedside is to reinstitute the centrality of the patient as both subject and object of the medical endeavor. It is also to modulate history's often overly neat divisions so as to become cognizant of its dynamic flow.

It is important to bear in mind the intrinsicality of such "layering," and with it the flux in styles of medical practice. Certainly from the 1830s onward the profession was in an incessant, excited commotion in the face of the reiterated revisions forced upon it by the challenges posed to its guiding premises by an avalanche of discoveries. Seen not in hindsight from the detached perspective of the contemporary historian but as an ongoing present experience of doctor and patient in the past century and a half, medical progress emerges less as the assured conquest of disease and death that is generally depicted and more as a bewildering onslaught of new assertions that undermined cherished beliefs and practices. Each innovation had to be scrupulously tested so that those with lasting worth could be sifted from those that raised only false, temporary hopes. For example, Louis Pasteur's public demonstration of the efficacy of his vaccine against anthrax in animals at the fair of the Agricultural Society of Melun in June 1881 vindicated what at the time seemed a far-fetched claim.[27] On the other hand, Robert Koch's tuberculin, submitted to the medical profession in 1890 as a treatment for tuberculosis, proved disappointing, although it did turn out to be a valuable diagnostic aid.

As scientific and technical advance brought an incrementally increasing number of therapies and procedures, it became ever more perplexing to steer the narrow path between inflated, possibly spurious claims and those that were revolutionary and legitimate. The reiterated dilemma of choice between the older methods, which were tried and known but perhaps marginally effective, and the newer, as yet little known ones, which held both greater promise and greater risk, was bound to arouse anxiety in patients and doctors alike. The antagonisms between the avant-garde and conservatives within the medical profession extended beyond it to heighten the tensions between patients and practitioners too. Some patients might be avid for the latest remedies, while others were suspicious of them. Physicians for their part were caught between the fear of doing harm to their patients and the hardly lesser fear of not doing all possible good. As medicoscientific matters quickly came to surpass lay understanding, patients had perforce to rely much more than previously on their medical attendants' judgment and decision-making skills. So the obverse to expansion of the doctor's authority—and responsibility—was a considerable intensification of the patient's dependence. As long as medical lore was so limited as to be open to common comprehension, physician and patient stood almost in parity, sharing assumptions and reaching agreement consultatively on the desirable treatment. That intellectual and social equilibrium terminated with the physician's ascendancy by virtue of command over a corpus of knowledge vastly more extensive, more technical, and therefore more arcane. It was thus that the doctor came to acquire (and to nurture) the reputation of always knowing best.

The purpose of this study is to chart the evolution of the changing balance of power in the wake of the advances made in medicine in the nineteenth and twentieth centuries, drawing on literary texts as sources. The pattern that emerges is a blend of continuity and change. The interaction between physician and patient has an archetypal constancy insofar as the patient always turns to the physician for advice and succor in coping with physical distress. The expectation of hopefulness with which the patient comes to the doctor has risen in the past one hundred and fifty years as a host of fatal or disabling conditions have become amenable to therapeutic intervention. Yet precisely through this tremendous extension of the physician's capacity to cure and to alleviate, the balance of power between the partners in the therapeutic alliance has changed significantly. Only through the inclusion of the missing patient can these changes be fully appreciated.

I make no attempt at the sort of complete, consecutive coverage to which historical scholarship aspires. Instead, within the overarching taxonomy of bedside, hospital, and laboratory I take a series of time frames, largely though not exclusively chronological in alignment, that offer insight into the etiquette of power at particular points. The first two frames, "Missionary to the Bedside" and "Seeing—and Hearing—Is Believing," are devoted to practice in the early to middle years of the nineteenth century, predominantly in England but also incorporating a sampling of parallel instances in other European countries and at subsequent periods. The third frame, "A Woman's Hand," moves to the United States in the closing decades of the nineteenth century, when intense controversy was triggered by the admission of women to the medical profession and the question of appropriate styles of medicine. The function of hospital medicine and its implications for patients in the nineteenth century is the subject of the fourth frame, "Diseases and Diseased People." The fifth, "The Questionable Sanctuary," examines the portrayal of laboratory medicine, while the sixth, "Eyeing the Institution," considers the perception of the contemporary hospital. Finally, "Balancing the Power" analyzes the confluence of factors that determine the current relationship between doctor and patient.

2.

"MISSIONARY TO
THE BEDSIDE"

— ∙ — ∙ — ∙ — ∙ — ∙ — ∙ — ∙ — ∙ — ∙ — ∙ — ∙ — ∙ — ∙ — ∙ — ∙ —

His patients are his friends. He goes from house to house,
and his step and his voice are loved and welcomed in each.
—ARTHUR CONAN DOYLE, *Round the Red Lamp*

— ∙ — ∙ — ∙ — ∙ — ∙ — ∙ — ∙ — ∙ — ∙ — ∙ — ∙ — ∙ — ∙ — ∙ — ∙ —

THE DESCRIPTION OF THE doctor as a "missionary to the bedside" was
coined by Henry C. Clarke in his M.D. thesis, "The Science of Medicine,"
submitted to the University of Pennsylvania in 1853.[1] The phrase is striking
and rather strange. It has a distinct religious resonance, for the word *missionary* generally denotes a person who preaches a gospel and tries to make
converts to it. His selfless devotion to his ideals wins admiration but scant
worldly rewards. In what ways, then, was the doctor the figurative equivalent
of the missionary? Nowadays the mission would include teaching the value
of exercise, a balanced diet low in fat and high in fiber, and of course not
smoking; however, such elements of modern preventive medicine were not
understood in the mid–nineteenth century. The closest common denominator between the normative connotations of *missionary* and *doctor* would be
the notion of succor, salvation, rescue from dismal circumstances. But there
is another fundamental convergence, at least for that period, in the root of
missionary in the Latin verb *mittere,* "to send." *Mission* is defined in the *Oxford
English Dictionary* as a "sending," a "calling," a "vocation," a "commission,"
a "duty," an "errand on which a person is sent." For the religious missionary
the sending would often entail a sortie into a distant, exotic realm to preach
to the heathen. For the doctor the calling would be into the patient's home.
Whereas the theological missionary is sent out, his physical counterpart is
sent *for* and *in.* The locus of medical attention through most of the nineteenth
century was predominantly the home.

What the missionary activity attributed to the doctor actually meant can be deduced from two English novels that portray the social scene: Anthony Trollope's *Doctor Thorne* (1858) and Elizabeth Gaskell's *Wives and Daughters* (1866). Nearly contemporaneous with Clarke's M.D. thesis, they can be read as illustrations and commentaries on his characterization of the doctor. The action of *Doctor Thorne* is close to that of its composition; 1854 is named as the year when Frank Gresham, the romantic "lead," comes of age and begins to be pressured to marry a woman of large fortune so as to restore his family's depleted coffers (11). The action of *Wives and Daughters,* on the other hand, is at a slight temporal remove: the first chapter, precisely sited as "five-and-forty years ago" and "before the passing of the Reform Bill [1832]" (36), can be dated to 1819 or 1820. Since the heroine is then twelve and the main part of the novel centers on her late teens, the time can be fixed as the latter half of the 1820s, about a quarter-century earlier than *Doctor Thorne.* In many other respects, however, these two novels show extensive parallels. Both take place in the English provinces in a semirural village setting, whose exact location is not specified but is not too far from London. Various characters travel on occasion to the capital, and in *Doctor Thorne* London is the source for medical consultants in problematic cases. Both enact complicated, multilayered plots of courtship and marriage that involve issues of money and social status, pertaining in *Wives and Daughters* particularly to Molly Gibson, the doctor's daughter, and in *Doctor Thorne* to Mary Thorne, his niece and ward. In the context of matchmaking, the two narratives raise fundamental questions about the doctor's social position and about his power in the well-defined hierarchies of the time. The images that emerge are fundamentally alike, albeit with some variations as a consequence of divergences in the professional standing of Mr. Gibson and Dr. Thorne.

In both works the doctor is the central figure. The titular character in Trollope's novel, Dr. Thorne is designated in the opening sentence as destined to be its "chief personage," although his stature is simultaneously undercut by the description of him as "a modest country medical practitioner" (5). What is more, his first appearance is postponed in favor of an expansive preliminary concentration on "the locality in which, and the neighbors among whom, our doctor followed his profession" (5). Chapter 1 is devoted to the Gresham family of Greshamsbury, and chapter 2, "Long, Long Ago," to important family events preceding the action, so that by the point when Dr.

Thorne comes into the forefront, in chapter 3, entitled "Doctor Thorne," he is already firmly embedded in the community in which he practices as well as socially subordinated to its landed gentry. When he is referred to as "our hero" (20 and 267) it is with a tinge of irony, especially on the second occasion, when he has receded from the plot for several chapters "It was in the early pages of this work that Dr. Thorne was to be our hero," the narrator remarks wryly; "but it would appear very much as though he had latterly been forgotten." Yet Trollope insists on Thorne's priority over Frank Gresham when he writes: "He [Frank Gresham] would have been the hero of our tale had not that place been pre-occupied by the village doctor" (10). The nature of Thorne's "heroism" in the dual sense of his pivotal role in the novel and of his boldness is one of the issues explored in the plot. By comparison, Mr. Gibson is made to seem rather more subsidiary in *Wives and Daughters,* partly because the title directs the main attention to the female protagonists. However, he is ubiquitously present throughout the novel, linking its diverse strands through his function as medical attendant. Although never openly hailed as a hero in the way that Dr. Thorne is, Mr. Gibson certainly possesses a good many of the positive qualities associated with that term. Morally he comes across as a far stronger character than the romantic "hero," young Roger Hamley, whom Molly finally marries. In *Wives and Daughters,* as in *Doctor Thorne,* the doctor is the preeminent male figure.

Despite Thorne's position as "our hero," more information is given about Gibson than about Thorne. He had been brought to Hollingford sixteen years before the start of the action as the successor to Mr. Hall, who had decided to retire. The title "Mr.," given to both Hall and Gibson, indicates that they are surgeons, a rank of healers whose training was mostly practical, whereas those called "Dr." were physicians educated at Oxford or Cambridge. Physicians, the top category, were regarded as gentlemen; apothecaries, the lowest on the scale, were considered tradesmen; surgeons were rather precariously situated between the two. This stratification of the medical fraternity echoed and coincided with established class distinctions, so that "doctors" were more likely to attend the aristocracy and the upper middle class, not least because their fees were the highest, whereas apothecaries cared for the poorest. Some flexibility was beginning to become apparent at about this time, especially in regard to surgeons, whose training and manners ranged from superior to barely mediocre. As a group they had broken away from the Company of

Barber-Surgeons in 1745 to form a separate Company of Surgeons, which became the Royal College of Surgeons when a charter was granted in 1800.
Nevertheless, the functions and status of surgeons remained ambiguous, still
smacking of trade on account of the use of hands and the dispensing of
drugs, though by no means confined to the craftsmanship of the knife. With
the rise of the middle classes concomitant on industrialization, surgeons became more prominent and the boundaries dividing the three categories of
medical men became somewhat less rigid.[2] Legally surgeons were supposed
to treat only "outward" disorders, "internal" ones being in the physician's
domain. The distinction was upheld in 1828 when a member of the Royal College of Surgeons was deemed in a lawsuit "non-suited in his claim for charges
for medicines supplied to and attendance upon a patient who had contracted
typhus fever, since it was ruled that typhus was a medical and not a surgical
disease."[3] But as *Wives and Daughters,* and also *Middlemarch,* shows, by the
early 1830s well-qualified surgeons were already on the way to becoming the
newly emergent breed of general family practitioners. Gibson certainly treats
internal diseases, although it is hard to say exactly which ones because Gaskell
is more specific about the doctor's function as a healer than about the maladies
themselves. This silence can be seen as indicative of the rather rudimentary
level of diagnostics at the time.

At the outset Gibson is consistently focalized through the eyes of the inhabitants of Hollingford. They recognize immediately that he is a cut above
the average surgeon: "his professional qualifications were as high as his moral
character" (61). Like his patients' diseases, those qualifications remain unstated.
That "he had been in Paris" is mentioned (61), raising the possibility of his
having taken advanced training in that preferred destination for British and
American doctors in the first half of the nineteenth century. But, significantly,
his link to Paris is esteemed by his prospective patients in Hollingford for its
social rather than its professional implications, for they are patently far more
concerned with his pedigree than with his knowledge. So the Paris episode
is interpreted in relation to his parentage: "His mother must have been a
Frenchwoman" (61). Conjecture "as to his birth, parentage, and education"
is rife in Hollingford, as Gaskell records with gentle but pointed irony:

> He was the illegitimate son of a Scotch duke, by a Frenchwoman;
> and the grounds for this conjecture were these:—He spoke with

> a Scotch accent; therefore, he must be Scotch. He had a very gen-
> teel appearance, an elegant figure, and was apt—so his ill-wishers
> said—to give himself airs; therefore, his father must have been
> some person of quality; and, that granted, nothing was easier than
> to run this supposition up all the notes of the scale of the peerage—
> baronet, baron, viscount, earl, marquis, duke. Higher they dared
> not go, though one old lady, acquainted with English history, haz-
> arded the remark, that "she believed that one or two of the Stuarts—
> ahem—had not always been—ahem—quite correct in their—
> conduct; and she fancied such—ahem—things ran in families." But
> in popular opinion, Mr. Gibson's father always remained a duke;
> nothing more. (61)

Through recourse to indirect discourse Gaskell here enters into the thoughts
of "Hollingford society" (61), clearly poking fun by overstatement, while
maintaining a skeptical detachment from these speculations, which are neither
denied nor confirmed. The outcome of this way of introducing Gibson is
to make him a slightly mysterious, almost romantic figure whose social level
is left open. The rumors continue to circulate about "his aristocratic connections" and his origins as "the son of a Scotch duke, my dear, never mind on
which side of the blanket" (69), always in reported speech. It is as if Hollingford society wants to make its doctor socially as well as medically acceptable
by investing him with a family background it considers desirable. Yet the ambiguity is underscored by such observations as, "For his station in life, Mr.
Gibson had an unusually good library" (65), which reminds us of his relatively
modest position even as he is extolled.

Hollingford's assessment of Gibson devolves entirely from his appearance
and speech. On his first day he is seen as "tall, grave, rather handsome than
otherwise; thin enough to be called 'a very genteel figure'" (61). The note of
irony surfaces again here, and once more it is in reported discourse, recording
how he is perceived by others. His "leanness, . . . a great way to gentility" (69),
is one factor in making him "perfectly presentable" (70) even at dinners for
"the grandest circle of visitors" (69) at Lord and Lady Cumnor's mansion.
Still more important is the fact that Gibson's "accent was Scotch, not provincial" (69), which reinforces the postulate about his putative father and also
suggests a possible basis for his professional competence since Edinburgh was

in the forefront of medical education at the time. Gaskell chooses not to explore his professional qualifications, thereby showing that his acceptance within the community is dependent on his personal appeal rather than on his expertise. Yet there is considerable evidence of his competence and certainly of his shrewdness in his interactions with his patients: within a year of his arrival in Hollingford his skill has earned him "as much welcome respect" (62) as his predecessor had ever enjoyed. He is also much sought after as a teacher at a time when professional training was often by apprenticeship: "his reputation as a clever surgeon had spread so rapidly that his fees, which he had thought prohibitory, were willingly paid, in order that the young man might make a start in life, with the prestige of having been a pupil of Gibson of Hollingford" (64). He shows unusual enterprise in beginning, under the stimulus of Lord Hollingford's scientific research, to send contributions "to the more scientific of the medical journals" (70). The very casual mention of this intellectual pursuit serves as a reminder that Gibson is evaluated through the eyes of the people of Hollingford, on whom such activity would make little impression. It is probably his high professional ability that is the foundation for his self-assured dealings with all strata of his patients. His "kindness," to which repeated reference is made, is tempered by his tendency to be "sarcastic" (61) or at least "slightly sarcastic" (70). By endowing her protagonist with her own quizzical irony Gaskell admits at least a degree of amused detachment on his part.

But Gibson's rather independent turn of mind does not prevent him from bowing to convention in the area of marriage. He had followed custom in his first marriage, to Mr. Hall's niece; marrying into the profession was an acknowledged way to get started. His wife had succumbed to tuberculosis several years previously, so that at the beginning of *Wives and Daughters* he is "a widower and likely to remain so" (63). This return to a kind of bachelorhood, with a small daughter, puts him in an awkward position, for marriage was considered extremely desirable in a doctor as a mark of stability. So one strand of the pervasive courtship and marriage plot of *Wives and Daughters* concerns Gibson's second marriage, to Mrs. Kirkpatrick, a widow who had been a teacher and who subsequently acts as companion to Lady Cumnor. The overt motivation for this alliance is the wish to provide his adolescent daughter with a mothering surrogate. At the same time, the married state would be regarded as a decided professional plus to Gibson. Yet his choice proves to be unwise: his second wife turns out to be a foolish woman lacking in understanding of her husband's professional obligations. Granted his limited options in his restricted circle, his poor judgment in this important decision in his own life is in paradoxical contravention to his astuteness in dealing with his patients' dilemmas.

Not to be married is also an "impediment" (36) to Dr. Thorne during his early years in Greshamsbury, but he resolutely resists societal pressures (at least for the duration of this novel) by remaining a bachelor. We hear that he had once been in love, though not formally engaged, and that the young lady had withdrawn during a period of trouble for the Thorne family. Clearly hurt, he thereafter "never again made matrimonial overtures to anyone" (30). Until his niece comes to live with him he leads a makeshift existence in the smaller of two decent, commodious private houses in the village, which he refurbishes and furnishes to provide a comfortable home for young Mary. Thorne's eschewal of marriage is just one of the ways in which he shows himself to be tougher than Gibson. It is easier for him to maintain a somewhat unorthodox stance because he has the then enormous advantage of lofty "connections." These are explicitly expounded by the narrator, who, unlike the voice in *Wives and Daughters,* is totally omniscient, with full knowledge of the hero's background and history. The very first trait mentioned in the characterization of Thorne is that "Dr. Thorne belonged to a family in one sense as good, and at any rate as old, as that of Mr. Gresham; and much older, he was apt to boast, than that of the De Courcys" (22). That interpolated "he was apt to boast" reveals his great pride in his lineage, a pride that is conceded as "the weakness for which he was most conspicuous" (22). This is obviously a facet of Thorne that has to be handled with tact and caution; on the one hand, Trollope has to avoid giving the impression that his hero is a snob, yet on the other hand, the very real importance of his family background to his sense of self and his functioning in this environment must be adequately conveyed to readers. "He was the second cousin to Mr. Thorne of Ullathorne, a Barsetshire squire living in the neighbourhood of Barchester, and who boasted that his estate had remained in his family, descending from Thorne to Thorne, longer than had been the case with any other estate or any other family in the county" (20–21). Thorne's boasting comes to seem less grave a flaw in light of what is apparently a family tradition of immense pride in its past.

But like Gibson, Thorne is in an essentially ambivalent situation for, as the narrator insists, he is "only a second cousin; and, therefore, though he was entitled to talk of the blood as belonging to some extent to himself, he had no right to lay claim to any position in the county other than such as he might win for himself if he chose to locate himself in it" (21). That sentence draws a crucial distinction between laying claim to a position, as a hereditary aristocrat can, and winning a position by one's own efforts, as a physician must do. That Thorne's father had been a clergyman places him on a respectable but fairly modest rung on the social ladder, and he is further hampered by the adventures of his younger brother, who was killed by Roger Scatcherd, the wealthy upstart, in revenge for the seduction of his sister, Mary. Nor did the clergyman leave more than a pittance, so that the youthful Thomas Thorne has to fend for himself as well as care for his niece. His capital is thus precisely "his Ullathorne connexion," which induces him "to establish himself in Barchester, very mainly in expectation of the help" it would afford him (22). Such "connections" among extended family and friends were often a foremost consideration in a young doctor's choice of location.[4]

Long after he has successfully established himself, Thorne's pedigree is a salient factor in his practice. Since he is, certainly in his own eyes, the social equal of the Greshams and even of the De Courcys, he can speak to them without the deference that would be expected from a person of lower rank. As "a graduated physician" (31), he also has "the dignity of a learned profession" (32). This combination of professional and social self-confidence fosters a rather high-handed personal style: "He was brusque, authoritative, given to contradiction, rough though never dirty in personal belongings, and inclined to indulge in a sort of quiet raillery, which sometimes was not thoroughly understood. People did not always know whether he was laughing at them or with them" (35). Stern and strict with "trifling ailments" (36), he reveals a "loving, trusting heart" and an "almost womanly tenderness" (35) to those in "real suffering": "no patient lying painfully on a bed of sickness ever thought him rough" (36). A more complex personality than Gibson, Thorne is admitted to be "far from perfect" largely on account of his "inner, stubborn, self-admiring pride, which made him believe himself to be better and higher than those around him" (28).

Apart from pride, Thorne's other besetting flaw is defined as "that of combativeness. Not that the doctor was a bully, or even pugnacious, in the usual sense of the word; he had no disposition to provoke a fight, no propense love of quarreling; but there was that in him which would not allow him to yield to attack" (33). Here as in most of the introduction it is the voice of the omniscient, controlling narrator that is the source of intelligence. The sole exception to this method in the opening chapters is the section where Dr. Fillgrave's perception of Thorne is recorded (31–34). As his Dickensian name suggests, Fillgrave, Thorne's counterpart in neighboring Barchester, is cast as the villain among the medical men. His complaints against Thorne provide the opportunity to air some of the controversies besetting the profession. His main objection to Thorne seems trivial unless it is taken in the context of the stratification of nineteenth-century British medicine. For Fillgrave decries Thorne as "a compounder of doses" (34) because he had "added the business of a dispensing apothecary to that of a physician" (31). The words "business" and "apothecary" are keys to the nature of Thorne's transgression against an unwritten professional code: it was beneath the dignity of a physician to dispense drugs to patients, a task assigned primarily to apothecaries connected to trade and carried out by surgeons too. Thorne breaks this unwritten law out of consideration for the "comfort" of his patients, but "in doing so, he was of course much reviled. Many people around him declared that he could not truly be a doctor, or, at any rate, a doctor to be so called; and his brethren in the art living around him, though they knew that his diplomas, degrees, and certificates were all *en règle,* rather countenanced the report" (31). Fillgrave is thus voicing a widespread disapproval of Thorne for infringing the conventional proprieties and lowering what were considered the proper standards for physicians, however benign his motivation might be.

Fillgrave also accuses Thorne of "always thinking of his money" (32). This is surely a case of the pot calling the kettle black. Well into the novel, Trollope states that "Dr. Thorne was still a poor man; the gift of saving money had not been his" (95). His charges are modest because he lacks a sense of acquisitiveness, especially as long as he has no one to care for beyond himself. It transpires that Fillgrave's censure of Thorne's fees is directed precisely at their modesty, which again makes his practice seem more like an apothecary's than a graduated physician's:

> That fellow Thorne would lug out half a crown from his breeches
> pocket and give it in change for a ten-shilling piece. And then it was
> clear that this man had no appreciation of the dignity of a learned

profession. He might constantly be seen compounding medicines
in the shop, at the left hand of his front door; not making experiments philosophically in materia medica for the benefit of coming
ages . . . but positively putting together common powders for rural
bowels, or spreading vulgar ointments for agricultural ailments.
(32)

Class consciousness and concern for the conventions appropriate at each level
are here shown to underlie every aspect of Fillgrave's behavior, including the
treatment of patients, in which "dignity" has priority even over the healing
mission. His interpretation of "the dignity of a learned profession" is uncovered as a hollow pretense when he expounds his guiding tenet: "A physician
should take his fee without letting his left hand know what his right hand was
doing; it should be taken without a thought, without a look, without a move
of the facial muscles; the true physician should hardly be aware that the last
friendly grasp of the hand had been made more precious by the touch of
gold" (32). This is a masterful way of obliquely exposing Fillgrave's hypocrisy,
using the same means as Gaskell, indirect discourse laden with irony, which
leads the speaker unwittingly to unmask himself.

The extent of Fillgrave's hypocrisy is brought out in the grotesquely comic
episode in which he is called in by the testy Sir Roger Scatcherd, who has
fallen out with his regular attendant, Thorne, because the latter has warned
him with utmost bluntness of the dangers of continuing his excessive drinking
(which does indeed soon thereafter kill him). In a fit of alcohol-induced rage
Sir Roger sends for Fillgrave without bothering to tell—and to dismiss—
Thorne. When Fillgrave eventually arrives the next morning, full of swagger-
ing self-importance, he takes offense first at being kept waiting and then at
being refused access to the patient, who has meanwhile recovered from his
hangover. "Then did Dr. Fillgrave seem to grow out of his boots, so suddenly
did he take upon himself sundry modes of expansive altitude;—to grow
out of his boots and to swell upwards, till his angry eyes almost looked down
on Lady Scatcherd, and each erect hair bristled up towards the heavens" (145).
The unmistakable exaggeration of the overwriting here undermines Fillgrave,
making him appear ridiculous in a transformation reminiscent of *Alice in
Wonderland,* not to mention echoes of the expression "too big for his boots."
The scene comes to a climax when Lady Scatcherd tenders Fillgrave a five-

pound note—for services *not* rendered. Fillgrave faces an acute dilemma: he must choose between his love for a five-pound fee and his commitment to dignity. With the arrival of Thorne to visit what he still takes to be *his* patient, an angry confrontation ensues between the rivals, which makes Trollope wish he had "the pen of Molière" (147). It ends, ludicrously, with Fillgrave flinging at Thorne the infamous note, which Lady Scatcherd had "put into his hat while he was in his tantrums" (151). So both fee and dignity are forfeited. That this unseemly collision is instigated by an insult to Fillgrave's *dignity* intensifies the implicit indictment of his petty-mindedness. Thorne's alleged "combativeness" assumes quite another complexion when it is seen to take the form of opposition to Fillgrave and the arrogance and vanity he represents.

None of the several other doctors in *Doctor Thorne* is drawn as blackly as Fillgrave, although all are "far from perfect." Mr. Rerechild of Barchester, "a follower and humble friend of Dr. Fillgrave," had often expressed "his abhorrence of Dr. Thorne's anti-professional practices" (277). But "prudent" and "discreet," not to say timid, "knowing that he could make more by medical friends than by medical foes" (277), he takes the first good opportunity for a reconciliation with Thorne, becoming as submissive to him as he had been to Fillgrave. The surgeon's humble reverence for the physician, the obsequiousness with which he poses questions and listens for crumbs of knowledge, aptly conveys the discrepancy in accomplishment and authority between the two estates. Two other physicians are brought in as consultants to Lady Arabella during the time when she too, in a fit of pique, has switched from Thorne to Fillgrave. Dr. Century, a colleague of Fillgrave's, is another figure of fun, though he is merely inept and indecisive, not mean or ill-tempered. The suggestion of agedness in his name is confirmed by his noncommittal passivity: he says little and looks grave. He is firmly put in place by the narrator with a single, reductive, repeated word: "Dr. Century came and slowly toddled into her ladyship's room" (367), and afterwards, "Dr. Century had toddled downstairs to see the squire" (368). The disparity between the assumed air of gravity and the toddling, that is, walking with the short, hesitating, uncertain steps of a young child, suffices to envelop Dr. Century in ridicule. The London specialist Sir Omnicrom Pie is likewise the butt of some mockery, notably in his extravagant name, but on the whole he is accorded respect because he shows sound medical judgment in recommending to Lady Arabella that she return to Thorne and abide by his guidance.

The peripheral doctors in *Wives and Daughters* are fewer and less precisely delineated. Here too "the great physician of the county" (231), Dr. Nicholls, is called in to supplement Mr. Gibson, although he is not introduced in person, only by hearsay. Similarly, Mr. Hall, Gibson's predecessor, appears indirectly through the opinions voiced by the inhabitants of Hollingford and the narrator. The former are dismayed at news of his retirement because he is familiar as "the skilful doctor . . . who could heal all their ailments" (60). His omnipotence is diminished by the interjected phrase "unless they died meanwhile" (60), a sardonic barb on the narrator's part. Mr. Hall, we deduce, was socially inferior to Mr. Gibson: "He had always been received with friendly condescension by my lady" (69). On the rare occasions when he had been invited to dine at the Towers he had felt "discomfort," for which he was, however, recompensed by the pleasure of being able to impress the squires he was in the habit of attending by referring to what "the earl" or "the countess" had said (69). Class consciousness and snobbery are as pronounced in *Wives and Daughters* as in *Doctor Thorne,* and in both the doctor is particularly vulnerable because of his intermediate status not only as a member of the emergent middle class but also as one who, through his profession, has to be able to move with some ease between the classes.

Whatever their standing or their temperament, all the doctors in these two novels have in common their role as missionaries to the bedside. The center of medical practice in the nineteenth century was still the patient's home, to which the doctor was summoned whenever necessary. Often self-help and domestic remedies were tried first, for basic diagnostics and medical care were an integral part of the woman's nurturing function. Instructional works such as William Buchan's *Domestic Medicine; or a Treatise on the Prevention and Cure of Diseases by Regime and Simple Medicine* (1772), John G. Gunn's *Domestic Medicine; or Poor Man's Friend. In the Hours of Affliction, Pain and Suffering* (1830), and *The Maternal Physician* (1818) by "An American Matron," popular reference books, were aimed mainly at mothers.[5] Buchan's *Domestic Medicine* was "the most widely read—nonreligious—book in English during the half century following its Edinburgh publication in 1769,"[6] running to 142 separate editions between 1769, its last English-language edition appearing in Philadelphia in 1871.[7] Sections on medical matters were also a feature of such housekeeping manuals as Cora-Elisabeth Millet-Robinet's *La Maison rustique des dames* (1844–45, The ladies' rustic home), *Mrs. Beeton's Book of Household Man-*

agement (1861), and Mary Mason's *Young Housewife's Counselor* (1871). The precepts extended far beyond hygiene, first aid, recipes for invalid foods, and directions for preparing plasters, "blisters," and leeches. Mrs. Beeton is outstanding for the guidance she offers on the handling of quite serious medical conditions and emergencies. This dissemination of medical knowledge among patients empowered them to discuss their symptoms and treatment with their doctors because they regarded themselves as rather well informed.

The established tradition of domestic medicine had its natural extension in doctors' visits to the home, which have been called "the basic unit of the physician's work day,"[8] even in the closing decades of the nineteenth century. The location of the medical consultation in the home was decisive in shaping the balance of power. The interference of family, relatives, friends, and local healers, all of whom felt entitled to express their opinions, was a fertile source of disagreements. The doctor's authority and the utility of his advice could be challenged and undermined, especially during the earlier half of the century, before the rise of the scientific method, when medical lore was still considered common property. In the domestic setting, the doctor would have to forge an alliance with those present there because he had to rely on their reports and cooperation. The ambivalences inherent in the doctor's visit are well conveyed in the performative metaphor, "The physician and his prescriptions were thus constantly on stage; the sick room was a social context that could serve to focus and mobilize the patient's emotional resources."[9] Although the input of family and friends could provide support, it was more likely to create disharmony, to disturb the patient's rest, and, above all, to contaminate the intimate personal rapport between doctor and patient through the intervention of others' views and prejudices. The meeting of doctor and patient in the home was not the private, confidential communication to which we are accustomed but a more or less public forum with multiple participants. In other words, it was a ritual with conventions very different from those of today. Even if others were not present at the actual bedside, members of the patient's family and circle would await the doctor after the examination in expectation of diagnosis, prescription, and prognosis. So the doctor was held immediately and continuously accountable for the patient's state and for his conduct of the case.

While intimacy between doctor and patient could be jeopardized by the home setting, it could also be enhanced by it. Just to see the patient in his own surroundings enables the alert doctor to assess the patient's situation and personality. The value of the house call for an understanding of the patient is emphatically articulated in Robertson Davies's novel *The Cunning Man* (1994). The rather unconventional, holistic physician who is the narrator of this novel set in Canada explains why he continues what used to be known as "Domiciliary Attendance" even after World War II. He wants to see where and how his patients live: What is in the medicine cupboard, where are the lights in the house, what books are there, or are there artificial flowers? Does the furniture look freely used, or is it protected by plastic covers and lace curtains? The home setting is seen as representing a telling semiotic text from which to read the patient's circumstances.

The later substitution of office for home decontextualizes the patient in a leveling effect that is completed by the stripping of personal clothing for the anonymity of the paper—or hospital—"gown," the uniform of the sick supplicant. The absence of an office on the doctor's premises is a striking feature of mid- and later-nineteenth-century portrayals of healers: neither Gibson nor Thorne, nor indeed Lydgate in *Middlemarch* or Dr. Leslie in Sarah Orne Jewett's *Country Doctor* (1884), has facilities for seeing patients other than at the patient's home. Usage in this respect varied from place to place. In Flaubert's *Madame Bovary* (1857), Charles Bovary, who practices in rural Normandy in the 1830s as a "health officer," a rank equivalent to but rather lower than that of the British surgeon, does have a room in his house to which patients come.[10] Its adjacency to the kitchen allows his wife to hear the patients' coughing and whispering; it also suggests the contiguity of domestic and professional medicine at that time. The local squire brings his servant to the Bovary residence when he needs to be bled. Just as the poor were the earliest users of hospitals because they lacked suitable care at home, so they were more likely too to go to the doctor, or later in the century in the city to a dispensary, than to be visited, for cost was another consideration. The doctor's office does not really come into the forefront in literary texts until the opening chapter of Sinclair Lewis's *Arrowsmith* (1925) with its vivid evocation of Doc Vickerson's chaotic, insalubrious central room, which serves in Elk Mills, Winnemac, in 1897 as "business office, consultation-room, operating-theater, living-room, poker den, and warehouse for guns and fishing tackle" (7).

The prevalence of home visits meant that the doctor normally spent most of his day making rounds. The obligation on the doctor to do the traveling, especially in bad weather or at night, imposed the burden of fatigue and so disadvantaged him in relation to the patient, who could stay put. In the country in the early nineteenth century horseback was the usual mode of travel. Dr. Benassis in Balzac's *Le Médecin de campagne* (1833; *The Country Doctor*, 1911) has been given a magnificent steed by a grateful patient. In a more urban area in the 1870s Dr. Pascal Rougon in Zola's *Le Docteur Pascal* (1893; *Doctor Pascal*) can visit on foot. Mr. Gibson in *Wives and Daughters* is "a great deal out—almost constantly" (262), his wife laments in complaining about the solitary life she has to lead. Because of the pressure of his visits as his reputation grows and he is summoned to "various halls, courts, and houses" (213), the Gibsons' dinnertime has to be postponed to a later hour. Likewise Dr. Thorne, who has the advantage "of being a good horseman" (115), has an exceptionally long working day: "his hours of labour extended much beyond those usual to the upper working world, the hours, namely, between breakfast and dinner" (89). As a result of his erratic schedule and his liability to calls at any time, he has no fixed hours for his meals. As was customary, his charges correlate to the distance he has to travel: "seven-and-sixpence a visit within a circuit of five miles, with a proportionately increased charge at proportionately increased distances" (31). To be called to a distant location, though inconvenient, was welcome as a sign of prestige and recognition of expertise. When Dr. Thorne goes to see an old woman at Silverbridge, Dr. Century's territory, his niece, Mary, has mixed feelings: "She did not like her uncle going off so late on such a journey; but it was always felt as a triumph when he was invited into the strongholds of his enemies" (100).

To arrive in a carriage rather than on horseback was definitely a mark of status and prosperity. When Dr. Fillgrave is summoned to Sir Roger Scatcherd, he decides that the occasion warrants the use of post-horses: "Dr. Fillgrave's professional advancement had been sufficient to justify the establishment of a brougham, in which he paid his ordinary visits round Barchester; but this was a special occasion, requiring special speed, and about to produce no doubt a special guerdon, and therefore a pair of post-horses were put into request" (141). Similarly in *Madame Bovary* the celebrated Dr. Canivet of Neufchâtel, who is sent for to attend a leg turned gangrenous after surgery, appears "like a whirlwind" (153), driving his own gig. Before seeing the patient, he gives orders for his horse to be unharnessed and himself goes to the stable to make sure it is properly fed. With characteristic irony, Flaubert implies that the horse's health takes precedence over the patient's. Where roads permitted, the horse- or dog-drawn carriage became the preferred form of transport. Dr. Leslie in Jewett's *Country Doctor* makes his rounds in a carriage, so Nan, his young protégée, who herself aspires to be a physician, can drive with him day by day, initially as his companion and soon as his assistant. In *Dr. Zay* (1882), by Elizabeth Stuart Phelps, the doctress is first glimpsed boldly and elegantly guiding her fly through the Maine countryside.

Although doctors generally did not travel more than ten miles from home before the construction of better roads, their range expanded greatly with the advent of the motor car. Not surprisingly, they were among the first in the United States to buy automobiles between about 1906 and 1912.[11] For Martin Arrowsmith, in his general practice in Wheatsylvania in 1910–11, the purchase of a car for his country calls is a major step forward from "the flapping buggy" (139). Indeed, "it is possible that half of the first dozen patients who drifted into his office came because of awe at his driving" (151). He uses the car to drive forty-eight miles in seventy-nine minutes, according to the report in the local newspaper, to fetch antitoxin for a child suffering from diphtheria. He is summoned by a telephone call, which replaced the slow method of sending for the doctor by a hand-carried note or a verbal message. The telephone made it far easier to track down the ever peripatetic practitioner. As early as 1877 the first rudimentary telephone exchange was inaugurated in the Capital Avenue drugstore in Hartford, Connecticut, linked to twenty-one doctors.[12] So Arrowsmith takes a mere eighty minutes to reach his patient despite losing his way in the dark, whereas Dr. Fillgrave can respond to Sir Roger's message only the next morning because he had been some five or six miles out of town in the opposite direction and did not get back till late.

Delay in reaching the doctor by note might contribute to the patient's death, as in the case of Guido in Italo Svevo's *La coscienza di Zeno* (1923; *The Confessions of Zeno,* 1964), although Dr. Mali lives not far away. A "practical doctor who had always done his duty as best he could" (334), the fifty-five-year-old Mali has just returned home and succeeded in drying and warming himself by the fire when he is called out again. While he waits for the soaking rain to abate somewhat the poison that Guido has ingested takes effect. His history of previous suicide attempts has deterred the doctor from taking this one sufficiently seriously. Black humor is injected into the incident when Dr. Mali mutters furiously: "It ought to be illegal to pretend one has committed suicide in weather like this!" (335). He explains his reluctance to go out again to the narrator in this strange apologia: "It was impossible, he said, for a layman to realize how used the doctor becomes to protecting himself against his patients, who are continually making attempts on his life, in their selfish insistence on saving their own" (335). So while Guido takes his life the doctor perversely sees him as attempting to take *his*. Dr. Mali's power play in putting his own welfare before that of his patient not only results in the latter's death but also represents a parodistic inversion of the ideal expected of the missionary to the bedside.

That ideal, as conceived by the mid–nineteenth century, included, to cite Worthington Hooker's phrase in *Physician and Patient* (1849), the doctor's act-ing as a "confidential *friend*" (384). This function derives, according to Hooker, from both the duration and the intimacy of the interaction: "If he has been the physician of the family for any length of time, and has been with them in many scenes of suffering, ready to relieve, so far as lay in him the power to do it, this feeling of affectionate reliance is deep and ardent"—especially in females, he adds. One factor in the development of such closeness was cer-tainly the doctor's easy access to the patient's home, the fact that he was re-ceived in "the very bosom of their families" (385) and entrusted with their secrets and anxieties. The doctor's responsibility transcended the treatment of immediate ills: "it was considered quite normal for a physician to visit homes for relatively minor complaints, to vaccinate, for example, and in the-ory even to advise on matters such as the location of a new house, proper plumbing, or an appropriate diet."[13] In the ideal practice, then, performed by a practitioner in the home, a personal as well as a professional rapport was established between the family and its doctor. In this context, the family doctor was one who provided care based on a comprehensive understanding of all the medical, emotional, and social problems that beset an extended family entity through successive generations.[14]

If in some respects the mid-nineteenth-century doctor had less power than his modern successor, in other ways he was in a position to exert a wider im-pact on the overall welfare of his patients and their families. The practice of medicine within the home could, on the one hand, create friction between the doctor and the patient's entourage but also, on the other hand, be con-ducive to the spread of his influence. The doctor's visit has been described as "both a social and a medical event. He was customarily invited to dine, and if the illness was serious, he might reside for several days in the patient's home."[15] Both Dr. Thorne and Mr. Gibson stay overnight in times of crisis: the former maintains a vigil over Sir Roger's deathbed, while the latter hardly leaves the bedside of the squire's wife during her last days. Intimacy was fostered too by the kinds of cases that nineteenth-century doctors faced, notably acute infectious diseases that entailed frequent visits, grave responsibility, and apprehension shared with the family. One example is Lydgate in *Middlemarch,* who succeeds in pulling Fred Vincy through an attack of typhoid fever by meticulous supervision of the in-home nursing and is drawn by this sustained contact with the family into marrying Fred's sister. In Thomas Mann's *Buddenbrooks* (1901; trans. 1952) Dr. Grabow is among the guests at all family events, and with his junior partner, Dr. Langhals, he is in constant attendance during Elisabeth Buddenbrooks's dying of pneumonia.

This exceptionally close bond between doctor and patient stemmed in part from the holistic assumptions underlying nineteenth-century medicine. The foundations and implications of this view are explored with finesse by Charles Rosenberg in his essay "Body and Mind in Nineteenth-Century Medicine."[16] He stresses the prevalence of "holistic pathology" in a period when "specific diseases played a relatively small role in a scheme that emphasized the body's unending transactions with its environment" (77). Hence, "no one doubted the causal relationship between situational stress and disease etiology, and, in particular, the dangers of emotions unchecked" (76). This unitary approach to the patient is the major advantage of old-style bedside medicine as still practiced in the mid–nineteenth century, before the increased discrimination of discrete syndromes, the primary outcome of advances in pathology, initiated the trend to specialization and fragmentation. Commanding less scientific expertise and fewer means to attain it, mid-nineteenth-century doctors relied perforce on pragmatic observation and intuitive insight into what ailed their patients. They compensated for the vagueness of their diagnostic terminology and the shortcomings of their therapeutic capacity by offering compassionate care. Although we never hear, for instance, what is wrong with Lady Arabella in *Doctor Thorne* nor what causes the death of the squire's wife in *Wives and Daughters,* in each of these cases the doctor responds with empathetic appreciation of family dynamics as well as with palliative physical measures. These examples illustrate well Rosenberg's contention that "until the mid–nineteenth century . . . all medicine was necessarily and ubiquitously 'psychosomatic'" (77) because no boundaries were drawn between the realms of body and mind. If "there were no specialists in disorders of mood, cognition, and behavior, . . . every clinician had to be something of a psychiatrist and family therapist" (78). Parsons's assertion that "all good medical practice . . . is to some degree psychotherapy"[17] has never been more true than in the early to mid–nineteenth century.

The doctor's position as confidential friend is a major theme in *Doctor Thorne* and *Wives and Daughters,* in both of which he is seen in his medical and personal interactions with several families. In each work one family is aristocratic (the de Courcys in Trollope's novel and the Cumnors in Mrs. Gaskell's) and one upper middle class (the Greshams in *Doctor Thorne* and the Hamleys in *Wives and Daughters*); in addition, *Doctor Thorne* also contains an upwardly mobile, nouveau riche family in the Scatcherds. In their conversations with their patients the two doctors do not substantially vary their tone according to their interlocutor's social level; they maintain a uniform style, though it differs considerably in conformity with their respective personalities. Mr. Gibson, gentle and reassuring by temperament, extends his paternal concern for his daughter, Molly, to his patients. He is a constant visitor to the Hamley home to see Mrs. Hamley, whose chronic invalidism has over the years made the family turn to him increasingly. As a result of the long and intimate association, he has acquired a subtle understanding of their intrafamily problems, notably the discord between the eldest son, Osborne, and his father, from which he wants to protect the fragile Mrs. Hamley. Without overt manipulation, Mr. Gibson acts as a diplomatic intermediary between the family members in an endeavor to attenuate their disputes. In a series of crises he plays the idealized doctor's role of rescuer: to Mrs. Hamley, who is said to be "craving for the wisdom which might fall from the doctor's lips" (153), he brings solace as she moves toward death; to Squire Hamley he gives comfort and support during his bereavement through his quiet tact, succeeding in "strengthening him physically, and encouraging him mentally" (615). With Osborne, the profligate son, he takes the lead in an understated yet decisive manner, trying to draw out the troubled young man, examining him with "a comprehensive look" from his "sharp and observant eyes" (368) and soon discerning that "there was some mental cause for this depression of health" (367). The coalescence of the mid-nineteenth-century doctor's twin functions is plainly articulated when Gibson tells his wife that he "didn't want him [Osborne] to consider me as his doctor, but as a friend" (608). Gibson is perhaps at his best with Osborne's forlorn wife, whose trust and cooperation he is able to elicit by addressing her in her native French in "low tones of comfort and sympathy" (632) as he feels her pulse and supervises her rest. This dual sensitivity to his patients' physical and psychological needs is equally evident in his dealings with Lady Cumnor, who has chosen him as "our family doctor" because "he's a man of sense" (157). That collective term "sense" here denotes a multitude of virtues, not the least of which is sensibility. Lady Cumnor's reliance on Mr. Gibson is revealed by her readiness to confide in him and to turn to him for guidance rather than to her husband, who actually stands in some awe of her strident personality. Through his tact and probity, Mr. Gibson occupies a responsible and singularly privileged place in the lives of these patients even though as a surgeon he does not occupy a high social station. His power derives primarily from his sterling personal qualities, which earn him universal respect from patients of every class.

Dr. Thorne can draw on his prestige as a graduated physician to exercise authority. His bluntness, however, is a source of tensions that erupt periodically in open strife, most often with Lady Arabella. Through shifts in viewpoint we are enabled to know exactly what she thinks of him: "Though she thought the doctor to be arrogant, deficient as to properly submissive demeanour towards herself, an instigator to marital parsimony in her lord, one altogether opposed to herself and her interests in Greshamsbury politics, nevertheless, she did feel trust in him as a medical man" (162). In contrast to the lesser qualified but urbane Mr. Gibson, Dr. Thorne is valued for his medical advice notwithstanding what are perceived by her ladyship as his deficiencies in due etiquette in his attempts to place her in his power. His "utter disregard of Lady Arabella's airs," together with "his subversive professional democratic tendencies" (38), eventually irks her so acutely that she leaves him for a while. It is Sir Omnicrom Pie, the London consultant, who conveys to her via her husband that she "was foolish to quarrel with her best friend" (469). Despite his usual astringency, Dr. Thorne is generous in his reconciliation, although "Lady Arabella felt that the doctor kept the upper hand in these sweet forgivenesses" (469).

He certainly keeps the upper hand with Sir Roger Scatcherd, on whom he uses what would nowadays be called tough love in trying to shock him into stopping or at least reducing his drinking. Sir Roger's immediate response is angry invective coupled with a threat (which he does fulfill) to leave Dr. Thorne. But as their regular medical attendant and one who knew the Scatcherds long before their rise to wealth and eminence, the doctor is too crucial to their well-being to be easily cast off. He alone is fully aware of the current degree of Sir Roger's alcoholism and also understanding of his aggressive-defensive stance. He maintains a tacit entente with the pathetic Lady Scatcherd, who implores him to continue to "slip in as a friend" (122) even after the most recent quarrel between him and her husband. That word "friend" had previously been applied to Dr. Thorne's relationship to Sir Roger, and the nature of this friendship precisely defined: "Scatcherd had but one friend in the world. And, indeed, this friend was no friend in the ordinary acceptance of the word. He neither ate with him nor drank with him, nor even frequently talked with him. Their pursuits in life were wide asunder. Their tastes were all different. The society in which each moved very seldom came together. Scatcherd had nothing in unison with this solitary friend; but he trusted him, and he trusted no other living creature on earth" (113). The peculiarities of this friendship are further elaborated in the following paragraph, where the narrator explains that Sir Roger's trust in Dr. Thorne resided in his character not in his theory or practice: "He disliked his friend's counsel, and, in fact, disliked his society, for his friend was somewhat apt to speak to him in a manner approaching severity" (113). Sir Roger's attachment to Dr. Thorne differs, therefore, from Lady Arabella's insofar as he does not value his medical advice yet at some deeper level recognizes his wisdom and integrity. The conflicted "friendship" with Dr. Thorne encompasses abusive hostility and deep faith alike. While thwarting Thorne's efforts to stop him from drinking, Sir Roger nonetheless begs him to act as guardian to his delinquent son, Louis: "Use the power that a strong man has over a weak one. Use the power that my will will give you. Do for him as you would for a son of your own if you saw him going in bad courses. Do as a friend should do for a friend that is dead and gone" (294). Sir Roger here openly acknowledges Thorne's "power," not, however, in his capacity as a physician but as "a strong man." Thorne's willingness to accept this troublesome charge against his inner inclinations tells us much about the doctor's sense of obligation from generation to generation toward those families to whom he is a "confidential friend." Though Louis proves arrogant, defiant, and stupidly self-destructive, Dr. Thorne stands by him to the best of his ability with sound medical and per-

sonal advice. His loyalty, perseverance, and selflessness fully earn him the title
"hero." He shows the same extraordinary commitment to his calling as Mr.
Gibson, the same readiness to sacrifice his own convenience to the needs of
others. But he is less idealized than his counterpart in *Wives and Daughters* because of his pride and his tendency to outspokenness. Nor do his relationships
with his patients go as smoothly as Mr. Gibson's; as a graduated physician,
he claims greater authority than the lowlier surgeon and so arouses a curious
amalgam of recalcitrance and devotion.

The difference may also be a matter of time: in the twenty years separating
Dr. Thorne from Mr. Gibson the prestige of medical opinion had begun to
rise and to claim priority over patients' self-diagnosis and self-prescription. As
long as doctors possessed relatively few diagnostic or therapeutic tools they
could not command significant superiority over their patients, whose lay
experience of domestic medicine equipped them to participate in decisions
concerning their care. For in the early nineteenth century "the best doctors
could do was to assist the healing powers of nature."[18] Even more pessimistic
evaluations have been put forward. It has been asserted, for example, that before the twentieth century scarcely more than half a dozen truly rational
medical agents existed that could materially alter the natural history of a disease.[19] Consequently, "citizens two hundred years ago fully expected to diagnose and treat a host of diseases, certainly at their onset and often until
their resolution,"[20] for "a good portion of the actual therapeutic practices of
formally trained physicians overlapped with those employed by untutored
laypersons."[21] What is more, patients and medical men shared the same concepts of the body's functioning and disturbances in a set of overarching theories that empowered patients as much as doctors. This common base had the
effect of blurring the distinctions between qualified and unqualified practitioners; the public had difficulty in discriminating between the categories in
the days before legal regulation, which took effect in Great Britain only in
1858 with the Medical Registration Act. Unable to judge by verifiable objective criteria, "patients wisely preferred to trust reputation as transmitted by
word of mouth. As a result, the general public frequently placed greater faith
in domestic practitioners than in university-educated physicians."[22] This habit
is very evident in *Wives and Daughters,* the earlier of the two works being
discussed here, in the spread of Mr. Gibson's repute by hearsay in reported
speech. While individual practitioners who had proven their worth might be

accorded respect, medicine in general was held in rather low esteem. It was in defense of medicine against accusations of charlatanism and superstition that the famous treatise by Pierre-George Cabanis, *Du degré de certitude de la médecine* (On the degree of certitude in medicine) was published in 1797. It is less an assertion of certainty than an attempt to circumscribe the uncertainties of medicine's epistemological status and indirectly to raise medical expertise, however limited it still was at the time, above domestic lore, not to mention sheer quackery.

This rather low regard for medical men is the context for Lady Arabella's and Sir Roger's resistance to Dr. Thorne, which stems from their belief in patients' right not only to question the doctor's prescriptions but also actively to suggest their own therapies. In a chapter entitled "Every Man His Own Doctor"—which should surely be amended to "Every Man and Woman" in light of women's command of domestic medicine—Murphy argues that "the optimum healing situation" was "one characterized by cooperation among all parties involved."[23] Expertise derived from personal experience in the application of herbal and folk remedies warranted due recognition. "No hard-and-fast delineation of lay and professional responsibilities was possible," Murphy adds. Doctors sought full obedience from patients and their families, who, however, felt entitled to withhold or to moderate such complete compliance. This tension between doctor and patient in the early part of the nineteenth century prefigures in some respects the power struggle latent in the relationship today as patients demand to be allowed more voice in decision-making. But today that means a measure of choice among the alternatives put forward by the physician, whereas in the time of Trollope and Gaskell, that is, before the elevation of medicine to a science, patients assumed a more radical posture that devolved from their conviction of their own capacity to select the best therapeutic course on the basis of merely lay advice. Paradoxically, opposition to the doctor's prescriptions, especially if they were disagreeable, like Thorne's exhortation to Sir Roger to stop drinking, did not prejudice the doctor's position as confidential friend. Trollope makes this clear in the passage cited above in expounding Sir Roger's contradictory attitude toward Dr. Thorne. Unbounded faith in his rectitude mingles with an obstinate self-assertion that becomes manifest in a querulous rejection of unwelcome directives.

The dominance of the patient in the consultative relationship most com-

monly took the form of switching to another doctor readier to make concessions to the patient's wishes. This is what both Lady Arabella and Sir Roger
do in turning to Dr. Fillgrave, who is certainly more tractable than Dr. Thorne.
At his most cantankerous Sir Roger is not above reminding Dr. Thorne that
he is in his employ. When Thorne admonishes him, "We must turn over a
new leaf, Sir Roger; indeed, we must," and adds, "I must do my duty to you
whether you like it or not," Sir Roger testily counters with, "That is to say, I
am to pay you for trying to frighten me" (118). Ignoring the insult and the
barely concealed bid for control, Thorne continues to focus on his patient's
welfare rather than nurturing a grievance. Though he may be "far from
perfect," in his firm and fair handling of his patients he shows great nobility
of spirit. He is as generous toward Lady Arabella, who sends for Dr. Fillgrave
on more than one occasion. She first comes to "hate the doctor" and to quarrel with him when she has a series of weakly babies and Thorne "sternly forbade the mother to go to London," and with each child he becomes "more
imperative than ever as to the nursery rules and the excellence of country
air" (38). As with Sir Roger, Dr. Thorne is here advocating proper care with
proper authority, to which the patient takes unreasonable and selfish objection.
While "she found Dr. Fillgrave a great comfort to her" (38), obviously because
he is lenient in yielding to her desires, the four frail little ones all die, and "the
mother's heart then got the better of the woman's pride, and Lady Arabella
humbled herself before Dr. Thorne. She humbled herself, or would have
done so, had the doctor permitted her. But he, with his eyes full of tears,
stopped the utterance of her apology, took her two hands in his, pressed
them warmly, and assured her that his joy in returning would be great, for
the love that he bore to all that belonged to Greshamsbury" (39). Nevertheless,
this experience and Dr. Thorne's magnanimity do not deter Lady Arabella
from again resorting to Dr. Fillgrave years later when she is exasperated by
a chronic ailment.

The petulant behavior of Sir Roger and Lady Arabella illustrates just
how tricky the doctor's work could be in countering patients' whims and persuading them to accept his opinions at a time when medicine did not enjoy
the privileged status of a well-founded science. It is no coincidence that Dr.
Thorne's difficulties are most acute with patients of high social class. Although
we do not hear very much about his visits to the local country people, he
clearly has far less trouble and reaps more gratitude from those lower on the

social scale, who would appreciate too the modesty of his fees. Mr. Gibson in *Wives and Daughters* seems to be universally liked. Several reasons can be put forward for the widespread favor he enjoys: it is a facet of the idealization to which he is subject in the novel; it is also an outcome of his temperament, which is more placid than Dr. Thorne's; above all, it is connected to his own humbler professional standing as a surgeon, which prevents him from expecting as much power as Dr. Thorne does and from speaking in so authoritarian a manner. Significantly, he is especially complimented on the fact that he "always managed my lady [Cumnor] so beautifully" (136).

Mr. Gibson's tact is again revealed in his handling of consultations. Recourse to a second opinion occurs in both these novels. When Dr. Nicholls, the venerable old physician in the county, is brought in to see Osborne in *Wives and Daughters* and reaches a different diagnosis, Mr. Gibson, who, we are here pointedly reminded, is only "the country surgeon" (409), says nothing—but is proven right by the outcome. Consultations are frequent in *Doctor Thorne*. Dr. Fillgrave calls in his colleague Dr. Century, as well as Mr. Rerechild as an assistant. In such instances the consultation is not so much for the patient's benefit as for the doctor's self-confirmation and aggrandizement when another physician endorses the proposed line of treatment. Ironically, Fillgrave's strategy misfires when he summons from London Sir Omnicrom Pie, whose unequivocal advice is that, though Fillgrave is "a very good man" (370), and Century too, Lady Arabella should go back to Thorne.

His reasoning for this recommendation raises a very important issue in the early-nineteenth-century relationship between doctor and patient: Thorne, he argues, "has known her ladyship so long" (370). Deep, personal knowledge of the patient was a paramount necessity for doctors then because treatment was patient-specific, not disease-specific, as it has since become. Indeed, until the 1860s disease-specific therapeutics were considered professionally illegitimate and suspect as characteristic of itinerant quacks who hawked a single blanket remedy for any affliction irrespective of the patient's needs. The principle of specificity as still understood in the first half of the nineteenth century mandated that treatment had to be specific to the particular patient's constitution, temperament, locale, and age and even to the prevailing season. Such an individualized match between the medical therapy and the singular patient in his physical and social environment could be achieved only by a doctor who knew not merely the patient's but also the family's idiosyncrasies. So "the physician best able to know what was natural for the patient and most capable of restoring the system to a natural balance when it was disrupted was a practitioner well acquainted with the patient's personal history and with the peculiarities of the locality and its diseases."[24] Since each patient possessed a unique physiological and psychological identity, the skilled practitioner would have to evaluate a great variety of factors in order to tailor the prescription to a particular patient at a particular time and in a particular place. No inconsistency was perceived in bestowing divergent or even opposite treatments on two persons suffering from the same disturbance because it was thought that they might require other means to restore the natural balance. This approach was indebted to the humoralism formalized by Galen in the second century A.D., which taught that health resulted from the natural balance of four bodily humors (yellow bile, blood, phlegm, and black bile) and their manifested qualities (cold, heat, moistness, and dryness). According to the relative proportions of the humors a person's temperament could be melancholic, sanguineous, phlegmatic, or choleric. In order to be effective, treatment had to fit the patient's predominant humor and temperament. The impact of these beliefs was an empiricism intent on meticulous observation of each patient in reaction against eighteenth-century speculative, theoretical systems, which had aligned medicine with philosophy.

Patient-specific therapeutics fostered a highly individualized type of medical practice. The notion of a family doctor took on a special significance in this context when wide-ranging familiarity with the patient formed the basis for care. Patient specificity obviously held special appeal at a time when the diagnostic potential was as yet quite primitive. Direct observation, accumulation of information about the family, and insight into its problems were all accessible through intelligent looking and listening without scientific instruments. The scarcity of diagnostic means in fact forced clinicians to develop their powers of observation to the utmost. Dr. Thorne and Mr. Gibson feel the pulse, but mainly they concentrate on scrutinizing the patient and drawing on longstanding knowledge of the diverse determining circumstances. Again and again in *Doctor Thorne* and *Wives and Daughters* the point is made that the most successful doctor is the one who best knows the patient. So Lady Arabella's son, in concurring with Sir Omnicrom Pie's advice that she return to Dr. Thorne, comments that he "has known my mother's constitution for so many years" (468) that he has learnt by experience how to deal with her symptoms. This style of medicine compensates for its scientific tenuity by emphasis on the holistic understanding of the patient. Like Dr. Thorne's attendance on Lady Arabella, Mr. Gibson's attendance on Mrs. Hamley in *Wives and Daughters* is predicated not on a physical diagnosis but on a shrewd appreciation of her position in the family and its psychosomatic consequences for her health. The decisive advantages of detailed knowledge of the patient and family are affirmed even more categorically in two other cases when Mr. Gibson, a mere country surgeon, comes nearer the mark than the graduated physician who is summoned from outside for consultation. With both Lady Cumnor and Osborne Hamley, Mr. Gibson's practical bedside grasp is a surer guide than the theoretical conclusions of Dr. Nicholls. During Lady Cumnor's recovery from surgery in London Mr. Gibson is "frequently consulted and referred to," his opinion holding "in opposition to that of one or two great names" in the city (557). The message is unmistakable: scholarly expertise in medicine is therapeutically less efficacious than the kind of alliance between patient and doctor that develops through long years of confidential friendship. Such friendship in turn, as a source of knowledge about the patient, gives the doctor an irrefutable power base.

On the other hand, the closeness to the patient essential to the doctor's optimal functioning can lead to problems for him and, by extension, for his family. Predicaments consequent to "friendship" occur in both *Doctor Thorne* and *Wives and Daughters* when Mary Thorne and Molly Gibson come under scrutiny as potential wives for patients' sons. Exceptionally charming, kind, good, sensible, well mannered, pretty, and adequately educated, each of these young women would seem to be a desirable match for any man. They are nonetheless unacceptable to the Greshams and the Hamleys as brides for their sons because they are deemed wanting in social status. As Squire Hamley openly tells Mr. Gibson: "Your Molly is one in a thousand, to my mind. But then, you see, she comes of no family at all—and I don't suppose she'll have a chance of much money" (438). In *Doctor Thorne* Lady Arabella goes so far as to dismiss the doctor lest his presence encourage her son's attachment to his niece, a connection she regards as ruinous to the young man.

As comedies of manners the two novels are brought to a happy end with the marriages duly contracted after the initial opposition has been overcome. But not before the iniquities of the social system have been uncovered: in addition to rampant hypocrisy and snobbishness, a self-seeking materialism also prevails. The obstacles to the marriages turn out to be pecuniary as well as class-related: Mary Thorne is welcomed by the Greshams with open arms after she inherits a large fortune, while Molly's lack of resources can be overlooked once her suitor makes good as a research scientist. In their mixture of cynicism and idealization these happy endings reiterate the well-to-do patients' conflicted posture toward their doctors. The social systems in *Wives and Daughters* and *Doctor Thorne* appear to be governed by a clearcut etiquette, yet the fictional happenings reveal a larger measure of improvisation and compromise than might be anticipated.

Through the objections to the marriages of Molly Gibson and Mary Thorne into the Hamley and Gresham families, respectively, the doctor's equivocal position in the first half of the nineteenth century is brought into sharp relief. Neither professionally nor socially was he granted the recognition automatically accorded to him today by virtue of his calling. Medicine itself was still an ill-defined field that encompassed folklore, amateurishness, and charlatanism alongside a limited amount of sound knowledge. The doctor's acceptance was, therefore, primarily a matter of personal consonance between him and the patients who employed him. Success depended on the ability to attract the interest and approval of a client or patron, and the crucial factor in that ability was the development of personal empathy between the parties. So the doctor's gifts as a psychologist were de facto more important than the actual treatment he gave. In the absence of effective pharmacological remedies, psychotherapeutic support was often the best, and sometimes the only, help the doctor could offer. This limitation suggests that patients were less capricious than is generally thought in choosing their doctors for their personal qualities rather than for their professional qualifications. It was not *what* the doctor was but *who* he was that ultimately mattered most to patients, and that lent him power. Exemplary moral character was the most highly prized trait in a man who would, ideally, become a confidential friend. That word *moral* was invested with meanings wider than its specific connotation today for it was taken to denote a whole range of positive attributes. The moral influence of persuasion was regarded as an active force, a major source of the doctor's healing effect. Despite its primitiveness, early-nineteenth-century medicine here foreshadows contemporary belief in psychotherapeutic healing as an integral part of any treatment.

Moral character was not, however, readily ascertainable, especially in a newly established doctor. The "connections" that were instrumental in winning acceptance come into a new light in this context as the equivalent to personal recommendations from those whose opinion was valued and who were able to vouch for the newcomer's moral character. Where such testimonials were lacking, doctors were likely to be judged first by their appearance and manners. Mr. Gibson's leanness and Scottish accent are held in his favor, while Dr. Thorne's somewhat negligent self-presentation is barely neutralized by his aristocratic affiliations. Likewise, Mr. Gibson's soothing, circumspect manner is clearly more pleasing than Dr. Thorne's tendency to outspoken directness. Significantly, none of Mr. Gibson's patients thinks of leaving him for any other medical attendant, whereas Dr. Thorne's do, not out of dissatisfaction with his care but out of exasperation at his style.

Good manners were considered a cardinal desideratum in a doctor, not merely as an expression of the proper etiquette but indeed as a surrogate for competence. Long after the medical profession had already instituted formal regulation so that qualifications could be checked, manners continue to be stressed as the royal road to success. "Manners help to make the majority of medical fortunes," Cathell proclaims on the opening page of his *Book On the Physician Himself,* which might be described as a sort of charm school for doctors. Cathell was convinced that physicians fail to achieve success not for want of knowledge, but "because they lack professional tact."[25] While he notes too that knowledge of "the family constitution, temperament, and tendencies" is "a powerful acquisition" (92) for any doctor, as it was in the earlier part of the century, he dwells almost compulsively on the indispensability of appearance and manners:

> The neglect of neatness of dress and the want of polite, refined manners might cause you to be criticised and shunned. You will sometimes see spruce little Dr. Tact, whose head is comparatively empty, succeed in getting extensive and lucrative practice, and paying heavy bills for horseshoes, almost entirely by attention to the outer trappings and affability of manner, while Dr. Talent, much better qualified, will languish, and never learn the price of carriages and oats, by reason of defects in these apparently trivial matters. Clean hands, a well-shaved face, polished boots, neat cuffs, gloves, fashionable clothing, cane, sun-umbrella, all relate to personal hy-

giene, and indicate gentility and self-respect, and naturally give
their possessor a pleasurable consciousness of being well dressed
and presentable.

The majority of people will employ a tidy, well-dressed physician
of equal, or even inferior, talent more readily than a shabbily dressed
one; and they will also accord him more confidence, and expect
from and willingly pay to him larger bills. (19)

Yet even with the best appearance and manners the early-nineteenth-century
doctor is constrained by the prevailing etiquette into an uncomfortable social
limbo. As a missionary to the bedside he is received into the home, and as a
confidential friend admitted into family secrets, but he is not regarded as an
equal by the upper middle class, let alone the aristocracy. His ambivalent
situation is vividly illustrated in the eating arrangements mentioned in the
two novels. As part of the social aspect of the doctor's visit, refreshment was
frequently offered, especially if the doctor had come some distance on horseback. Mr. Hall in *Wives and Daughters* has the "custom of taking his meals, if
he needed refreshment, in the housekeeper's room, not *with* the housekeeper,
bien entendu" (69). This information is imparted in reported speech, filtered
through Lady Cumnor's mind; the class hierarchy between the housekeeper,
the surgeon, and her ladyship is underscored by her slightly pretentious, obviously distancing use of a French phrase. In *Doctor Thorne* Dr. Fillgrave is given
a glass of sherry and lunch, which he takes alone; Thorne himself, with his
usual gruffness, invariably refuses even sherry or a cordial, perhaps to avoid
the humiliation of being made to eat alone. Gibson's difficulty in finding a
second wife is another pointer to the doctor's rather dubious place. For his
country clientele falls into "two classes pretty distinctly marked: farmers,
whose children were unrefined and uneducated; squires, whose daughters
would, indeed, think the world was coming to a pretty pass, if they were to
marry a country surgeon" (135). The woman he marries, Mrs. Kirkpatrick, a
clergyman's widow, is, like him, astride the classes. Twenty-five years later, in
Doctor Thorne, there are indications of incipient change: "The doctor used
his surgical lore, as he well knew how to use it. There was an assured confidence about him, and an air which seemed to declare that he really knew what
he was doing" (469). Here the increase in professional expertise clearly marks
the beginning of the medical man's elevation to greater prestige and power.

The role of missionary to the bedside was beset by equivocation that required a precarious balancing act on the doctor's part. On the one hand, he was expected to maintain the appearance and bearing of a gentleman and to be able to manage any crisis with equanimity. On the other hand, however, he was treated as a social inferior and had to defer to his patients' wishes even if they were foolish or injurious to their own health. Perhaps the true heroism of Mr. Gibson and Dr. Thorne lies in their remarkable dexterity in steering between these conflicting demands. The apparent ease with which this difficult task is carried through in *Wives and Daughters* bespeaks the idealization in which the surgeon is enveloped; he makes mistakes, for sure, particularly in regard to his second wife, but toward his patients he is a model of empathetic responsiveness and astute judgment. His modesty, affability, and humor enable him to sustain a sense of proportion and of detachment and very cleverly to wield power without seeming to. In other words, he is adept in negotiating etiquette by his discretion, his unassuming self-presentation, and his receptiveness to his patients' predilections. Without ever openly claiming power, he is nevertheless a powerful figure in his world. Dr. Thorne's dilemma is parallel but more intense. Far greater tension permeates the etiquette of power between doctor and patient in *Doctor Thorne* than in *Wives and Daughters*. Although Dr. Thorne shows an almost saintly streak when his patients are in need, at other times he can be roused to acerbity by their willful disregard of his advice. Because he is of loftier professional and social status than Mr. Gibson, Dr. Thorne expects to be able to exercise greater authority. He is therefore irked by the contrariety of the headstrong among his clients, who exact a degree of self-determination as their right. This self-assertiveness is most pronounced in his wealthiest and most upper-class patients, who challenge Thorne's professional prerogatives on the basis of their financial and social prominence. A clash occurs here between an older etiquette that acceded more readily to patients' privileges and an emergent one in which the physician projects a more assured sense of self and so aspires to more affirmative compliance from patients. But in mid-century Dr. Thorne cannot yet command the extensive professional expertise necessary to impose his will. Much less willing than Gibson to compromise, he goes through a series of battles, particularly with Lady Arabella and Sir Roger, over the issue of control. Since he proves right in every instance, his suzerainty is ultimately, though grudgingly, conceded.

The charge of being a missionary to the bedside persists through a long line of nineteenth-century literary works. The doctor's archetypal rescuing function is performed within a variable power structure. In Balzac's cycle *La Comédie humaine,* one of the recurrent characters is Dr. Bianchon, who was modeled on Jean Bouillard (1796–1881), author of a treatise on encephalitis. Bianchon is summoned to the bedside of the dying old man in *Le Père Goriot* (1835; *Old Goriot,* 1975), where he watches attentively, alleviating the suffering as best he can, although it is plain even to the still inexperienced medical student that Goriot is beyond help. Here it is sheer compassion that prevails, since the moribund pauper and the student are alike outside the sphere of social or professional power. Madame Grandet too, in Balzac's *Eugénie Grandet* (1833; trans. 1968), is already on her deathbed when the town's most celebrated physician is brought in. He observes the courtesies while making laconic comments, but he recognizes, probably from long experience, that in the face of Grandet's obsessiveness moral intervention would be just as futile as medical remedies. He is obviously privy to the dire regime of miserliness in this family since he cannot repress a smile when asked whether the care will be expensive and require many medications. By contrast, very active directives, particularly in personal and public hygiene, are dispensed by the energetic Dr. Benassis, the titular figure in Balzac's *Médecin de campagne.* He is both friend and missionary to his country patients, whom he visits in their homes. Poor peasants, they reverence and obey him unconditionally even when his orders conflict with their folkloric beliefs. Charles Bovary too rides the countryside to attend to local farmers; he gladly partakes of their meals and inspects their wounds, but mostly he refrains from doing much because he is dimly aware of his own limitations. His lack of intelligence and vision preclude him from any power.

By the late nineteenth century the doctor is regularly accorded growing respect by virtue of his professional knowledge, but the element of friendship still remains strong. Dr. Pascal Rougon, in Zola's *Docteur Pascal,* set in a small country town in the south of France in the early 1870s, is as devoted to his patients as to his research. Like Mr. Gibson and Dr. Thorne, he is fully conversant with his patients' personal and family histories. His involvement in their lives comes close to threatening the detachment and objectivity necessary to a physician because of the unusual circumstances of his work: he experiments with innovative therapies of his own devising so that he experiences his patients' setbacks as his own. Despite the failure of some of his cures, his humble patients trust and admire him boundlessly. A more conventional relationship is represented by old Dr. Kittredge in *Elsie Venner* (1861), by Oliver Wendell Holmes. He is described as "a model for visiting practitioners. He always came into the sick-room with a quiet, cheerful look, as if he had a consciousness that he was bringing some sure relief with him" (520). With Elsie, who is prone to agitation, his manner is calculated to have a calming effect: "He came to her bedside in such a natural, quiet way, that it seemed as if he were only a friend who had dropped in for a moment to say a pleasant word" (521). Under the guise of friendship, Dr. Kittredge exercises a positive psychological influence on his patient.

The most consummate missionary to the bedside is Dr. Leslie in Sarah Orne Jewett's *Country Doctor*. On his first appearance he immediately proves himself "the wielder of great powers" (26), instinctively taking command through "his sagacity and skill" as well as "his true manhood, his mastery of himself" (27). He is in many ways reminiscent of Mr. Gibson, though at a more advanced professional level: a widower, he gives his entire life to his practice and goes so far as to accept responsibility for the upbringing of a patient's orphaned granddaughter who has been entrusted to him. The adverbs repeatedly applied to him are *kindly, warmly, patiently,* and *compassionately*. On an "errand of mercy and good fellowship" (49) he visits lonely old Captain Finch, a retired sailor, "more from the courtesy and friendliness of the thing than from any hope of giving professional assistance" (43). He drives a great distance "to see a dying man, who seemed to be helped only by this beloved physician's presence" (171), and he is welcomed by a seriously ill child who "smiled as her friend came in" (249). The "repository of many secrets, he was a friend who could be trusted always" (93). Again like Mr. Gibson, Dr. Leslie derives his power above all from his personal qualities, mainly his sincere concern for the welfare of his patients. The strain of idealization in this portrait is even more pronounced than in that of Mr. Gibson, perhaps because Dr. Leslie is based on Jewett's memories of her own father, who was a country doctor.

This idealization contrasts with the impishness of the elderly doctor in Theodor Fontane's *Effi Briest* (1895; trans. 1956), which is set in northern Germany at the time of Bismarck. The rapport between him and his young patient is instantaneous; on his side it springs from his recognition of her resemblance to her mother, who had been his patient twenty years before, and on hers it is trust in a longstanding family confidant (she had rejected the suggestion of a young doctor as embarrassing). The reasons for her preference soon become apparent: she is putting on a show of indisposition so as to avoid having to return to the remote place where she had been living with her much older husband and had been guilty of an indiscretion with a dashing officer. In light of her wholesome color and her vague, changing symptoms, the shrewd doctor quickly sees through her pretense but decides to play along on the assumption that she has good reasons for her behavior. The ordained sickness ritual is then instituted, just as if there were a genuine illness, with a medication to be taken every two hours and follow-up visits from Dr. Ruhmschüttel the next day and every subsequent third day. The delicate transactions between physician and patient are traced through the shifts of perspective from one to the other: Effi knows that he is countering her pretense with his own, but each upholds the charade in an unspoken collusion that is presumed to be for the patient's welfare. The silent entente between them is buttressed by the doctor's wish to respect his patient's needs as well as by the social alliance between those who observe the conventions of polite conduct. The etiquette at this point is like an intricate dance in which doctor and patient engage in an unvoiced accord. Later in Effi's life, when she has been banished from her husband's and her parents' home after the accidental discovery of her brief liaison long ago, Dr. Ruhmschüttel asserts his authority in a decisive manner. Now in his seventies, the old doctor still pays house calls whenever she sends for him by letter. He is in fact the only person whose attitude toward her is unchanged; his quiet friendly manner is balm to her in her ostracized state. As a physician he has the privilege of exemption from society's moral judgments, and he makes full use of this. When Effi is dying of consumption, he takes the initiative of writing to her parents to intercede for her. Though apologetic for this interference, he is firm and outspoken in upholding the physician's duty to his patient. Dr. Ruhmschüttel has a small yet significant role in *Effi Briest* as "peace-maker" within the family.[26] The effectiveness of his plea in persuading her parents to override the normative objections to receiving their daughter in their home provides strong evidence of the power that a physician could command even within the rigid Prussian social code.

In the twentieth century the home visit to the bedside has more and more been superseded by the consultation in the office or hospital, where the doctor has high-tech equipment at hand. Now it is the patient, however debilitated or indeed infectious, who has to do the traveling. The role of missionary to the bedside in the literal sense becomes the exception. One such exception is portrayed in John Berger's *Fortunate Man* (1967), a documentary record of a country doctor in a still rural, rather isolated part of England. Dr. John Sassall has access to a cottage hospital and a modicum of modern equipment, but his practice conforms mainly to an older pattern. He himself is embedded in his community and is able consistently to contextualize his treatments in his intimate knowledge of his patients' circumstances. His holistic methods, which include simple reassurance and therapeutic interviews, grow out of his comprehensive grasp of his patients as struggling human beings whose illnesses are interconnected to the predicaments and crises in their lives. *A Fortunate Man* is remarkable for the absence of tension through the reciprocal respect that doctor and patient show each other.

The negative opposite to this harmonious cooperation is found in Virginia Woolf's *Mrs. Dalloway* (1925) in the fatuous general practitioner Dr. Holmes. His repeated insistence that "there was nothing whatsoever the matter" with Septimus Smith, despite his headaches, sleeplessness, fears, and dreams, becomes a parodistic refrain that exposes the almost criminal incompetence and insensitivity behind his "amiable way" (141). It is the sound of Holmes coming upstairs to see him that precipitates Smith's suicidal leap from his bedroom window. The missionary here turns into an executioner whose power is destructive because of his own utter blindness. Not quite as nefarious but rather sinister is Dr. Stern in Doris Lessing's *Proper Marriage* (1952), which takes place in South Africa in 1939. Dr. Stern, though he sees his patients primarily in his office, strives to be an old-style family doctor and cultivates the image of being his patients' friend and confidant. However, he turns out to be a manipulative friend when he assures Matty that she is not pregnant in order to prevent her from seeking an abortion. Gradually, as her rebellion gathers momentum, she comes to see him as an instrument of the social establishment. She rejects his bland phrases about the ubiquity of marital strife and tears up his prescription for a tonic—clearly a symbolic action that denotes the dissipation of her trust in him as well as of his power over her. Yet his will is accomplished insofar as she does bear the child she does not want.

By a curious twist, the doctor has very recently begun to resume the function of missionary to the bedside thanks to the modern technology of telemedicine. By means of two-way video and telephone doctors can reach out to see and interact with patients in their own locations, following their progress, for instance, after specialized surgery or providing emergency advice, as in the clinic at Logan airport, Boston, which is linked to the Massachusetts General Hospital.[27] What is lost, of course, in this new version of the doctor's traditional missionary activity is the intimate, long-term familiarity with patients and their environment that was the keystone of nineteenth-century practice. The new technology will have to evolve its own appropriate etiquette to deal with the disappearance of any direct physical contact between doctor and patient.

3.

SEEING—AND HEARING —IS BELIEVING

▪ ▪ ▪ ▪ ▪ ▪ ▪ ▪ ▪ ▪ ▪ ▪ ▪ ▪ ▪ ▪ ▪ ▪ ▪

The symbol of the doctor from the Middle Ages to the eighteenth century was the urinal. The symbol of the modern doctor is the stethoscope.—ERWIN H. AKERKNECHT, *Medicine at the Paris Hospital*

▪ ▪ ▪ ▪ ▪ ▪ ▪ ▪ ▪ ▪ ▪ ▪ ▪ ▪ ▪ ▪ ▪ ▪ ▪

WHEN LYDGATE, THE NEW SURGEON in Middlemarch, uses a stethoscope to diagnose Casaubon's heart disease a new phase is inaugurated in clinical medicine and, indirectly, in the balance of power. George Eliot's novel appeared in 1872, when the stethoscope had become ubiquitous, but the time of its action spans the years 1829–31, when the instrument was still quite a novelty.

The stethoscope was devised in 1819 by René-Théophile-Hyacinthe Laënnec (1781–1826), one of a coterie of brilliant French physicians who made Paris the foremost center for experimental medicine from the second decade of the nineteenth century onward. The Parisian method was praised by foreign students as "sensualist"; they were referring to the fact that Parisian physicians abandoned purely theoretical conjecture and chose instead to rely on such indications of disease as they could cull from the visible, the palpable, the audible, even the tastable and sniffable realities available. While this marked important progress toward the formation of more accurate diagnoses, the scope of the new approach was limited by the constraint on patients, especially women, to maintain their modesty and dignity. Their refusal to permit examination of their bodies was an expression of their power over the doctor, but it led in the early nineteenth century to a common and serious neglect of this now central facet of medical practice. Doctors were obliged to heed primarily patients' subjective accounts of their symptoms, so much so, indeed, that practice by mail was countenanced, not least because of the difficulty of travel.[1] This usage also demonstrates both doctors' and patients' confidence in anecdotal descriptions of illness as well as doctors' readiness to bow to the will of patients in regard to the means to be used to arrive at a diagnosis and to prescribe treatment. Mr. Gibson in *Wives and Daughters* and Trollope's Dr. Thorne at most feel their patients' pulse occasionally in a stylized interaction, depending largely on the acuity of their evaluative gaze and assessing the efficacy of their remedies by their visible effects.

Neither uses percussion, a mode of examination by auditory resonance communicated by the Austrian Leopold Auenbrugger (1722–1809) in his brief but notable monograph *Inventum Novum* (1761). Auenbrugger, a skilled musician and composer of several operas, applied his knowledge of resonance, pitch, and tonal quality to the sounds emanating from patients' chests when they were tapped. He is said to have hit on this mode of examination while tapping the contents of his father's beer barrels. Since fluids and air spaces emit different tones, Auenbrugger was able to make inferences about his patients' condition from the nature of the sounds he discerned. He spent seven years investigating the potentialities of percussion, conducting experiments on both patients and cadavers and confirming the results he obtained from the living by collating them with the findings at autopsies. Useful though Auenbrugger's technique was, it did not attract much attention partly because he himself was a remarkably modest man and partly because physical evaluation of the chest in the later eighteenth century concentrated on visual observation of breathing together with pulse count. Auenbrugger suffered the double misfortune first of being before his time and then of seeing percussion superseded by the stethoscope.

The stethoscope was a great advance over percussion because it gave access to far more extensive and differentiated information and also because it precluded the necessity of direct touch. Called "mediate" or "indirect auscultation," it had the advantage of placing an intermediary object, that is, a tube, between the patient's body and the physician. So by alleviating patients' antipathy to excessively close contact it was a significant tool in changing the balance of power as the patient's objections no longer determined the physician's methods. Like Auenbrugger, Laënnec was a musician, a player of the flute, a wind instrument that likely alerted him to the sounds he heard in his patients' chests.[2] The story goes that Laënnec first had recourse to such a buffer in trying to examine an obese girl with symptoms of heart disease whose corpulence was an impediment to percussion. The age and sex of the patient forbade him the direct application of the ear to the precordial region.[3] Seeking a way to overcome this obstacle, he remembered the well-known acoustic phenomenon that when one puts one's ear to the end of a beam, one hears quite distinctly a needle scratching at the other end. He applied this principle by shaping an exercise book into a tight cylinder, then putting one end on the girl's precordial region and the other to his ear. To his surprise and satisfaction, he could hear the heart's sounds much more clearly than by direct application of his ear to her chest. Three years later, in 1819, he published a nine-hundred-page treatise in two volumes, *De l'auscultation médiate, ou traité du diagnostique des poumons et du coeur, fondé principalement sur ce nouveau moyen d'exploration* (On mediate auscultation, or a treatise on the diagnosis of the lungs and heart, based principally on this new method of exploration).

The spread and adoption of the stethoscope was patchy in those days of halting communications. Foreign travelers to Paris in 1823 and 1825 reported that it was on exhibit in all the shops and used by all students.[4] On the other hand, it was not in service at the main hospital in Clermont-Ferrand, a provincial capital some two hundred miles south of Paris, before 1850. Laënnec's opus received a lengthy review in January 1820 in the *Medico-Chirurgical Journal,* a progressive London periodical,[5] and an English version, translated very freely by Sir John Forbes, was issued in 1821 under the title *Mediate Auscultation.* In the same year an Edinburgh M.D. thesis on auscultation was presented by a young Englishman, Charles Locock, at the behest of Andrew Duncan Jr. (1773–1832), a Scottish professor and early champion of auscultation. Reviews also appeared in American, Dutch, Italian, Russian, Spanish, Polish, and Scandinavian medical journals, and a German translation was published in 1822. But it would be erroneous to jump to the conclusion that the stethoscope was rapidly hailed and assimilated into general practice. It remained the prerogative of elite physicians just as physical diagnosis retained the aura of high-level practice. In fact, the lag between the academic acceptance of auscultation and its introduction into routine practice has been cited as evidence of "the gap that existed in the period between the 'best' practice and the day-to-day round of the average practitioner."[6] The first note of the physical examination of a patient in the records of Guy's Hospital, London, is found on 10 June 1836, but it was not until 1859 that the printed instructions for medical students actually started with guidelines for physical examinations and details of the scrutiny of the various bodily systems.[7] The conservatism of the majority was fostered by teaching through apprenticeship, in which the pupil was enjoined to imitate his preceptor and to repeat tasks. Similarly, textbooks played safe by reiterating established lore, and journals, the current vehicle for the rapid dissemination of new ideas, were in their infancy as yet.[8]

How, then, does Lydgate, a provincial surgeon like Mr. Gibson and a contemporary of his, come to be using a stethoscope as early as 1829? George Eliot validates his exceptional enterprise by making him have spent some time in Paris for professional education. He is neatly contextualized in medical history as one of the many ambitious young doctors who flocked to Paris at that time when it was the unrivaled mecca for advanced study and exciting research. Laënnec in particular attracted numerous foreign students since his stethoscope had immediate clinical applications.[9] Apart from his theoretical lectures at the Necker Hospital (1816–23) and at the Collège de France (1822–26), Laënnec imparted practical instruction in auscultation at the Charité Hospital (1824–26). His habit of speaking Latin at the bedside fulfilled a dual purpose: it prevented patients from learning their diagnosis, and it was a means of communication with those whose French was scant. It also had the incidental side effect of raising the doctor's prestige and heightening his mystique. The British contigent was noticeably large, drawn to the Paris clinic by innovative practices that were seen as "guides to the cognitive and social transformation of medicine" in their own country.[10] The complaint, summarized in Charles Babbage's *Reflections on the Decline of Science in England* (1830), that British medicine had fallen behind French, certainly in the theoretical nosology of disease, if not in practical treatment, had by then been circulating for more than a decade. With the end of hostilities after the defeat of Napoleon at Waterloo in 1815, the influx of British medical students to Paris mounted sharply. The name Gallomaniacs was coined for British converts to French medical ways on account of their tendency to proselytism.[11] Prominent among them were Scottish practitioners who formed an important and somewhat radical element in the movement for medical reform in Great Britain. Edinburgh, where Lydgate had studied before going to Paris, had special ties to France through James Thomson (1765–1846), first holder of the chair of pathology and a key figure in the development of pathological and surgical teaching, who encouraged Edinburgh students to pursue further studies in France.[12]

The training with which Eliot invests Lydgate therefore makes it wholly credible that he should be wielding a stethoscope in Middlemarch in 1829.

Besides Laënnec, several other leading French medical researchers are
named in *Middlemarch* as having made a great impression on Lydgate: Marie-
François-Xavier Bichat (1771–1801), the pioneer in pathological anatomy;
Pierre-Charles-Alexandre Louis (1787–1872), the inventor of the numerical
method that became clinical statistics as well as an expert on typhoid fever;
François-Joseph-Victor Broussais (1772–1832), a brilliant physician and surgeon
who aggressively sponsored the localistic orientation of medicine that led
to disease specificity; and François Raspail (1794–1878), a chemist who advocated
camphor as a disinfectant to stave off cholera. Of these the most influential
by far for Lydgate is Bichat, whose *General Anatomy Applied to Physiology and
Medicine* (1801) not only classified symptoms characteristic of disturbed organs
but also introduced the concept of tissue, of which organs are composed,
as the primary site of pathology. Bichat's work was of enormous significance
in instigating one of the most momentous contributions made by the French
school: the turn away from patient specificity to disease specificity in diagnosis and treatment. His new theory was grounded in his extensive research in
pathological anatomy; he is credited with having autopsied six hundred
corpses in one winter alone. Pathological anatomy was the foundation for
the revolution in medical treatment that resulted from the understanding of
diseases as discrete entities whose categoric ravages could be seen in the cadaver. With the introduction of the stethoscope, the various sounds heard in
the living person could be directly related to the pathologies uncovered at the
autopsy to form a diagnostic taxonomy based on what was heard and then
seen. The combination of pathological anatomy with auscultation opened
up totally new vistas in medicine; the stethoscope, by providing at once a confirmation and an extension of the findings of pathology, created a vital link
between research on cadavers and clinical practice. The crucial transition was
thereby accomplished from the older speculative medicine to the modern
pragmatic method. Diagnosis and therapeutics, instead of being directed at
restoring the systemic balance in the body's total economy and natural harmony, focused on complexes of signs and symptoms that could be analyzed,
measured, and remedied separately and differently for each syndrome. The
gateway to this shift from essentialism to the localization of lesions was
pathology: "about 1829 the dark territories of Pathology were a fine America

for a spirited young adventurer" (*Middlemarch*, 177). The attraction of the new science was so intense that between 1822 and 1824 courses in normal and pathological anatomy were taught in Paris in English in dissecting rooms near the teaching hospital.[13]

What most fascinates Lydgate about Bichat's work is his descriptive catalog of the systems common to all organs, which were then called "cellular tissue" and are now known as "connective tissue." "Enamoured" of the potential continuation of Bichat's investigations, Lydgate wants to grasp "the very grain of things" (178), "the primary webs or tissues, out of which the various organs—brain, heart, lungs, and so on—are compacted" (177). If this project smacks of a quixotic overreaching, it must be seen in the context of the immense enthusiasm generated by the striking advances then being made. Lydgate also draws inspiration from another model, Edward Jenner (1749–1823), like himself a country doctor, who had succeeded in discovering a safe method of vaccination against smallpox by simple observation and experimentation. For his research Lydgate has a microscope, another piece of basic medical equipment not used by Mr. Gibson and Dr. Thorne. However, it is highly unlikely that the instruments available in Lydgate's day would have been at all adequate for what he hopes to do. While magnifying lenses had been employed certainly since the Renaissance,[14] the modern achromatic microscope, which eliminates the visual aberrations of the more primitive instruments, became current just a little too late for Lydgate. After the theoretical solution to the problem of distortion was discovered in 1829 by Joseph Jackson Lister (1786–1869), father of Joseph Lister, the initiator of antiseptic surgery, vastly improved microscopes began to be made, which in turn spurred interest in the analysis of minute elements of the body. In 1843, for example, the microscopic department at Guy's Hospital in London examined phlegm from lungs, blood, urine, and mother's milk,[15] and instruction in its use for medical students was inaugurated in 1845.

With his stethoscope and his progressive French ideas, Lydgate practices a different style of medicine than Mr. Gibson or Dr. Thorne, although the continuities should not be underestimated. One salient difference, in keeping with the evolution of medical thinking, is in disease specificity. While no diagnosis is ever pronounced on the patients in *Wives and Daughters* and *Doctor Thorne* (except for Sir Roger's and his son's alcoholism), those in *Middlemarch* suffer from identified syndromes. Casaubon has "fatty degeneration of the

heart" (461),[16] Fred Vincy typhoid fever, Nancy Nash cramps, Trumbull pneumonia, and Raffles delirium tremens. In none of these cases does Lydgate
base his diagnosis on the patient's subjective description of symptoms; his
criteria are the signs, that is, perceptible marks of the disease that he can objectively observe with the help of the stethoscope on Casaubon, the thermometer on Trumbull, by questioning and examining Nancy Nash, by
recognizing "the pink-skinned stage of typhoid fever" (293) in Fred as a result
of clinical experience, and by thoroughly examining and evaluating Raffles.
This centrality of the doctor's independent physical examination of the patient
distinguishes Lydgate radically from his predecessors and empowers him as
a diagnostician and in some cases as a healer.

Because "careful examination of the body by the physician is the act that
grounds the patient-physician encounter" for us nowadays,[17] it is hard to realize that "only in relatively modern times have patients and physicians learned
to accept physical intrusion upon the body as necessary to the diagnostic
process."[18] The introduction of the stethoscope had a curiously paradoxical
impact on the relationship between doctor and patient by simultaneously in-
terjecting greater physical distance between them and vouchsafing the doctor
more intimate information and hence greater power. But the struggle for
control was by no means over. The innovative methods of examination were
at first more acceptable than the older modes of listening to chest sounds because of the distancing; however, innocuous surface instruments such as
the stethoscope, the thermometer, and the opthalmoscope were eventually
followed by an increasingly invasive set of "scopes" (the laryngoscope, the
bronchoscope, the endoscope, and so forth), which aroused renewed resistance. Patients felt resentment—and fear—at inroads on their most private
spaces by intrusive means of investigation. The present law that requires "informed consent" to examination by invasive instruments not only protects
the doctor from lawsuits in case of injury or even death; it also represents a
form of negotiation between doctor and patient for control. Although doctors
are predominant as a result of their expertise and patients are likely to comply
out of their desire for relief, theoretically at least patients have the last word
in agreeing (or refusing) to sign the consent.

The stethoscope and its successors made possible a wholly new, disease-
specific precision in diagnosis by enabling doctors to describe "what for centuries had remained below the threshold of the visible and the expressible."[19]

The priority of physical examination, backed from the late nineteenth century onward by laboratory tests of biochemical functions, unquestionably changed the prevalent mode of practice, and, as a consequence, the balance of power between doctors and patients. The identification of diseases by the only means previously known, patients' subjective narration of their major symptoms, gave way to the evidence deduced from the growing panoply of instruments inaugurated by the stethoscope. In this process of change Laënnec was of decisive importance: "From the date of Laennec's discovery the criterion of objective diagnostic findings has been the hallmark of clinical examination."[20] With the probing capacity of their instruments and their cumulative scientific understanding of disease, doctors' power swelled, whereas that of patients was inevitably diminished when their word came to have lesser significance. What doctors found took unquestioned precedence over what patients believed.

The beginnings of this metamorphosis are portrayed in *Middlemarch*. The struggle for medical reform that animates Lydgate's hope "to do good small work for Middlemarch, and great work for the world" (178) is one facet of the political, social, and economic transformation that England was undergoing in the transitional years around the Reform Act of 1832. As "A Study of Provincial Life," to cite its subtitle, *Middlemarch* encompasses various aspects of change as they impinge on and determine the lives of its protagonists. Eliot's capacious concern with public affairs endows her novel with greater breadth and depth than either *Wives and Daughters* or *Doctor Thorne*. The similarity of their provincial, semirural setting and the relative proximity of the time of their action serves to underscore the distinctions. Parallel themes are handled in different ways. For instance, courtship, marriage, and money are pivotal to the plots of all three works, but whereas Gaskell's and Trollope's novels have a palpable romance strain, especially in their happy endings, *Middlemarch* is quite muted. Marriages, however romantically they start, are troubled by a gradually worsening clash of personalities, as with Lydgate and Rosamond, or result in acute disappointment, as in Dorothea's union (or, rather, nonunion) with Casaubon. Ultimately, all the characters in *Middlemarch* have to learn that life entails compromise and renunciation through acquiescence in the middle marches of existence. So Lydgate is forced, under financial duress, to give in to Rosamond; Dorothea becomes a Victorian wife and mother with only scant participation in lofty projects; the Bulstrodes forfeit wealth and power; Fred Vincy becomes a working land manager instead of a gentleman; Brooke does not get elected to Parliament; and Farebrother is not appointed chaplain to the new hospital, nor does he win the hand of Mary Garth. This blunting of heroism and thwarting of desire give expression to the essential realism of *Middlemarch* in its steady, unvarnished contemplation of the frustrations that human beings have to face in the ordinary course of life. The reiteration of a like fate in having to settle for second best among a very large and diverse cast of characters lends an inescapable universality to the theme and an impressive stature to the novel.

Included in this panorama of provincial life in Middlemarch is a spectrum of medical men. Five others appear alongside Lydgate, and although they are episodic figures, each is concisely placed professionally and socially. Two are dignified by the title "Dr.," so they are presumably physicians. Dr. Sprague and Dr. Minchin "enjoyed about equally the mysterious privilege of medical reputation, and concealed with much etiquette their contempt for each other's skill" (212). Dr. Minchin likes to cite Pope's *Essay on Man* and has a preference for "well-sanctioned quotations" and "refinements of all kinds" (212). His standing in Middlemarch is boosted by the common knowledge that "he had some kinship with a bishop" (212), a connection that lifts him, like Dr. Thorne, in rank. But Minchin's misdiagnosis of Nancy Nash's cramps as a tumor suggests that he has more social grace than medical acumen. This incident also hints through irony at the waywardness of Middlemarch opinion, for Dr. Minchin "was usually said to have more penetration" (285), a quality singularly lacking in this instance. Dr. Sprague, "hard-headed and dry-witted" (211), author of a treatise on meningitis thirty years back, "was considered the physician of most 'weight'" (185). The quotation marks here suggest the same kind of irony as is directed at Dr. Minchin's "penetration." These two senior physicians are called only when danger is extreme because of their high charges. Normally the inhabitants of Middlemarch resort to one of the town's surgeons, primarily Mr. Wrench or Mr. Toller. Mr. Wrench's ignorance is exposed when he dismisses Fred's typhoid fever as "a slight derangement" (292), while his social level is revealed by his wretched home: "the doors all open, the oil-cloth worn, the children in soiled pinafores, and lunch lingering in the form of bones, black-handled knives, and willow-pattern" (389). Mr. Toller has "lazy manners" but makes up for this defect by being very "active" in his treatments, favoring such heroic methods as copious bleeding, blistering, and starving (486). The fifth medical man in Middlemarch, Mr. Gambit, is of still lower standing, being "especially esteemed as an accoucheur" (484).[21]

Lydgate stands out markedly from his peers—Wrench, Toller, and Gambit— in his background, education, expertise, and interests. The portrait of him gains subtlety and complexity from its dual derivation from the views of the inhabitants of Middlemarch and those of the omniscient narrator as Eliot fuses the heterogeneous narrative techniques that prevail in *Wives and Daughters* and *Doctor Thorne,* respectively. The Middlemarchers soon grant that he "was not altogether a common country doctor," for he quickly creates the impression that he "was something rather more uncommon than any general practitioner in Middlemarch" (171). The recurrence of the words *common* and *uncommon* in the introduction of Lydgate is significant; if he has spots of commonness in his character, as the narrator asserts, they do not impinge on him professionally. From the outset he is immediately recognized as "a gentleman" (117) who is "clever" and "talks well" (128). In short, he has the style of a physician, although his qualifications are those of a surgeon. His diagnostic acumen is particularly remarkable since surgeons were supposed to be skilled operators, possessing speed and dexterity, but to have relatively little need for diagnostic capacity as they worked on the body's surface. His social background too is at least the equivalent of that of the higher type of medical man: "He is one of the Lydgates of Northumberland, really well connected. One does not expect it in a practitioner of that kind," Lady Chettam remarks, adding: "For my own part I like a medical man more on a footing with servants" (117). This condescending attitude divulges the extent to which medicine was at that time "a dependent occupation," not a "liberal profession."[22] Well-informed, self-assured, and independent-minded, Lydgate breaks rank by a bearing above his station as a surgeon. His nonconformity is partially explained by his social pedigree, which greatly impresses Middlemarch. Even his Latinate name, Tertius, denotes a certain superiority to the more ordinary Fred, Peter, Ned, and Will of the other characters.

Lydgate's singularity extends back to his origins, for he is rather unusual in coming from a family with no medical tradition at a time when practices were often passed down from generation to generation. The son of a military man who had made little provision for his three children, orphaned at an early age, Lydgate expresses the wish for a medical education, which his guardian grants through apprenticeship to a country doctor despite "objections on the score of family dignity" (172). The interpolated reference to "family dignity" points once more to the still relatively low social standing of medicine as a profession. It is likely that Lydgate's guardian accedes in his wish because he is an orphan, that is to say, a somewhat tangential member of the family, whereas he might well have refused the same request from his own son. Lydgate's "decided bent" (172) for medicine is prompted by his reading of encyclopedias, which arouse his curiosity about the "finely adjusted mechanism in the human frame" (173). His initial medical education was probably haphazard, as was the norm even in many early-nineteenth-century medical schools, which had no set curriculum, compressed too many subjects into too short a time, let pupils "walk the wards" at will, and even issued certificates on payment of fees without heed to attendance.[23] It says much for Lydgate's intelligence and ambition that he goes on to choose for himself the best medical training then available by selecting London, Edinburgh, and Paris. In London, Charing Cross Hospital was founded in 1821 with the specific purpose of providing a university (i.e., liberal) education for medical students. Previously the combination of liberal and medical education was limited to Oxford and Cambridge, where the medical side was, however, very scanty compared with the classical component.[24] Edinburgh is a wise continuation for "it offered a medical education of a type quite new in Britain involving the integration of a wide range of medical and allied subjects,"[25] including anatomy, surgery, botany, chemistry, pharmacy, and midwifery. Scottish graduates, though not formally recognized in England, were allowed to practice without interference, partly owing to the chaotic multiplicity of licensing bodies.

Lydgate's subsequent experience of French medical methods is decisive for his reformist impetus. The innovative French principles were most readily espoused precisely by men like Lydgate, ambitious provincial practitioners, often involved in building institutions such as infirmaries. The appeal to a scientific argument could bolster support for their own program, and this correlated well with an ardent dedication to the redistribution of power within the profession. For the contest for power, as *Middlemarch* shows, was not solely between doctor and patient but equally among the various types of practitioners. The thrust for medical reform, illustrated in *Middlemarch,* had two main prongs: it comprised attempts both to introduce more scientific methods into diagnosis and treatment and to revise the structure of the profession by legitimizing the status of the emerging breed of general practitioners such as Lydgate.[26] Despite vociferous pressure from the physicians to uphold the validity of the traditional demarcation between the three ranks of the medical hierarchy (physicians, surgeons, and apothecaries), the boundaries separating the categories were becoming more porous by about 1830, especially in the provinces. Yet the labels persisted throughout the ever more bitter disputes, however little relation they might bear to what practitioners actually did. So Lydgate is introduced as the "new young surgeon" (117) but successfully handles internal diseases with Casaubon's heart condition (460), Nancy Nash's cramps (489), and Trumbull's pneumonia (490), in addition to Fred's fever. This reflects the situation in the early 1830s, when so many surgeons were acting in the role of physicians that the limits were becoming undefinable, if not untenable. Conversely, some physicians were taking on the degrading manual tasks of surgery and even of midwifery and pharmacy to supplement slender incomes. At stake was not merely money but even more so status as the College of Physicians endeavored to combat the incursion of manual and trade practices, while the College of Surgeons in turn became hostile to midwifery as a lower branch. This dichotomization of medicine and surgery was the target of Thomas Wakley's attacks in the *Lancet,* where he argued for the need for greater flexibility and unity in order to extend the usefulness of both fields. Throughout the 1820s the two colleges were locked in an unceasing battle over this issue.[27] In addition, within the Royal College of Surgeons dissent was rife between 1826 and 1831 about the possible establishment of a new institution to enfranchise surgeons in general practice such as Lydgate, a hybrid class in an anomalous position. The upcoming generation of respectable, educated general practitioners, who provided a powerful stimulus to reform, were at best tolerated and more often distrusted as a threat to physician and apothecary alike for trespassing on their turf and subverting the established order of the profession. It is important to grasp that Lydgate in his work in Middlemarch is transgressing the accredited professional structure that still held sway. He is as avant-garde in his defiance of rigid compartmentalization as in his use of new instruments and his advocacy of new approaches.

To ground professional identity in scientific knowledge, as Lydgate does, entailed an advancement of the initiated that not only bestowed additional power and prestige on them but also served the purpose of distancing them from dispensing druggists and irregular practitioners. Expertise in the scientific bases of medicine could confer a substitute status to the trappings of gentility as well as access to patronage enjoyed by elite physicians. Not surprisingly, it was that elite who were most resistant to change and most opposed to foreign notions. A direct connection therefore exists between Lydgate's desire to pursue tissue research and his wider commitment to medical reform. However, his idealism is such that he envisages his research not in strategic terms as a means to his own furtherment but in an exalted, altruistic light as directed at the future benefit of mankind.

Why does so exceptionally well qualified a doctor opt to settle in Middlemarch? The question is made more pointed by the fact that Lydgate has no family or other ties to the place. Generally young doctors would start up where they already had a base of connections since these were so crucial to building a practice. Failing a generational tradition, they might enter into a junior partnership with a doctor in whose practice they had been apprenticed or perhaps marry into a practitioner's family, as Mr. Gibson in *Wives and Daughters* had done in his first marriage. It is characteristic of both Lydgate's boldness and his lack of a sense of expediency that he follows none of these conventional routes. He makes a deliberate decision to "keep away from the range of London intrigues, jealousies, and social truckling" (174). Because he regards the medical profession as "presenting the most perfect interchange between science and art, offering the most direct alliance between intellectual conquest and the social good" (174), he plans in Middlemarch to engage in both "the assiduous practice of his profession" (176) and basic research in cell theory. His highest hope is "that the two purposes would illuminate each other" (176). He is motivated too by his perception that medicine "wanted reform" (174). With his small capital he buys a retiring surgeon's practice that is said to bring in eight hundred pounds per year, then a handsome income. But in setting up in Middlemarch Lydgate is taking a considerable risk: he has no friends or connections there, competition from several established practitioners, and no partner with whom to share the responsibility and to whom to shift fickle patients. As events prove, he makes a misjudgment in setting too great a store in the value of his own professional proficiency and in underestimating the force of custom and convention, particularly in a small provincial town such as Middlemarch. As in *Wives and Daughters* and *Doctor Thorne,* personal qualities such as tact take precedence for patients in their choice of medical attendants over knowledgeability, perhaps because scientific understanding of disease was as yet fairly rudimentary. Lydgate's outstanding ability does not protect him from the capriciousness of paying patients, at whose mercy he is. The potency of science is held in check by human folly.

That folly is as evident in Lydgate's fellow practitioners in Middlemarch as in his patients. They aggravate his problems by their instinctive mistrust, temporarily setting aside their own feuds to unite in obstructive and maligning opposition to him. His scientific expertise and the success he reaps from it at first, ironically, militate against him. In the treatment of Fred Vincy Lydgate ousts Mr. Wrench, although he is careful to observe due etiquette by getting the Vincys to inform Wrench of the switch. His refutation of Dr. Minchin's diagnosis in the case of Nancy Nash causes even more trouble because it is an affront to the hierarchical system: "it was indecent in a general practitioner to contradict a physician's diagnosis in that open manner" (490). He is castigated, too, for "a certain showiness as to foreign ideas" (186), for a disposition to "flighty, foreign notions" (295), as well as for siding with "the *Lancet's* men" (186). So Lydgate antagonizes the Middlemarch medical establishment through his superior knowledge, his innovative practices, and his disregard for the professional pecking order, in short, through his disturbing nonconformity and his commitment to reform. If his patients and fellow practitioners are guilty of folly, so is he in his naive assumption that attitudes toward progressive methods would be as favorable in Middlemarch as in Paris. His stance is conveyed in a vivid metaphor: he eschews "the broad road which was quite ready made" in order to make "a good clear path for himself" (121).

The "growing though half-suppressed feud between him and the other medical men" (305) comes to a head over the issue of dispensing drugs. Like Dr. Thorne, Lydgate is trespassing on a hallowed convention, and his infraction becomes so inflammatory because of its substantive entanglement in professional status and dignity. There is a curious chiasmus here between Lydgate and Dr. Thorne: the one is censured for dispensing medications, while the other is castigated for not doing so. The explanation lies, once more, in class distinctions: elite physicians never dispensed drugs, a practice that approximated to trade. On the other hand, surgeons were fully expected both to prescribe and dispense drugs; indeed, it was customary for them to submit bills not for medical attendance but for drugs, possibly as a way to circumvent the prohibition on internal medicine by surgeons since technically their charge was for drugs: "their only mode of getting paid for their work was by making out long bills for draughts, boluses, and mixtures" (483). This question of dispensing drugs looms so large in *Middlemarch* because of its association with initiatives for reform and its fundamental challenge to the dominant structure of medical rank. Lydgate, a surgeon, is arrogating the privilege of a physician, and he does so on the basis of his medical convictions, which devolve from his insights into science. Lydgate's adamant refusal to dispense drugs must therefore be understood not only as a provocative flaunting of medical usage but also as an essential part of his endeavor to raise the level and power of the profession by dissociating it from trade. Mr. Wrench is right in prophesying that Lydgate's "attempts to discredit the sale of drugs by his professional brethren would by-and-by recoil on himself" (295). His stand on this matter arouses extreme ill will, offending medical men and laypeople alike, and leads to the gossip that he believes "physic was of no use" (485), which alarms patients. Lydgate ignores the gentle advice given to him by his friend the minister Farebrother that "a young doctor has to please his patients in Middlemarch" (204). From his own experience of poverty, Farebrother knows all too well the power of the affluent and the painfulness of dependence on their pleasure. Young and idealistic, Lydgate insists on sticking to his principles of sound practice even at the risk of losing popularity— and income.

Lydgate's inflexible stand against dispensing drugs is so badly received by the inhabitants of Middlemarch because their conservatism makes them wary of any amendment to the status quo. As a newcomer who is an unknown quantity he is greeted with a mixed reception. His quality as a gentleman is a major asset to him; like Mr. Gibson and Dr. Thorne, he is judged less on his knowledge, scientific interests, or even intelligence than on his personal characteristics: "it was individual face-to-face encounters that tipped the balance between distrust and confidence."[28] Lydgate gains Lady Chettam's approval by showing himself to be a good listener, by displaying "a certain careless refinement about his toilette and utterance," and above all by concurring with her views "with an air of so much deference accompanying the insight of agreement, that she formed the most cordial opinion of his talents" (118). It is important to note here the striking dearth of logic and discrimination that leads her to form "the most cordial opinion of his talents" simply on account of his "deference" (and it is only "an air" of deference!). The men value him on more rational grounds. Mr. Brooke, who has received a letter about him from an uncle of Lydgate's, thinks "he is likely to be first-rate—has studied in Paris, knew Broussais, has ideas, you know—wants to raise the profession" (118). Mr. Bulstrode hails Lydgate's advent because, as he acknowledges, "medical knowledge is at a low ebb among us" (119), and he immediately sees Lydgate's potential usefulness for the new hospital he is planning. Lydgate's reputation as a clever doctor, initiated by his cure of Mrs. Bulstrode from a chronic ailment by his new regimen, is confirmed by his treatment of Fred Vincy and of Casaubon. When Nancy Nash recovers spontaneously from her cramps, he is credited with the capacity to cure cancer since Dr. Minchin had thought her to have a tumor. Lydgate's misjudgment of Middlemarch is in this incident matched by Middlemarch's misreading of him; ironically, he is esteemed for powers he does not possess, as he will subsequently be stigmatized for failings of which he is not guilty.

Lydgate encounters mainly suspicion among the general public, in part because of Middlemarch's ingrained distrust of "a stranger" (153), a "new settler" (170), a "new-comer" (479 and 491). He is never allowed to forget his somewhat dubious status as an outsider, which is contrasted unfavorably with that of Mr. Toller, who "belonged to an old Middlemarch family" (486). Gambit is preferred to Lydgate for employment by the medical "Clubs," company insurance schemes that provided a modest but steady income (778). On account of his research in cell theory, he is imputed by Mrs. Dollop, landlady at the Tankard, of intending "to let people die in the Hospital, if not to poison them, for the sake of cutting them up" (481). Lydgate's training in Paris, where autopsies were routine in the study of pathological anatomy, turns into a decided liability in Middlemarch. In the ensuing discussion a topical reference is made to Burke and Hare, who were notorious for murdering at least fifteen people in order to supply anatomical specimens, a crime for which Burke was hanged in 1829. It was not until the Anatomy Act of 1832 that the secretary of state for the Home Department was empowered to issue licenses for the lawful acquisition of corpses for dissection.[29] The charge that Lydgate is "for cutting up everybody before the breath was well out o' their body" (778) is brought up again later and contributes to the decline of his practice.

Although Lydgate does not manage to cultivate a favorable image in Middlemarch, in individual encounters with patients he is much more successful.

Apart from his emphasis on physical examination, his interactions with patients show several resemblances to those of Mr. Gibson and Dr. Thorne. Like them, he is a missionary to the bedside, making home visits to all except Nancy Nash, a poor charwoman who is an outpatient at the dispensary. He acquires patients primarily by word-of-mouth recommendation, which is quite natural in a place where gossip plays so major a role. When Casaubon suffers an acute "fit," Dorothea's brother-in-law, Sir James Chettam, promptly suggests that she send for Lydgate because his mother had called him and "found him uncommonly clever" (318). Just as Mr. Gibson's attendance on Lady Cumnor at the Towers in *Wives and Daughters* is a distinct asset, so here the approving patronage of the local gentry is precious capital to the young physician in a society that still has a streak of feudalism in its respect for the opinions of the aristocracy. Lydgate is summoned to Trumbull following his success with Nancy Nash and to Raffles by Bulstrode, who has got to know him on the hospital board. He is called to Fred Vincy as an emergency while passing by on the street at the urgent plea of the scheming Rosamond; although she cites Lydgate's cure of Mrs. Bulstrode, her own attraction to the dashing newcomer is no doubt as strongly implicated as her concern for her brother. If hearsay initially builds Lydgate's reputation, it is equally forceful in later destroying it. The crux of the objection to him is, significantly, not any lack of professional competence but his infringements of traditional usage.

In making home visits, Lydgate habitually confers with the patient's family about diagnosis, therapeutics, and prognosis. With Casaubon, after examining him with his stethoscope he sits quietly by his side and watches him. To Casaubon's inquiries about the seriousness of his attack he gives soothing, mildly evasive replies. With Dorothea, on the other hand, seeing "the unaffected signs of intense anxiety in her face and voice," he decides "that he was only doing right in telling her the truth about her husband's probable future" (321). But it is she who presses categoric questions in order to get beyond his general, reticent statement: "Such cases are peculiarly difficult to pronounce upon" (322). When she beseeches him "to speak quite plainly," he does so on the grounds that "it is one's function as a medical man to hinder regrets . . . as far as possible" (322). Lydgate is at his best here, showing courage, tact, and consideration, wishing that this obligation was not necessary yet convinced of the ethical propriety of his course. With the Vincys Lydgate's task is both easier and trickier: easier because Fred's case, though serious, has a more positive prognosis than Casaubon's but trickier on account of Mrs. Vincy's volatile temperament. As with Casaubon, Lydgate makes sure that he is "out of Fred's hearing" (293) before dealing with Fred's weeping, "convulsed" mother, whom he has to comfort and support. He adopts a different tone with Mrs. Vincy than he had with Dorothea, focusing above all on such concrete matters as Fred's food, where he can make her feel useful, thereby scotching her tendency to a frenzied, sterile effusiveness. Lydgate is clever in empowering both Dorothea and Mrs. Vincy, and at the same time making them his allies, by involving them in the therapeutic process.

Lydgate's conversations with Dorothea and Mrs. Vincy reveal his appreciation of the psychological dimensions of patient care. The narrator comments that "a medical man likes to make psychological observations" (321), in this instance correctly gauging Dorothea's capacity to tolerate the truth in contrast to Mrs. Vincy's need for reassurance only. He also heeds the interdependence of body and mind in agreeing with Dorothea to keep the facts from Casaubon since "anxiety of any kind would be precisely the most unfavourable condition for him" (323) at this point. Later, however, when Casaubon himself asks "to know the truth without reservation" (460), the physician responds with a frankness moderated by prudence and caveats about the uncertainty of predictions in diseases of the heart. Following these reservations, he goes ahead with an honest disclosure: "Lydgate's instinct was fine enough to tell him that plain speech, quite free from ostentatious caution, would be felt by Mr. Casaubon as a tribute of respect" (461). With Trumbull, Lydgate again makes a shrewd personal assessment of his patient, surmising "that he would like to be taken into his medical confidence, and be represented as a partner in his own cure" (491). He does have an ulterior motive in enlisting this patient's active cooperation, for he sees in the robust auctioneer "a good subject for trying the expectant theory" (490). Lydgate scores a signal therapeutic success here thanks to his perspicacity in selecting the most suitable candidate for the experiment: Trumbull "went without shrinking through his absistence from drugs, much sustained by application of the thermometer which implied the importance of his temperature, by the sense that he furnished objects for the microscope, and by learning many new words which seemed suited to the dignity of his secretions. For Lydgate was astute enough to indulge him with a little technical talk" (491).

In drawing Trumbull into this therapeutic partnership Lydgate is continuing the old established convention of consultation and agreement between physician and patient as to the optimum treatment, but beneath the surface concurrence he is really modifying it substantially; there can be no doubt that it is the physician who has the upper hand. His scientific knowledge gives him incomparable superiority over Trumbull in the decision-making process. This is an early prototype of the contemporary situation, in which patients are involved in making their own choices though the partnership is extremely uneven on account of the physician's supremacy by virtue of expertise. Lydgate is wholly preeminent with Nancy Nash, whose situation is unique among the medical encounters in *Middlemarch* insofar as she is a charity case, socially much inferior to the physician, who confers with his colleague, not with her. In any event, she is so relieved to be spared surgery (in the days before anesthesia) that she is only too happy to accept his more conservative and milder prescription. Lydgate is holistic and caring in his approach, advocating rest in addition to a blister and some steel mixture and giving her a note to her best employer "to testify that she was in need of good food" (489).

Lydgate's interaction with his other patients conforms more closely to the traditional model of a large measure of control on the patient's part. The patient's dominance is connected to the prerogative of choice, which in turn devolves from the patronage derived from payment. So wealthy old Featherstone switches to Lydgate because he "had taken the new doctor into great favour" (155). The reasons for this "favour" are not disclosed, but the word itself seems to suggest an emotional response of liking rather than a rational decision based on Lydgate's expertise. The vagaries of patients' choices are again revealed when the Vincys dismiss Wrench and engage Lydgate for mixed motives, not all of which by any means are considerations of health. The balance of power is illustrated once more in the case of Raffles; since Bulstrode calls Lydgate in and foots the bill, it is with him that Lydgate discusses the treatment and prognosis. Lydgate strives to assert his authority, but he is overshadowed by the banker, who has a "native imperiousness" (757) and who is, moreover, aware of Lydgate's financial distress, which relegates him to a dependent position.

With Casaubon and Dorothea the balance of power is more delicate. They both clearly acknowledge and defer to Lydgate's proficiency in seeking information about Casaubon's condition; in other words, they grant him respect for his medical knowledge. However, analysis of the meeting between Lydgate and Dorothea, and the later interview between him and Casaubon reveals the extent to which the patient and family member orchestrates and controls each encounter. Socially above the young surgeon, Dorothea takes the lead, for instance, by enjoining him to sit down. Lydgate is placed, as it were, in a responsive role in having to reply to the questions she poses. He is neither cowed nor forward, answering with a forthrightness and sensitivity rooted in his empathy for her predicament as well as his admiration for her personally. The rather formal exchange is infused with feeling on both sides and characterized by a directness noticeably missing in Dorothea's conversations with her husband. She counters Lydgate's unadorned closing words, "I wish I could have spared you this pain," with the equally frank assertion, "It was right of you to tell me. I thank you for telling me the truth" (323). Lydgate's parallel meeting with Casaubon is considerably more ritualized, the underlying emotion deliberately deflected by the elderly scholar's dry tone. He at once signals his dominance in his opening phrase, "I am exceedingly obliged to you for your punctuality" (459), which expresses a certain condescension under the veneer of politeness. It is Casaubon who has explicitly sent for Lydgate, who chooses the location and mode of the interview while ambulating in the Yew Tree Walk, who formulates his demands in a manner that is peremptory, though unusually plain for him, and who abruptly terminates the colloquy with a brusque "I thank you" before "proceeding to remark on the rare beauty of the day" (461). Who is master in this visit is quite obvious.

While there are resemblances between *Wives and Daughters, Doctor Thorne,* and *Middlemarch* in the interaction of patients and doctors, the scope of the medical work is wider in Eliot's novel through incorporation into the plot of a community hospital. When Lydgate arrives in the town, a new hospital is being planned under the sponsorship of Bulstrode, who coopts the young surgeon onto the board. In later-eighteenth- and early-nineteenth-century England provincial hospitals were "founded by persons of high standing in their local communities and governed by persons at the top or keen to approach the top of the social pyramid."[30] The governance of the hospital thus replicates in microcosm the town's social structure. Prominent laymen, such as Bulstrode, expected to call the tune in all matters as they were the ones who paid the piper. Their duties covered every aspect of hospital administration, from the construction and repair of the physical plant to appointments at all levels. They had the right not only to nominate patients but also to pass judgment on the work of the medical men, who rarely served on the boards and had no say in the choice of senior colleagues. Their claim to the prerogative to interfere personally and professionally had the ill effect of making doctors subject to and dependent on lay employers.[31]

Hospital staffs were unanimous in wanting reform of the appointments system with open applications, nominations from leaders in the field, and examinations, but boards were unlikely to adopt voluntarily any changes that would result in removing control from their hands. Although positions were indeed advertised, local candidates were always strong favorites. Letters of recommendation habitually emphasized such qualities as personal character, good conduct, and exemplary rectitude while making little reference to professional skills. In fact, as in private practice, knowledge and merit counted for far less than connections to members of the board: "the non-professional standards of the lay world continued to be the standards by which medical men were judged and appointed."[32] Nepotism and the calculations of cliques and parties therefore dominated appointments, often through the presence of relatives and certainly friends among the governors. "In general," Lydgate laments, "appointments are apt to be made too much a question of personal liking" (185). In its investigation of the procedures for the selection of medical staff at St. Thomas's Hospital, London, in the 1830s, the thirty-second *Report of the Charity Commissioners* (1840) openly commented on the role played by some "influential governors, if not by personal favour and connection."[33] Such appointments, though unpaid and seen as the doctors' own contribution to the relief of the poor, were eagerly sought as a source of status and indirectly of income. To be asked to be a member of the honorary staff was an empowering mark of confidence from the town's leaders. The authority of office enhanced the respect of patrons, not to mention the lucrative possibility of becoming medical adviser to board members and their families.

Through his insistence that the new hospital "be the special destination of fevers" (152) Lydgate is in danger of alienating the board as well as his fellow practitioners long before the episode of his refusal to dispense drugs. Once again the young newcomer transgresses the social code by voicing so emphatic and rather unwonted an opinion. Isolation was not standard at this time, when hygienic conditions were primitive and the chain of cause and effect between the transmission of infectious diseases and such factors as poor ventilation, polluted water, and rudimentary sanitation was not understood. As late as 1834 A. F. Chomel, in the first volume of his *Leçons de clinique médicale, faites à l'Hôtel Dieu de Paris* (Lectures on clinical medicine given at the Hotel Dieu Hospital in Paris), contended that nostalgia was one of the main origins of typhoid fever.[34] Indeed, typhoid fever is a good example of the slow beginnings of disease specificity, particularly in infectious diseases, for in the first third of the nineteenth century it continued to be bracketed with typhus, a blanket designation applied to all enteric fevers. In 1835 the differentiation between what the British called typhus and the French called typhoid fever was on the agenda of the French Academy of Medicine. The answer had actually already been provided by Pierre Louis and his pupils in a work published in 1829 under the title *Recherches anatomiques, pathologiques et thérapeutiques sur la maladie connue sous les noms de fièvre typhoïde, putride, adynamique, ataxique, bilieuse, muqueuese, gastro entérite, entérite foliculeuse, dothiénenthérie, etc.* (Anatomical, pathological, and therapeutic research on the disease known under the names of typhoid, putrid, adynamic, ataxic, bilious, mucous fever, gastroenteritis, folicular enteritis, dothienentheria, etc.). The range of names given to the syndrome shows the confusion surrounding it. On the basis of autopsies, evidence was given for the differential diagnosis between typhus, a louse-borne infection induced by the microorganism rickettsia, and typhoid fever, induced by the salmonella bacillus, although it was only in the late 1830s and the 1840s that the two diseases were properly separated, and the typhus bacillus was not actually identified until 1880.

In his championship of a fever hospital Lydgate is, however, contending, not with typhoid fever (he makes no attempt to isolate Fred Vincy), but with the far more devastating and very imminent threat of cholera, which had never been endemic in Britain but was then advancing rapidly from China and Japan through eastern and central Europe. By 1829 Poland, Germany, Austria, and Sweden had all been affected, so that it was merely a matter of time before the pestilence struck England. The first English cases, probably carried by ship, occurred in the harbor town of Sunderland in 1829, but it was not until 1831, when the disease hit Hamburg, a port of regular communication with Great Britain, that the danger was seen to be acute. A central board was set up which encouraged the formation of local boards and the organization of ad hoc isolation hospitals for the sick.[35] Eliot carefully notes the progress of the epidemic in the *Quarry for "Middlemarch,"* beginning with

"Cholera in Russia. Oct. 1830" (23), going into some detail about its incursion into England, including the first cases in Sunderland on 4 November 1831 (25); its outbreak in "Dantzic" is mentioned in the novel too. "And yet there are people who say that quarantine is no good!" Lydgate exclaims with utmost indignation (483). He works indefatigably at the New Fever Hospital, preparing "a new ward in case of the cholera coming to us" (689).

Is Lydgate here showing an almost visionary foresight, far ahead of the "mixture of jealousy and dunder-headed prejudice" (481) with which the inhabitants of Middlemarch obstruct the fever hospital, or does a strain of anachronism enter into *Middlemarch* at this point? That cholera is a water-borne infection was proven in 1849 by the London physician Dr. John Snow in his monograph *On the Mode of Communication of Cholera*. Before then the spread of most diseases was attributed vaguely to "miasma," conceived as foul exhalations emanating from swamps and marshes and lingering pestilentially in the atmosphere. The problem of public health, especially in the newly populous urban districts, was addressed by an active band of Victorian writers led by Charles Kingsley (1819–75) who campaigned for sanitary reform. But they were a tiny minority who did not begin to make an impact for some twenty years after the period of *Middlemarch*. Germ theory too was evolving during the time of the novel's composition, though not during the time of its action. In 1840 the German Jacob Henle (1809–85) argued in his treatise *On Miasma and Contagion* that minute living creatures, animalculae, caused infectious diseases. The concept of fermentation, basic to bacteriology, was authoritatively reviewed by the British physician Thomas Watson (1792–1862), whose *Lectures on the Principles and Practice of Physic* appeared in five successive editions between 1843 and 1871 as the chief textbook of British medicine. The 1850s and 1860s brought vast expansion in many diverse areas of bacteriology, culminating in the fundamental breakthroughs of Louis Pasteur (1822–95) in France and Robert Koch (1843–1910) in Germany. Yet these developments took place decades after the action of *Middlemarch*. Lydgate, if we see him as very up-to-the-minute, might conceivably have been cognizant of Louis's 1829 distinction of enteric fevers, but he could not possibly have had accurate information on cholera. In the early 1830s disagreement was rife concerning its contagiousness and the need for quarantine; curiously, the common populace was more inclined to believe in contagion, while the medical community argued against it.[36] Discussion of cholera was also vitiated by a pronounced

moralistic strain in the belief that it was a scourge almost exclusively of the
thoughtless and immoral.

Another apparent anachronism occurs in Lydgate's treatment of Raffles
by a new method described by Dr. John Ware in his *Remarks on the History
and Treatment of Delirium Tremens,* published in Boston in 1831. The argument
is compelling that "however advanced Lydgate is as a doctor, it seems im-
probable that he would have heard of this work at that time."[37] Although this
is a lesser issue than his understanding of cholera, it does again raise the question of Lydgate's extraordinary grasp of the latest medical thinking. Eliot obviously wants to portray him as absolutely on the cutting edge professionally,
but in so doing she strains historical credibility. These minor anachronisms
suggest a more fundamental one insofar as the cell research to which Lydgate
aspires was in fact carried out in Germany almost thirty years later. Rudolf
Virchow's *Cell Pathology* (1858) achieves exactly what Lydgate wants to do by
proving the cell to be the primary site of sickness. Such anachronisms, however, it must be emphasized, are rare in *Middlemarch,* which is by and large
very true to the medical conditions of the time. Eliot took utmost pain to ensure accuracy by engaging in extensive research; the first half of the *Quarry
for "Middlemarch"* (21–36) is devoted exclusively to notations of medical facts.
The few anachronisms do not affect Eliot's and our reading of the situation
in a provincial English town around 1830. They concern solely the image of
Lydgate, who comes across as excessively prescient, unbelievably (literally)
enlightened, in short, a highly idealized medical man. Such idealization is
more disturbing in *Middlemarch* than in *Wives and Daughters* or even *Doctor
Thorne,* where it can more easily be accommodated alongside the romance
tendencies; by contrast, within the essential realism of Eliot's novel Lydgate's
perfection as a doctor goes against the pervasive grain of human fallibility.

Admittedly, Lydgate is idealized solely in regard to his medical wisdom. As
a man he suffers the same sort of weaknesses as the other protagonists in
Middlemarch. They are subsumed by the narrator as his "spots of commonness," which "lay in the complexion of his prejudices, which, in spite of noble
intentions and sympathy, were half of them such as are found in ordinary
men of the world: that distinction of mind which belonged to his intellectual
ardour, did not penetrate his feeling and judgment about furniture, or women,
or the desirability of its being known (without his telling) that he was better
born than other country surgeons" (179). Here limits are set to the "distinction"

of his mind, which does not extend beyond the intellectual arena into the every-day conduct of his life. As the narrator later amplifies, "He would have liked no barefooted doctrines, being particular about his boots; he was no radical in relation to anything but medical reform and the prosecution of discovery. In the rest of practical life he walked by hereditary habit; half from that personal pride and unreflecting egoism which I have already called commonness, and half from that naïveté which belonged to preoccupation with favourite ideas" (383). So Lydgate is fraught with paradox: the nobility of his dedication to his vocation and his exceptional professional excellence are counterbalanced by human failings that make him almost a tragic figure.

For the "naïveté," if not the "commonness," that ruins his personal happiness also adversely affects his professional profile. In a complicated symbiosis of the positive with the negative, Eliot suggests that the very qualities that make him so outstanding a doctor lead him astray in other areas of his life. His care "not only for 'cases', but for John and Elizabeth, especially Elizabeth" (174) is a manifestation of the same sensitivity that renders him vulnerable to Rosamond's tears and her quivering neck when she fears that he has no attachment to her. His emotional tenderness overcomes his resolve, reiterated more than once, to delay matrimony for several years, "until he had trodden out a good clear path for himself away from the broad road which was ready made" (121).[38] His surrender to his feelings in acquiescing in Rosamond's desires initiates a pattern in which he becomes a yielding prey to his wife's petulant obstinacy. Her willful extravagance, the product of her self-centered immaturity, drives Lydgate not only into debt but also into subjugation and ultimately to the reluctant recognition "that he must bend himself to her nature" (815). In this intimate relationship he becomes more and more powerless to control his wife in the way a Victorian husband was expected to do. He accepts "his narrowed lot with sad resignation. He had chosen this fragile creature, and had taken the burthen of her life upon his arms. He must walk as best he could, carrying that burthen pitifully" (858). The image of his walking down the road of life weighed down by this burden contrasts wrenchingly with his early aim of treading out "a good clear path for himself" and brings out in full the crushing foreclosure of his potential.

Lydgate's self-destructive "naïveté" surfaces again in his professional conduct in the public forum, though not in one-to-one dealings with his own patients, where he shows considerable psychological insight. His stand against dispensing drugs can be taken as a matter of principle, but his stance on the hospital board demonstrates that his medical sagacity is not matched by worldly wisdom. He is placed in the awkward position of having to cast the swing vote in the appointment of a new chaplain. He himself favors Farebrother, who has so far attended to the patients' spiritual needs, who could do with the additional income, and who has become Lydgate's friend, but Bulstrode unequivocally directs that he wants his candidate, Tyke, to be installed. Trying to be "circumspect," Lydgate first equivocates: "As a medical man I could have no opinion on such a point" (154), then expresses the hope that he need have "nothing to do with clerical disputes" (155). This attitude reveals his innocence and his ignorance of the complicated, interlocking intrigues that determine the functioning of the social organism. Bulstrode, though endeavoring to maintain at least a semblance of tact, impresses on Lydgate his expectation of submissiveness in return for his decisive support for Lydgate's appointment to the hospital staff: "What I trust I may ask of you is, that in virtue of the co-operation between us which I now look forward to, you will not, as far as you are concerned, be influenced by my opponents in this matter" (154–55).

In obediently casting his vote for Tyke over Farebrother, is Lydgate being cooperative or corrupt, prudent or weak? By the time of the ballot he has few illusions about the implications of "this trivial Middlemarch business. He could not help hearing within him the distinct declaration that Bulstrode was prime minister, and that the Tyke affair was a question of office or no office" (208). This incident clearly illustrates the medical man's direct dependence upon patronage for the position that will secure him income. The prudence of "cooperation" is incompatible with idealism in the Realpolitik world of Middlemarch. In the short run, Lydgate's compliance with Bulstrode pays off: he is appointed medical director of the New Infirmary. But he has the greatest difficulty in confronting "the entanglements of human action" (481), wishing, ideally, to separate politics from his calling: "What he really cared for was a medium for his work, a vehicle for his ideas" (210). Only very slowly does he dimly begin to sense "the hampering threadlike pressure of small social conditions, and their frustrating complexity" (210).

In the long run, Lydgate's close association with Bulstrode proves catastrophic; when the latter falls into disgrace, Lydgate too is tarnished, even though he returns the check for one thousand pounds that Bulstrode lends him to pay off his debts. To mentalities accustomed to crude trade-offs the loan can mean only conspiracy and bribery. At this juncture a series of ironies and ambivalences comes into play. Lydgate's unjust implication in the scandal surrounding Bulstrode and the unpopularity of the hospital contribute to the further decline of his practice, already seriously undermined by his unconventional medical beliefs and methods. He is even branded a "charlatan" because of his "arrogance" and his penchant for "reckless innovation" (494). In assessing his own situation, Lydgate concludes in a fit of self-recrimination that his problems "are all connected with my professional zeal" (736). Yet he escapes blame for his handling of the case of Raffles, whose death takes Lydgate aback and makes him feel uneasy. The sudden expression on his face, Bulstrode notices, "was not so much surprise as a recognition that he had not judged correctly" (765). Lydgate cannot know (or does he suspect?) that Bulstrode, anxious for the final removal of Raffles, has failed fully to convey his orders to the housekeeper, who has cared for Raffles overnight and given him brandy and a substantial dose of opium, the standard treatments at the time but absolutely contrary to Lydgate's prescriptions, which draw on the very latest therapeutic views. His deliberation that "he himself might be wrong" (765) suggests an erosion of his professional self-confidence. Such an interpretation is borne out by the narratorial comment that his playing billiards for gain "was one of several signs that he was getting unlike his former self" (766). Ultimately, Lydgate's reluctant semicomplicity with Bulstrode is one of the main sources of his downfall. Given the banker's power in Middlemarch and the necessity of a hospital appointment for Lydgate to further his practice, it is hard to see what alternative, if any, was open to him. To have him buck the town's entire social and medical system—and succeed—would entail converting *Middlemarch* into romance. Lydgate's "naïveté," like his spots of commonness, are the tribute this figure, idealized in his professional sphere, has to pay to the novel's realism.

Lydgate's final fate is nicely designed to take into consideration both his excellence as a doctor and his poor judgment in marrying Rosamond and in alienating the people of Middlemarch. Lacking the rootedness in the community that Mr. Gibson in *Wives and Daughters* and Dr. Thorne possess, Lydgate commits the error of assuming that his outstanding medical accomplishments will be a sure way to success. Although his expertise wins approbation in some quarters, it cannot compensate for his unwillingness to adhere to traditional expectations of a surgeon. Forced by the threat of bankruptcy to put income above all else, he divides his time, according to season, between London and a Continental watering place and builds an excellent, that is, profitable, practice. The very phrase "according to the season" (892) reveals how he has been driven to follow the dictates of convention. It was quite customary in the nineteenth century for doctors to resort to fashionable watering places in order to extend their practice and increase their income. Seaside towns and inland spas were equally lucrative since both were patronized by the well-to-do. The financial motif surfaces again in the fact that Lydgate writes a treatise on gout, "a disease which has a good deal of wealth on its side" (893). In London Lydgate has many paying patients who rely on his skill; nonetheless, "he always regarded himself as a failure: he had not done what he once meant to do" (893). In this disparity between success in the eyes of the world and failure in his own eyes, which no doubt precipitates his death at age fifty of diphtheria, the paradox of Lydgate's fate is captured to perfection. Although he has greater medical power than Mr. Gibson or Dr. Thorne, he is still decisively constrained by the social power not only of affluent patients but also of public opinion. Even Dorothea's faith in him and her offer to help him financially to avert impending bankruptcy cannot make him change his mind about leaving Middlemarch, admittedly to spare Rosamond further distress rather than for his own sake. He realizes that through his injudicious behavior he has forfeited respect in Middlemarch to the point where it is hardly redeemable. That this failure is attributable at least as much to the narrow-mindedness of Middlemarch as to his overconfidence does not lessen the tragedy.

The stethoscope, as the symbol of the newer style of medicine, appears in several other medical encounters in fictions of approximately the same period as *Middlemarch*. In Eliot's story "Janet's Repentance," published as one of the *Scenes of Clerical Life* (1859), Dr. Madely, the consultant brought in from the neighboring town, uses a stethoscope to examine a patient with advanced tuberculosis.[39] This well-qualified but impersonal physician is a complete contrast to the local surgeons, Mr. Pilgrim and Mr. Pratt, who are on familiar terms with their patients. Mr. Pratt, for instance, is asked to give the orphaned Janet away at her wedding, and when she later takes to drink, he, as "medical attendant," his sister comments, "can hardly fail to be acquainted with family secrets" (190). Like *Middlemarch*, "Janet's Repentance" shows the medical profession on the cusp of transformation: Mr. Pilgrim and Mr. Pratt represent the old-style practitioners, "confidential friends" with psychological power, whereas Dr. Madely, with his stethoscope, is one of the new breed of scientifically more advanced, specialized doctors, who have a merely episodic rapport with patients. The introduction of the stethoscope can be traced in Thomas Mann's *Buddenbrooks* too: the family doctor applies his black listening tube to Thomas's chest to ascertain death. The date of this incident is January 1875. Interestingly, use of the instrument is not mentioned at the time of his mother's death from pneumonia about five years earlier. Her pulse and temperature are taken, and the spread of the malady inferred, presumably through percussion. Here, however, the new is grafted onto the old in a nice continuity as the longstanding family physician adopts the novel methods while still remaining the trusted "friend."

The very protracted and detailed evocation of Elisabeth Buddenbrooks's dying is a prime example of the growing precision with which disease is recorded in literature in consonance with the increasing command of the specifics of various afflictions and their course. Lawrence Rothfield, in *Vital Signs,* draws attention to the difference in the presentation of smallpox in Laclos's *Les Liaisons dangereuses* (1782; *Dangerous Liaisons*) and Zola's *Nana* (1880): in the eighteenth-century novel it functions as a device for closure and carries definite moralistic connotations, whereas in the late-nineteenth-century work there is "excrutiatingly fine detail . . . that emphasizes the temporality of the disease" (7). A similar observation is made by Gian-Paolo Biasin in his study *Literary Diseases: Theme and Metaphor in the Italian Novel:* "The scientifically generic and poetically vague way in which the romantics treated the theme of disease was replaced after the second half of the nineteenth century by a cold and precise, clinical and positivist tone. Disease-passion inexorably became physical illness in all its terrible concreteness" (8).

The gulf between the old and the new conceptualizations of disease is central to Ivan Turgenev's *Fathers and Sons* (1862; trans. 1989). As its title implies, its theme is generational discord, and it is played out in the medical as well as the personal sphere. Both Bazarov and his father, Nikolai Petrovich, are doctors, but they are diametrically opposite in training, outlook, and method. The older man, "like all stay-at-homes, had studied simple cures and even ordered a homeopathic medicine chest" (30). The affinity of his style with domestic medicine is suggested by the fomentation he applies to a swollen, red eye, making it up himself with a torn handkerchief. For "surgical poison-

ing" he urges "cold pack—emetic—mustard plaster on the stomach—bleeding" (157). The similarity between these measures and folk medicine is underscored by the ministrations of another elderly man, Vassily Ivanovich, an
amateur medical attendant to his peasants, who gives "centaury and St. John's
wort" (100) to a case of chronic jaundice and recommends that the sufferer
eat more carrots and soda. A retired major too "doctors the people . . . out
of philanthropy" (94). By contrast, the young Bazarov is wholeheartedly committed to the natural sciences, which he is studying in preparation for a career as a country doctor. He uses a microscope to conduct experiments on
frogs, which he dissects to see, as he explains to his friend, "what's going on
in his insides, and then, as you and I are much the same as frogs, only that we
walk on legs, I shall know what's going on inside us too" (14). Though a declared nihilist, Bazarov has wide interests in botany, chemistry, and physiology
as well as in homeopathy. His experience of dissecting cadavers prompts his
cynical comment on Anna Sergeyevna: "What a magnificent body, . . . perfect
for the dissecting-table" (62). It is his fervor for dissection that causes his un-
timely death: he cuts his finger while performing an autopsy on a peasant
who had succumbed to typhus fever, and as the district doctor has no caustic
at hand, he develops poisoning and dies. The German doctor brought in by
Anna immediately recognizes the hopelessness of the situation even as Bazarov
warns him not to speak Latin for he knows the meaning of *jam moritur* ("now
dying" [160n]). The "most scientific, most modern method" (152) is in its own
way just as treacherous and destructive as the old.

The distrust of the new scientific medicine that is so salient a theme of
Middlemarch is the subject of "Behind the Times," one of the stories in Arthur
Conan Doyle's collection *Round the Red Lamp* (1894). Dr. Winter is "behind
the times": he prefers innoculation to vaccination, is suspicious of chloroform,
chuckles about germ theory, and considers the stethoscope "a new-fangled
French toy" (4). Yet "his patients do very well. He has the healing touch—that
magnetic thing which defies explanation or analysis, but which is a very evident fact none the less. His mere presence leaves the patient with more hopefulness and vitality. Dying folk cling to his hand as if the presence of his
bulk and vigour gives them more courage to face change" (5–6). So patients
flock to him as he doses the entire countryside with senna and camomel, leaving the young doctors with their modern instruments and latest alkaloids neglected. Assessing the new physician against the old, the patient in this story

concludes: "I thought of his cold, critical attitude, of his endless questions, of his tests and his tappings. I wanted something more soothing-something more genial" (7). This patient's preference for the "genial" over the "tests" and "tappings" recalls the resistance Lydgate encounters in Middlemarch. It also serves as a reminder that even after the advent of scientific medicine patients empower their doctors for their human qualities as much as—or perhaps, as in this instance, more than—for their technical abilities.

But Conan Doyle, himself a qualified physician, does not give the last word to the reactionary patient. In another of the stories in Round the Red Lamp, "A Question of Diplomacy," the authority of the doctor with his scientific instruments is forcefully asserted: "With a bishop one may feel at ease. They are not beyond the reach of argument. But a doctor with his stethoscope and thermometer is a thing apart" (169). He is "a thing apart," "beyond the reach of argument," as a consequence of the unquestionable certitude ascribed to the findings of the sciences. Still essentially a missionary to the bedside, the mid- to late-nineteenth-century doctor is both more and less than a confidential friend: more through the power bestowed on him by the series of instruments that began with the stethoscope, and less as a result of the physical and emotional distance between physician and patient inserted by those very instruments. The new relentless pursuit of diagnosis and cure supersedes the old compassionate troth of comfort and consolation.

4.

"A WOMAN'S HAND"

—·—·—·—·—·—·—·—·—·—·—·—·—·—·—·—·—·—·—·—

"But this is a woman's hand!"—ELIZABETH STUART PHELPS, *Dr. Zay*

—·—·—·—·—·—·—·—·—·—·—·—·—·—·—·—·—·—·—·—

THE DIGNITY AND SANCTITY of the medical profession," Nathanael West proclaimed in a commencement address in Cincinnati in 1877, "its chief excellence is, not that it is scientific, but that it is redemptive."[1] *Redemptive* is an adjective hardly likely to be applied to medicine today. It has an even more pronounced religious thrust than *missionary* in denoting, in a theological context, salvation from a state of sin and its consequences and so, by extension into the secular, deliverance from evil courses. As striking as West's championship of redemption as the crux of medicine is his concomitant disparagement of science, or at least his relegation of it to a secondary position. This dichotomy is of more than academic interest, for the physician's preference for the scientific or the redemptive clearly has important implications for the balance of power: the idea of redemption projects a model of moral persuasion as the doctor's major function, whereas the emphasis on science entails a cerebral, rationalistic way of reaching out to the patient. In addition, *redemptive* solicits the patient's cooperation far more immediately than *scientific,* which proclaims the primacy of the physician.

West's dictum articulates the tension between comfort and cure that had been developing since the emergence of scientific medicine, but it is also an expression of the controversies in the United States about the aims and approaches proper to medicine in the closing third of the nineteenth century, when pluralism was rife. Besides orthodox, conventionally educated "regular" physicians, there was a plethora of "irregulars." The term was by no means synonymous with mere quackery, for it embraced such sects as homeopathy, hydropathy, Thomsonianism, Grahamitism, and eclecticism, each of which adhered to a more or less coherent system; however, it could comprise too self-styled healers of obscure training who propagated cures of more than questionable efficacy. It was to combat this disorderly multiplicity that the American Medical Association was founded in 1847 with the purpose of raising and standardizing the requirements for medical degrees. Its political squabbles exasperated its younger, more active and ambitious members, so that in 1886 the more scientifically minded men split off to form a separate learned society, the Association of American Physicians, devoted to the pursuit of knowledge.[2] These associations were relatively powerless because they did not control licensing, which was in the hands of the individual states and was therefore open to considerable variation in both the date and the scope of its enactment.[3] The sheer size of the continent, the differing conditions in its diverse parts, and the autonomy of the states resulted in a teeming pluralism, in contrast to the strict regulation instituted in Great Britain by the 1858 Medical Registration Act. Apart from "irregulars" or "sectarians," "unauthorized" practitioners such as bonesetters and Indian doctors were a feature of the American medical scene. Because of their independence from any control, it is difficult to arrive at a reliable assessment of their incidence. Joseph Kett admits that his figure of one sectarian for every ten orthodox physicians between 1835 and 1860 is intended as no more than a rough but reasonable estimate based on three contemporary surveys and one of his own.[4] By 1871 the proportion had risen to 13 percent, and by 1880 it was approaching 20 percent.[5]

The freewheeling organization of the profession encouraged schisms such as the dichotomization between the proponents of the scientific conceptualization of medicine and those who gave greater allegiance to its redemptive qualities. The "irregulars" either ignored science or evolved theories of their own, which in many instances were pseudoscientific and idiosyncratic. But "regulars" too, especially in remote areas, were resistant to newer methods and instruments, preferring to play safe with time-honored usage. This split between the adherents to science and the advocates of redemption was not unique to the United States. Conan Doyle's Dr. Winter, who spurns vaccination, chloroform, germ theory, and even the stethoscope and yet is gifted with the healing touch, is obviously an exponent of the redemptive. But he is presented, with a certain whimsical humor, as an anachronism, an exception in his stubborn skepticism toward science. A stance such as his tended to be more prevalent in the United States for reasons connected to its history and geography, which helped to shape patterns of development.

That American medicine was at a low ebb around the mid–nineteenth century is the universal consensus among medical historians. Akerknecht maintains "that the situation as a whole grew increasingly unsatisfactory" after the Civil War furthered "the decline with the dissolution of the fine medical centers that had developed in the South, particularly in Virginia, Kentucky, Tennessee, and Louisiana."[6] Rosenberg, writing of 1849, asserts roundly that "never before had the status of the American medical profession been as low."[7] In 1838 South Carolina and Maryland and in 1844 New York removed all legal restrictions on the practice of medicine; by 1851 fifteen states had repealed such legislation, while others had never passed any.[8] Indeed, "starting in the 1820s and continuing until the outbreak of the Civil War, the medical profession in America came under aggressive popular attack."[9] The reorientation from rationalism to empiricism that had begun in the 1820s led to a fragmentation of the profession that was to persist until American medicine recovered strength in the 1890s. The bitter feuds between the different sects not only divided the profession internally but also had the effect of weakening the trust and respect it could elicit from the public as its disunity and instability undercut its authority. Paradoxically, "the most hopeful period . . . in the history of medicine was the one in which the public looked to medicine with the least hope."[10] Nevertheless, between 1820 and 1860 at least seven hundred American physicians pursued postgraduate study in Paris, where they embraced and celebrated the new empiricism. Back home, they tended to become professors and editors and contributors to learned journals, but the influence of this elite was restricted, in part precisely because it was an elite in a culture deeply committed to democracy, common sense, and experience and also antagonistic to monopoly.

The science these men espoused was regarded as an estimable pursuit but definitely secondary to what was considered the principal purpose of medicine. "The practitioner at the bedside of his patient does not care to indulge in medical metaphysics," a reviewer in the *Cincinnati Lancet and Observer* tartly asserted in 1876,[11] just one year before West's exaltation of the redemptive over the scientific. Like the missionary visit to the bedside, the notion of the redemptive attests to the perception of medicine as a practical service to the patient, to whom it implicitly continued to yield considerable power. Science, by contrast, thought to be an intellectual, speculative exercise, was suspect as redolent of rationalistic system-building. The same reproach was also leveled against laboratory medicine, which, together with basic science, was relegated to the fringes of the healing enterprise. The center was firmly held by traditional bedside practice, which remained the mainspring of the profession's role and identity. And its pivot in turn was an active interventionism that stemmed from faith in the physician's power to cut short or even alter the natural course of disease by large doses of drugs and/or copious bleeding.

But these literally murderous bleedings and purgings of heroic therapeutics, with their debilitating side effects, were increasingly dreaded by patients. "Fame for not being heroic and not giving much strong medicine is just now a splendid item in a physician's reputation," Cathell counsels in 1881.[12] In reaction against the havoc that could be wrought by regular medicine, a renewed faith in the restorative capacity of nature gained ground. The movement to trust nature, which saw much disease as self-limiting, favored therapeutic moderation. Healing could be supported by far gentler remedies such as those sponsored notably by homeopaths, with their minimalist dosages. Given the extremism of heroic depletive measures, it is hardly surprising that homeopathy, whose pleasant-tasting pills were devoid of distressing effects, attracted a sizable following, especially among the urban upper and middle classes.[13] Homeopaths occupy an interesting intermediary position on the scientific/redemptive scale: while they held themselves to be scientific and therapeutically active, they managed to be largely noninterventionist and redemptive. The high point of redemptiveness was reached in Mary Baker Eddy's (1821–1910) Christian Science, whose very name summarizes the attempt to fuse religion with science as a form of medical practice. The appeal of these organized "irregular" sects encouraged a massive efflorescence of quacks, who touted secret patent remedies, filling daily and weekly papers with advertisements for wares that claimed to do wonders of all kinds. These unscrupulous profiteers seized the opportunity afforded by the public's disaffection with regular practitioners to transform practice into business for their own gain.

One literary example of this type is Doctor Selah Tarrant, the mesmeric healer in Henry James's *Bostonians* (1886). This thoroughly dubious character, seen by his patients as "very magnetic" (58), is always given the designation "Doctor," although the hardheaded Olive Chancellor does not believe "that he had come honestly by this title" (93). In her eyes he is "a charlatan of the

poor, lean, shabby sort, without the humour, brilliancy, prestige which sometimes throw a drapery over shallowness" (94). Her view is confirmed by the
information that "Selah had addicted himself to mesmeric healing" (55) as a
result of his "inability to earn a living" (59). With "his habitually sacerdotal
expression" he "looked like the priest of a religion that was passing through
the stage of miracles" (82). His adherents are mainly well-to-do elderly ladies,
whose unlimited faith in him makes them totally dependent on him. For all
his peculiarity, Tarrant is acknowledged as one of "the great irregular army
of nostrum-mongers" (57), and what is more, he practices in the environs of
Boston, one of the leading centers of the most advanced medicine in the late-
nineteenth-century United States.

The hold exercised by such healers as Selah Tarrant perhaps explains the
explicit emphasis put on the fact that Dr. Austin Sloper in James's *Washington
Square* (1881) is not "the least of a charlatan" (2). He is at the opposite end of
the spectrum to the mesmerist: a successful, elderly "regular" physician,
who is presented by the narratorial voice in the opening pages in a favorable
light. He is "a clever man" who has become "a local celebrity" and whose positive reputation rests on the even balance of his skill and learning: "he was
what you might call a scholarly doctor, and yet there was nothing abstract in
his remedies—he always ordered you to take something. Though he was felt
to be extremely thorough, he was not uncomfortably theoretic; and if he
sometimes explained matters rather more minutely than might seem of use
to the patient, he never went so far (like some practitioners one had heard of)
as to trust to the explanation alone, but always left behind him an inscrutable
prescription" (1). In other words, Dr. Sloper skillfully manages to achieve a
combination of the scientific and the redemptive aspects of medicine that enables him to retain control while satisfying his patients' expectations. James's
use of the second-person "you" in this passage places us as readers among Dr.
Sloper's patients. Although he is described in an obviously complimentary manner as "very witty," "the 'brightest' doctor in the country," "an observer,
even a philosopher," and "a man of the world" (2), there is no mention of any
of the geniality or kindness that would make him a confidential friend; indeed,
he seems rather austere, as his name perhaps suggests. On the other hand, his
honesty as a medical practitioner is categorically underscored, in ironic contrast to the personal deviousness he shows in his relationship to his daughter.

Another category of medical practitioner in the 1880s is represented in *The*

Bostonians by Dr. Mary Prance. No information is given about her background or professional education, but her strong scientific interests make it evident that she has received "regular" training.[14] Dr. Prance is seen almost exclusively through the eyes of Basil Ransom, a young southern lawyer recently moved north. In decidedly unflattering terms he describes her as "a plain spare young woman, with short hair and an eye-glass" (23), a dry, laconic observer of the feminist campaign in Olive's circle. His initial impression of Dr. Prance is unpropitious: "The little medical lady struck him as a perfect example of the 'Yankee female'—the figure which, in the unregenerate imagination of the children of the cotton-States, was produced by the New England school-system, the Puritan code, the ungenial climate, the absence of chivalry. Spare, dry, hard, without a curve, an inflection or a grace, she seemed to ask no odds in the battle of life and to be prepared to give none" (31–32). Ransom is as put off by her appearance ("She looked like a boy, and not even like a good boy" [32]) as by her "flat, limited manner" (331), which makes casual small talk virtually impossible, for "she had no interests beyond the researches from which this evening she had been torn" (33). She keeps her distance—and her counsel—preferring to devote her time to her studies, which she pursues late into the night. From the little physiological laboratory she has set up in the back room that would normally be the bedroom, the sound of sharpening instruments comes through the open windows, giving rise to the "belief that she dissected" (31). She is vehement about not wanting "the gentlemen doctors to get ahead of her" (37) and also about not having anyone tell her "what a lady can do" (38). Her pointblank refusal to "cultivate the sentimental side" (33) shows not only detachment but even a certain contempt for the womanly norms of the period.

But once Ransom grudgingly recognizes that "this little lady was tough and technical" (33), she becomes more interesting to him as a specimen of a new species of womanhood he has never encountered before. Eventually he develops something akin to admiration for the way she conducts business "with the greatest rapidity and accuracy" (331) as well as for the lucidity of her mind, which is hardly short of "diabolical shrewdness" (319). He is glad to see her again on Cape Cod near the end of the novel, although he cannot imagine how to engage with her socially. "He wanted to express his good-will to her, and would greatly have enjoyed being at liberty to offer her a cigar. He didn't know what to offer her or what to do, unless he should invite her to sit with him on a fence" (288). On this occasion the undertow of comedy that suffuses all Ransom's meetings with Dr. Prance is apparent when he is at such a loss as to the appropriate behavior toward this young woman who fits none of his conventional images yet whose company he slowly comes to enjoy despite her eccentricities. The humor here is at his expense, not hers. He discovers, too, that her commitment to science, her habit of giving priority to facts, does not preclude a capacity for feeling. Toward the aged, dying Miss Birdseye, whom she attends through her last days, she displays a tenderness that goes beyond professional devotion. Her customary dryness is tempered by kindness as "this competent little woman indulged her patient" because "the good lady was sinking fast" (328). Although Dr. Prance is treated throughout *The Bostonians* as something of a curiosity, she actually turns out to be the only woman in the novel with significant achievements: "It was certain that whatever might become of the [feminist] movement at large, Dr. Prance's own little revolution was a success" (38). Amid all the fulsome and vapid grandiloquence of suffragettism "the sturdy little doctress" (37) has attained a considerable measure of independence and genuine accomplishments, perhaps precisely because she has distanced herself from the agitation of the movement in order to pursue her professional development. And while she maintains a cardinal allegiance to science, Dr. Prance also has the ability to be redemptive when the occasion and her patients' needs warrant.

Dr. Prance is one of a cluster of doctresses, as they were then called, who appear in American fictions in the decade between 1881 and 1891. In chronological order they are *Dr. Breen's Practice,* by William Dean Howells (1881); *Doctor Zay,* by Elizabeth Stuart Phelps (1882); *A Country Doctor,* by Sarah Orne Jewett (1884); *The Bostonians,* by Henry James (1886); and *Helen Brent, M.D.,* by Annie Nathan Meyer (1891). In all of these except *The Bostonians* the life, work, and status of the doctress is the main theme. Only in James's narrative is the figure of the female physician not the central heroine, though still an important persona in the spectrum of possible womanly roles.[15]

This sudden spate of novels about doctresses within a few years testifies to the extent that they had not only attained public visibility but also captured the imagination as part of the wider debate about the "woman question" in the late nineteenth century. Access to medical education for women had become a highly controversial issue on both sides of the Atlantic after the middle of the century, when they had begun to try to gain admission to regular medical schools. Women had traditionally functioned as informal healers within the kinship circle of family and neighbors, and they had always been particularly prominent as midwives. In the late nineteenth century they also became active in various sectarian health reform movements such as the then fashionable water cures and notably in the physiological societies, which taught the "laws of life" and especially hygiene to female audiences as a supplement to domestic proficiency.

The extensive incorporation of medical knowledge into domesticity is amply illustrated by the widely used, influential nineteenth-century manuals of household management. All of them include significant amounts of medical lore and enjoin women to acquire diagnostic and therapeutic knowledge for the well-being of those under their domestic care. For instance, the third part of Cora-Elisabeth Millet-Robinet's *Maison rustique des dames,* "Domestic Medicine" (2:1–101), covers in its ten chapters the following topics: instruments and medications to be kept in the home; the preparation and administration of medications (including infusions, enemas, pills, baths, leeches, etc.); indications for calling a doctor; infant and child care; children's diseases (convulsions, croup, scarlet fever, chickenpox, worms, etc.); the diagnosis and treatment of medical and surgical conditions ranging from weight loss to chillblains, bleeding, fevers, sciatica, fractures, and burns to epilepsy and urinary retention, reviewed in a lengthy reference section (2:48–86); animal and insect bites; poisonings; asphyxiation; and the establishment of death. An even more thorough primer is *Mrs. Beeton's Book of Household Management,* which has separate chapters entitled "Invalid Cookery," "The Rearing and Management of Children and Diseases of Infancy and Childhood," and "The Doctor." The latter deals with much the same ground as Millet-Robinet's "Domestic Medicine" but is more advanced, giving guidance on when and how to bleed (1065–66), how to distinguish between hemorrhage from the lungs and from the stomach (1066–67), how to handle concussion (1073) and cholera (1073–74), how to differentiate between apoplexy and epilepsy as well as between epilepsy and drunkenness (1077–78) and how to treat each of these conditions, how to set about trying to revive a drowned person (1091–92), and how to cure stammering (1089). "The Sick-Room" is the title of a similar section in Mary Mason's *Young Housewife's Counsellor.* Mrs. Mason offers general advice on hygiene, tact in handling the patient, recipes for the invalid's diet, and directions for preparing and applying various types of plasters, "blisters," and leeches. The woman who mastered the precise instructions in these manuals would clearly be a valuable medical resource.

But however broad and effective a woman's medical knowledge might be, it was to be exercised exclusively within the "woman's sphere," that is, within the confines of her domestic province. The deeply entrenched belief in the necessity for segregating the woman's from the man's sphere led to a fundamental paradox regarding the activity proper to women in the medical arts. On the one hand, their innate aptitude for healing within the domestic domain was endorsed and even systematized in the manuals of domestic management. On the other hand, their suitability for professional practice beyond the home was emphatically denied. While the most vociferous (and powerful) adversaries of medical education for women were male, the majority of Victorian women also subscribed to this view. This inconsistency reveals the two sides of the same ideological coin. The objections to the idea of women entering the medical profession were so strong because they stemmed from the basic assumptions about women, notably the concept of separate spheres of endeavor for men and women, that kept the woman locked into the domestic realm as "the angel in the house," "the queen of the hearth." Although individualistic, rebellious women did, of course, infringe social conventions, such behavior elicited dire censure as "unladylike," "unfeminine," that is, likely to entail the loss of the offender's social status and to incur painful ostracism. This penalty was imposed on any woman who dared to invade the male sphere and to compete with men by working outside the home at all, and worse yet, for pay. For example, Sophia Jex-Blake, a leading British pioneer of medical education for women, was categorically warned by her father that if she accepted a salary, she "would be considered mean and illiberal."[16] For a middle-class woman who failed to marry and who could not count on financial support from members of her family the only acceptable occupation was that of governess, precisely because it still assured her at least the protection of remaining within the woman's sphere by working in a home, albeit someone else's. The tribulations and humiliations of even this form of work have been vividly chronicled by both historians and novelists.[17]

Ironically, the opposition to women in medicine was reinforced in the United States by the profession's recovery from its low ebb after the mid—

nineteenth century. The gradual institution of regulatory organization consolidated its authority and enabled it to close ranks against women. As long
as instruction solely by apprenticeship had been an approved form of medical
training, women had in fact been able to get a rudimentary medical education,
as Harriot and Sarah Hunter did in Boston in the early 1830s. It was perhaps
the women's bad luck that their attempts to gain access to regular training
coincided with a major revision of the system of medical education, which
in the first half of the nineteenth century had been "an open market."[18] After
the war of 1812 medical schools began to proliferate, often with only tenuous
connections to universities and with primitive facilities. Much of the growth
after 1820 took place in the West and in rural areas, where costs could be kept
low. The "diffusion and degradation of emblems of status"[19] is symbolized
by the elimination of the bachelor's degree and its inflation into the M.D. By
1850 between 40 and 50 medical schools were in operation (compared with
just 3 at the same time in France), and from then on the numbers accelerated
rapidly: 75 in 1870, 100 in 1880, 133 in 1890, 160 by 1900. The enormous variations
in the quality of these schools were bound to temper lay people's trust in the
degree and even in the profession. "The profession of medicine," Paul Starr
comments, "did not endow its members automatically with public trust"—or
power.[20]

A concerted effort to improve medical education was initiated in 1870 by
Harvard President Charles Eliot. His aim was to transform medical training
into a rigorous professional course along the lines of the German model,
shedding its proprietary standing and integrating it into the university. The
previous two-year program, consisting largely of theoretical, didactic lectures
devoid of regular sequence, was expanded in 1871 into a three-year course in
which anatomy, physiology, chemistry, and pathological anatomy, that is, the
laboratory sciences, came to play an ever more important part. Experimental
science gained unprecedented prominence in the new curriculum, giving
each student practical laboratory experience. At about the same time hospitals
moved from the periphery to the center of medical education and practice,
transformed from refuges for the homeless poor and insane into the physician's
primary workshop. By the late 1880s medicine had become dependent on special technologies that required trained skills to achieve competence. It was
also in the 1870s and 1880s that medical men converged in agreement on the
need for licensing and proper regulation of the profession. This stiffening and

enforcement of the requirements is typified by the 1877 law in Illinois that empowered a state board of examiners to accept diplomas only from reputable
schools.

The reform and institutionalization of medical education militated against
women, who "were the casualties of medical professionalization."[21] Whether
such an oppression-victimization model is a simplification has been a matter
of argument among historians, some of whom see women's attempts to
enter into regular medicine as part of the larger nineteenth-century struggle
for female self-determination. It was obviously a rebuff to such aims that
women's repeated efforts to be admitted to medical schools met with scoffing
rejection under a profusion of pretexts, although Elizabeth Blackwell was admitted in Geneva, New York, in 1845 because students and faculty thought
the application a joke and voted for its acceptance in jest. She graduated at
the top of her class in 1849. Another exceptional case is that of Marie Elizabeth
Zakrzewska, who had been a brilliant midwife in Berlin and who graduated
in Cleveland in 1856. But by and large, specious objections and excuses were
put forward to exclude women from medical schools and hence from the profession. The very idea of a female doctor was considered to violate the norms
of feminine behavior; women were regarded as unfit, physically and temperamentally, for the "blood and agony" of medical practice, which would
compromise their innate delicacy. Indeed, they were deemed constitutionally
unfit for education after puberty, when all their energy should be directed to
the development of the "pelvic power" that would make them good mothers.[22]
That was the central argument of Dr. Edward H. Clarke in his 1873 treatise
with the misleading title *Sex in Education: A Fair Chance for Girls,* in which he
asserted that intellectual activity during menstruation would surely lead to
"neuralgia, uterine disease, hysteria, and other derangements of the nervous
system."[23] A vigorous rebuttal to this hypothesis appeared in England in the
April 1874 issue of the *Fortnightly Review,* where Elizabeth Garrett Anderson,
Britain's first licensed woman physician, asserted that

> it is difficult to believe that study much more serious than that usu-
> ally pursued by young men would do a girl's health as much harm
> as a life directly calculated to over-stimulate the emotional and
> sexual instincts, and to weaken the guiding and controlling forces
> which these instincts so imperatively need. The stimulus found in

novel-reading, in the theatre and ball-room, the excitement which attends a premature entry into society, the competition of vanity and frivolity, these involve far more real dangers to the health of young women than the competition for knowledge, or for scientific or literary honors, ever has done, or is ever likely to do.[24]

Beliefs such as these prompted courageous women to begin to organize their own medical colleges when they found the doors of established schools insolently slammed in their faces. The New England Female Medical College was founded in Boston in 1848, the Women's Medical College of Pennsylvania in Philadelphia in 1850, the New York Women's Medical College (homeopathic) in 1863, the Homeopathic Medical College for Women in Cleveland and the Women's Medical College of the New York Infirmary for Women and Children in 1868, the Woman's Hospital Medical College in Chicago in 1870, and the New York Free Medical College for Women in 1871.[25] None of these endeavors could have got off the ground without the support and cooperation of some male physicians who were willing to act as instructors until the women themselves had acquired sufficient expertise and experience to teach their successors. Hands-on case work was also essential to medical training. Since women were denied internships and residences, they founded first dispensaries and then hospitals for women and children, of which the earliest were the New York Infirmary for Women and Children, opened in 1857, and the New England Hospital for Women and Children, in 1862. From these institutions the pioneer women doctors were graduated, including three black women: Rebecca Lee in 1861, Rebecca Cole in 1867, and Sara McKinney Stewart in 1870. Some of the more affluent and ambitious went on to further training in those European universities, notably Paris and Zurich, that were open to women. Back home, well prepared to practice and intending to serve women and children, the doctresses faced more difficulties in obtaining membership in the state medical associations. Such membership was not strictly a prerequisite for practice; nevertheless, it had important practical ramifications as a symbol of legitimate acceptance as well as for referrals or admission to hospital staffs, in other words, for full integration into the profession. Curiously evasive terms such as *inexpedient* and *inopportune* were advanced for a while as grounds for rejection; the qualifications necessary for admission were declared to apply to males only. But in 1877 the state societies of Kansas, Michigan, and Rhode Island did take women; others followed, with Massachusetts, in 1884, among the last.

Opposition to the admission of women was probably motivated by economic considerations too. One consequence of the large number of medical schools was the grave overproduction of doctors that prompted Cathell's *Book On the Physician Himself.* Yet while much concerned about rivals, Cathell is extremely proper in recommending: "Do not refuse to consult with foreign physicians, doctresses, colored physicians, or any other regular practitioners" (214). The very need to issue such advice is an illuminating commentary on the marginalization of doctresses. If the position of doctors as a whole was "insecure and ambiguous" in the latter half of the nineteenth century,[26] that of women doctors was doubly so.

Although editions of Cathell's manual after 1885 bear the title *The Physician Himself and What He Should Add to His Scientific Acquirements* and he refers to his target audience as "a live, earnest-working, scientific physician" (5), his severely practical approach admits only halfhearted lip service to science, which is contravened by several passages of vehement warnings against science as anathema to "popularity," that is, financial success:

> I have often thought that the secret why so many truly scientific but dry-as-dust physicians of a statistical or hypothetical turn, to whom a patient is the same as a rock is to a geologist, or as a flower is to a botanist, who, more naturalists than physicians, love the rays of philosophy and the beams of science better than humanity; and who, with their eye at the end of the microscope, watch cases merely from a scientific point of view, or to study the action of medicine; very often decidedly and permanently lack popularity, and fail to get much practice; is that cold logic and rigid mathematics, chemistry, physiology, and other high theoretical attainments, however much admired abstractly, are not a certain guarantee of popular favor, since they are often attained at the expense of the endearing sentiments, and hence create none of those ties upon which many a successful practice depends. (10–11)

He advises physicians never "to be led from the practical branches of medicine for histology, pathology, microscopic anatomy, refined diagnostics, bacteria-

mania, comparative anatomy, biology, psychology, and other captivating subjects that merely interest and create a fondness or monomania for the marvelous" for, he reminds them, "the first question to ask yourself in everything
of this kind is, What is the use?" (75). Cathell here concurs with West in according priority to the redemptive over the scientific. As late as the 1880s he
still believes that the physician's power over patients springs from the "ties"
of "endearing sentiments" rather than from "high theoretical attainments."
The friendship offered by the missionary to the bedside is recommended as
the foundation for "favor" and "popularity." The worth of Cathell's argument
is, of course, undermined by his simple equation of success with a substantial
income.

The dichotomy between redemptiveness and science was particularly
troubling for the women physicians who were contemporaries of Cathell's
fledgling practitioner. To begin with, whereas he is pragmatic, they were essentially idealistic: the main reason they cited for seeking professional training was to enable them "to attend medically to those of their own sex who
need them," to give "sisterly help and counsel."[27] The need for doctors of
their own sex was rooted in Victorian women's modesty, which often led
them to shun examination by a male physician.[28] Accordingly the doctresses
showed little concern about either competition or income: for "the woman
who practises as a physician would probably confine her practice to women
only."[29] In 1889 Blackwell affirmed "emphatically that anyone who makes pecuniary gain the chief motive for entering upon a medical career is an unworthy student."[30] On the other hand, the pioneering women doctors were
deeply preoccupied with the search for the most appropriate style of medicine
for them *as women*. So the "woman question" surfaces here in a very specific
form: the concern of the late-nineteenth-century female physicians was not
whether they should practice medicine but *how*. In this debate, West's terms
"scientific" and "redemptive" are useful ciphers for the opposing positions.

The foremost advocate of the theory that women should practice an alternative to normative, that is, male, medicine was Elizabeth Blackwell (1821–1910).
Although she did not actually use the word *redemptive* in outlining the mode
she considered most fitting for female physicians, it is immanent to her ideas
because they bear the unmistakable imprint of the religious environment
in which she was brought up. As she recorded in her autobiographical sketch
Pioneer Work in Opening the Medical Profession to Women (1895), "a strong sense

of religion was early implanted" (7). The hypothesis that "one clue to Black-well's thinking lies in the fact that her interest in moral reform antedated her attraction to medicine" is a compelling one.[31] In describing how she envisaged "the idea of winning a doctor's degree . . . as a great moral struggle" (29), Blackwell twice uses the telling phrase "a moral crusade" (62 and 72). She makes her decision following a kind of epiphany; she describes how her "ter-ror of what I was undertaking" was suddenly dispelled by "a spiritual influence so joyful, gentle, but powerful, . . . that the despair which had overwhelmed me vanished" (34–35). What Blackwell here evokes is her sense of the calling to a mission, a term she herself later invokes.

Secure in "the necessity of my mission" (72), she lets her religious and moral convictions shape her attitude to medicine. In her essay "Scientific Method in Biology" (ca. 1880) she includes a section entitled "The Moral Ele-ment in Research," in which she argues for "Morality as a Guide in Biological Science" and against the vivisection of experimental animals as an "erroneous method in medical education" fraught with "moral danger."[32] She holds that "Religious or Unitary truth possesses invaluable guidance for Medicine" (2:49) and that "The Religion of Health" consists in "Obedience to Divine Law" (2:211). Blackwell's exaltation of the moral and the religious leads her to the same kind of deprecation of the scientific as West. She applies the ad-jective *abused* (2:43, 124) to science and the scientific and even inveighs against the "exaggeration of bacteriology" (2:73).

The priority Blackwell accords to the "spiritual life" (2:77) results in the elaboration of a feminist ethos. Her key concept is maternity, not in the literal sense of childbearing but in reference to the affective, redemptive effect of nurturing. In her autobiography she makes the crucial connection between maternity and theism: "I had always felt a great reverence for maternity—the mighty creative power which more than any other human faculty seemed to bring womanhood nearer the Divine" (*Pioneer Work*, 30). Blackwell here en-visages what she calls "maternity" as the particular power possessed by women. This notion is developed in the central piece of the *Essays in Medical Sociology*, "The Influence of Women in the Medical Profession," an address given at the opening of the winter session of the London School of Medicine for Women in October 1889. The "great essential fact of woman's nature" is here identified as "the spiritual power of maternity" (2:9), which confers on women physicians "special responsibility" and also enables them to make a "special contribution" (2:8). In contrast to "the onward rush of the male intellect" (2:8), which is perceived as a possible danger, women in the medical profession must be sure to exercise "the most beneficial influence" so as to have an "appreciable effect on future society for good" (2:4). This entails a constant awareness of "moral considerations," of "what is right or wrong for us, in medicine, both as human beings and as women" (2:6). Women, Blackwell continues, "must seek a high moral standard as their ideal" (2:10), must let "the Moral guide the Intellectual" because "the moral faculties are antecedent or superior to the intellectual faculties" (2:21). She associates the intellectual with the male mind, the spiritual with female maternalism. Consequently, "it is our duty and privilege, as women entering into the medical profession, to strengthen its humane aspirations" (2:43).[33]

The way in which women physicians were to accomplish this, according to Blackwell, is in a way very reminiscent of the mid-nineteenth-century ideal of the doctor as a missionary and a confidential friend. For women's special contribution lies in "those beneficent moral qualities—tenderness, sympathy, guardianship—which form an indispensable spiritual element of maternity" (2:12). Blackwell was by no means alone in this belief: in her valedictory address to the Female Medical College of Pennsylvania in 1864 Dr. Anne Preston pointed to the particular gifts of "tact and insight" and "quick sympathies" that women could bring to medical practice.[34] Harkening back to another, older view "that the body and the mind are inseparably blended in the human constitution" (2:5–6), Blackwell concludes that the woman doctor "must often be a confessor of her patient" (2:12) and "she must always be the counsellor and guide" (2:13). This self-conceptualization makes her recoil from the temptation to regard patients, especially poor ones, as "clinical material" (2:13), which she sees as implicit in the scientific experimental approach. Instead, echoing T. C. Minor's rejection of "medical metaphysics" at the bedside, she asserts that it "is not a brilliant theorizer that the sick person requires, but the experience gained by careful observation and sound common-sense, united to the kindly feeling and cheerfulness which make the very sight of the doctor a cordial to the sick" (2:14). The various strands of Blackwell's philosophy are linked in the closing words of her autobiography in an explicit restatement of the redemptive vision as she looks forward to the future influence of Christian women physicians, who will "apply the vital principles of their Great Master to every method and practice of the healing art" (*Pioneer*

Work, 254). So to Blackwell medicine is essentially a form of service to the suffering, and its practice by women is justified by their special capacity for the kind of self-sacrifice such work involves. Her ideology, which verges on a theology, can therefore be seen as an attempt to reconcile women's traditionally ordained position in society with their unconventionality in entering the medical profession.

Some twenty years younger than Blackwell, Mary Putnam Jacobi (1842–1906) took a much bolder line. After graduating from the Women's Medical College of Pennsylvania in 1863 and several years of clinical work at the New York Hospital for Women and Children, she studied for five years at the Ecole de Médecine in Paris, where she took her M.D. in 1871 with high honors and a bronze medal. Her early love of chemistry naturally drew her to the laboratory in Paris and to a lasting interest in the discoveries of the bacteriologists. Her letters to the *Medical Record* between 1867 and 1870, signed "P.C.M.," in which she reported on medical matters in Paris, mark the beginning of a series of nine books and 120 articles on diverse aspects of internal medicine, ending, poignantly, with "Description of the Early Symptoms of Meningeal Tumor Compressing the Cerebellum, from which the Author died. Written by Herself."[35] In contrast to Blackwell's mainly sociological writings, Jacobi's are devoted to medical topics except for a sprinkling of occasional addresses and a piece entitled "Shall Women Practice Medicine?" which appeared in the *North American Review* in 1882.[36] Her anonymously submitted essay "The Question of Rest for Women during Menstruation," a rebuttal of Dr. Edward Clarke's book on the harmfulness of education for girls after puberty, won the Boylston Medical Essay Prize in 1876. By then she was already well launched on a distinguished career as a private practitioner and professor of therapeutics and materia medica at the New York Infirmary of the Women's Medical College. On her return to New York in 1871 she was described by Sir William Osler as having "a Paris degree and a training in science unusual at that time even among men."[37] A member of eight medical societies,[38] she was the first woman admitted to the New York Academy of Medicine, whose section on neurology she chaired.

By temperament as well as by education Jacobi was a scientific rationalist who insisted on stringent adherence to empirical investigation and factual analysis. In her "Inaugural Address at the Opening of the Woman's Medical College of the New York Infirmary," on 1 October 1880, she takes the exam-

ple of a fractured skull to illustrate how essential the basic sciences are to medical practice; she underscores the need to know anatomy, physiology, physics,
chemistry, and pathology in order to be able to handle this case properly.
"Here, then, are four separate sciences, with entirely different methods, with
which the physician must be to a considerable extent acquainted before he
can in the least understand the condition of the patient we have imagined."[39]
Jacobi's language is as eloquent as Blackwell's, though more terse, hammering
at her target with a sharp aim. Her advocacy of science makes her dismissive
of the spiritual and moral dimensions underscored by Blackwell. "It is impossible to be a physician on the basis of personal sympathies alone. If the interest in the disease be not habitually greater than the interest in the patient, the
patient will not profit, but suffer. He may gain a nurse, but he loses a physician."[40] The distinction drawn here between the functions of a nurse and
those of a physician is of crucial importance in formulating the new decision-
making rather than merely caretaking obligations of women qualified as doctors. Ultimately, the divergence in attitude between Blackwell and Jacobi
transcends the controversy over medical style for women insofar as it reflects
and summarizes changes under way in the medical world at large. While
Blackwell upholds the doctor's traditional role as "confessor," "counsellor
and guide," that is, missionary to the bedside, Jacobi represents the newer
ideal that devolves from the laboratory and the application of scientific discoveries.

So much so indeed that the basic question that preoccupied Blackwell—how
to be a *woman* doctor—is almost a non-issue for Jacobi. In her "Address Delivered at the Commencement of the Woman's Medical College, of the New
York Infirmary" on 30 May 1883 she bluntly confronts "the topic which most
frequently suggests itself at our graduation exercises, . . . that of the sex of
the graduates" with this trenchant advice: "You are liable to be so much and
so frequently reminded that you are women physicians, that you are almost
liable to forget that you are, first of all, physicians. As a rule, I have always ad-
vised you to reverse this order; to so saturate and permeate your consciousness
with the feeling for medicine, that you would entirely forget that public opinion continued to assign you to a special and, on the whole, inferior class of
workers in medicine."[41] Jacobi tries here to shift the gender problem by projecting it onto "public opinion." To her the difficulty resides not intrinsically
in women's practicing medicine but extraneously in a "series of misconcep-

tions" (377) and "social bewilderments" (373) concerning the nature of both
medicine and women and the consequent false conclusions about their un-
suitability to each other. She contests the view that medicine is "dirty, horrid,
and irreverent" (372) or "coarse and disagreeable" (373) as well as ingrained
prejudices exemplified by the outcry "*Girls* don't play ball!" (377). She mentions
some of the conventional arguments in favor of women doctors, such as the
venerable tradition of women as healers; their admission to medical schools,
she points out, denotes "no innovation at all" (368), merely an adaptation "to
the changed condition of things" (369). Jacobi's position is parallel to that of
Sophia Jex-Blake, who asserted that the "innovation lies in the exclusion of
women" as a result of the 1858 British Medical Registration Act.[42] But rather
than pressing such pleas, Jacobi defiantly takes an absolute stand by minimiz-
ing the role of gender in medical practice. The weakness of her position lies
in a perhaps willful underestimation of the force of public opinion as she
seeks to discard the reservations that trouble Blackwell in order to affirm that
women have the right and the ability to "reenter" the mainstream of the
profession (369).

An ideological struggle parallel to that between Jacobi and Blackwell is
reenacted in the debate over the policies and modalities of the new hospitals
for women and children. This dispute centers on the conflict between integration and separatism: should a hospital governed by and for women adopt
the same methods as those run by men for all sections of the sick, or should
it develop its own characteristically feminine conventions? In her study of the
New England Hospital in Boston, with the revealing title *Hospital with a
Heart,* Virginia Drachman traces the confrontation between the proponents
of the two opposing systems. Those who favored integration argued that in
the long run it would open up more opportunities for women. Its adversaries,
led by Marie Zakrzewska (1829–1902), thought that separatism would help
women to acquire courage and self-reliance. Since she was the hospital's guiding force, her views prevailed. While certainly scientific in its methods, the
hospital also sought to be redemptive through attempts to recreate the cozy
atmosphere of a pleasant home.

A similar philosophy inspired the evening dispensary for working women
opened at Trinity Church, Boston, in 1886 and the evening clinic for women
founded the following year by the Women's Industrial and Educational Union
of Boston. Staffed by women physicians, both were expressions of practical

medical maternalism in Blackwell's sense. The moralist undercurrent implicit
in the redemptive concept of usefulness, so important to both real and fictional
women doctors, indicates their need to justify their unconventional lives as
service to others.

This tension between two heterogeneous styles of medical practice had
to confronted and resolved according to individual temperament by every
nineteenth-century practitioner, male or female, and it can be argued that it
still remains an issue today, though the divide is no longer seen as strictly gendered, and in the secularized late twentieth century the terminology would
not be imbued with a religious hue.[43] The pioneering doctresses, because they
had consciously to fashion their professional identity, openly discussed—and
agonized over—the dilemma that faced every physician: how to reconcile the
new medical technology with the traditional role of missionary to the bedside.
While most, men and women alike, would settle for a middle course in hopes
of doing some justice to both aspects, for women the choice was complicated
by the ascription to them of innate maternity. If this made them in some respects especially suited to medicine as caring, it could in other respects be
prejudicial through an imputed want of toughness. So besides the concrete
problems of gaining access to professional education, women were also
hampered by the ideological allegation that they were by nature not fitted to
medical practice. When Helen Brent, M.D., in Meyer's novel by that name
successfully completes difficult operations, "she had never been known either
to faint or to go into hysterics, as Dr. Manning had prophesied would be the
conduct of the woman physician" (15). But there is widespread evidence of
societal prejudice, not least among the male members of the profession itself.
Cathell warns in 1889: "Jealous midwives, ignorant doctor-women, busy
neighbors, and Job's comforters too often exert a malign influence."[44] Dr.
Silas Weir Mitchell, inventor of the rest cure, is more oblique yet potentially
more alarming to any young women contemplating entry into the profession:
"Personally, women lose something of the natural charm of their sex in giving themselves either to this or to other avocations until now in sole possession of man."[45] The references in Sinclair Lewis's *Arrowsmith* to the "co-eds"
are also unflattering: they are described as "virginal and unhappy" (23), "emotional and frightened in bacteriology" (35), and shuddering as a hypodermic
needle punctures the skin of a pig's belly in a laboratory demonstration.

The ideal of a conjunction of the scientific with the redemptive is summed

up in the title of Regina Morantz-Sanchez's *Science and Sympathy,* the authoritative history of women physicians in the United States. A plea for an alliance
of the two was the theme of Dr. Eliza M. Mosher's 1925 speech "The Humane
in Medicine, Surgery, and Nursing." Yet a certain contradictoriness pervades
the dualistic encomium of her as a physician with high standards *and* a gentle, courteous woman in the prefatory material and in Mosher's own speech.
Although she begins by extolling the "ideal that the human and the scientific
go hand in hand" (117), she actually devotes most of her address to the former.
Her conclusion is a resonant reiteration of Blackwell's ideas. "The opportunities to put something helpful and uplifting into the lives of our patients, while
administering to the purely physical, is too great and too precious to be lost.
One of the greatest responsibilities and privileges which comes to women in
medicine lies just here, for to women even more than to men comes by
heredity and training, a sympathetic understanding of the meaning of pain
and physical limitations" (119). So women are particularly able "with that
touch of the human" (119) to treat hurt souls as well as sick bodies. This is a
nice compromise: it allows women who do enter the male sphere as physicians
to follow, at least to some degree, the norms of behavior prescribed to women
of that period.

In what ways are these issues played out in late-nineteenth-century American fictions about doctresses? Are these novels, as one critic has claimed,
merely "personified arguments for or against a question thrust upon a reading world"?[46]

Undeniably, all the novels have a political dimension insofar as the contemporary polemic about women doctors is aired. None of them evades the
problem, although they vary in the degree of directness with which they
address it. The topic surfaces both internally in the opinions voiced by fictional
characters and extraneously in the narrator's implied posture. A good example of discussion within the fiction is the long conversation in Jewett's *Country
Doctor* between Dr. Leslie and an old neighbor, Mrs. Graham, just as Nan's
resolve to become a doctor takes shape. Later, when she has already embarked
on her apprenticeship and visits her aunt in the little Maine town of Dunport,
the conventional ladies in Miss Prince's circle are deeply shaken by her non-
chalant announcement that she is studying medicine. "What do you mean?"

demands the aunt coldly before dismissing the idea as "Nonsense, my dear" (185). Nan is reminded that it is "proper for young women to show an interest in domestic affairs" and that "a strong-minded woman was out of place" (208); she is further rebuked that it is totally unnatural for "a refined girl who has an honored and respected name to think of becoming a woman doctor!" (209). Nan has sufficient self-assurance to brush these reproaches aside, but Grace Breen is undone by other women's "distrust of a physician of their own sex" (*Dr. Breen's Practice,* 22). The young Mr. Libby's astonished question to Grace's sole patient "You don't mean *that's* your doctor!" (17) is less hurtful to her than the rejection by her fellow women. This recurrent disapprobation of a woman's practicing medicine reflects the rigid belief system governing the conduct of women, especially of the middle and upper classes, in the late nineteenth century. The unwritten rules of proper behavior for a lady were firmly laid down. All the doctresses are transgressing fundamental codes of their time by working outside the home, by supporting themselves financially, and by trespassing into the male sphere of science. Their lifestyle would certainly have been perceived as an arrogation of powers unbecoming, indeed forbidden, to women. This is underscored by the contrast with what James calls "sweet *home-women*" (*The Bostonians,* 27). The foil to Dr. Zay is Mrs. Butterwell, with whom she lodges and who represents the venerated ideal of the devoted housewife. Similarly, Helen Brent stands out against the socialites at New York tea parties; she realizes that "her hopes, her aims, her theory of life were so irrevocably different from those of the women about her" (93). Yet these average, upper-class women are unmasked as hypocritical, shallow, and unscrupulous social climbers. Less pernicious but equally empty-headed are the conservative friends of Nan's aunt in *A Country Doctor.*

The motif of surprise at a woman's practicing medicine recurs in one guise or another in all five novels, often linked to the underlying question of the propriety of such a way of life for a woman. The limits of propriety were most gravely challenged by medicine because it involved exposure to the body and could be surreptitiously linked to the taboo on sexuality. The quality that redeems the doctresses from utter disgrace and goes some way toward neutralizing their ambiguous social position is the acknowledgment that every one of them is a lady and that their purpose in taking up medicine is service to their peers. Curiously, the former appears to be the more important of the two in attaining social acceptance, for it is categorically mentioned in every instance. Even Dr. Prance in *The Bostonians,* despite her want of conventional femininity, is unequivocally recognized to be a lady. Grace Breen has "a ladylike manner" (96), moderating her "business-like alertness" with "ladylike sweetness" (10). The adventurous Nan of *A Country Doctor* is, it is emphasized, by no means "mannish" (160); "a young lady," she should, according to one of her elderly neighbors, "be made to look like the little lady she is" (129). That Dr. Zay "was unmistakably a lady" (17) is a great consolation for her patient, Waldo, as he comes to terms with the revelation that his physician is female. It is reassuring to him that she has "the dress and carriage of a lady" (44). Her dress is given close attention: on calls she is unobtrusively modest in "blue, or black, or blue-black, or blue and black" (18) in winter and cream or white in summer. But on social occasions her colors are brilliant: on one occasion she wears a "parlor dress" of violet muslin with lace and satin ribbons at wrists and neck (155), on another a ruby dress with a plush jacket and white lace. Likewise, Helen Brent, who wears a plain, stiff black alpaca dress and large, wide, flat shoes in her professional guise, can, when she chooses, blossom into "a queenly lady" in a gown with a graceful train, a profusion of soft lace, and pretty kid slippers (175–76). She and Dr. Zay are idealized figures projected by a woman's imagination, able to combine "the decisive step" of "women of business" with "grace of movement and curves of femininity" (*Doctor Zay,* 97).

Just as being a lady makes social amends, so being useful acts as an ideological justification and seems to override overt concerns with power. The urge to be useful is prominent in all the doctresses, as is their conviction that their service will have a decisive impact on their patients' lives. The necessity of asserting themselves as *women* doctors subsumes the issue of power, which is displaced onto the criterion of usefulness. Grace Breen, for example, is obsessed by a Puritan sense of duty and a "severe morality" (39) that impels her to be "more useful to others" (12). Disappointed in love and rich enough not to have to work, she has chosen medicine "in the spirit in which other women enter convents, or go to heathen lands" (12). These words clearly evoke the concept of the doctor as missionary, but perhaps Grace is the least successful of the doctresses precisely because her vocation is vaguely to be of service to womankind rather than specifically to study medicine, which she has found in part "almost insuperably repugnant" (12). Such hesitations are unknown to Nan Prince in *A Country Doctor,* who is strongly motivated by her drive to be useful: "she was filled with energy and a great desire for use-fulness" (159), excited by the "renown some women physicians had won, and the avenues of usefulness which lay open to her on every side" (193). Her final riposte to her aunt's objections is simply that to study medicine "is the best way I can see of making myself useful in the world" (283). Dr. Zay is impelled by the personal experience of having watched her mother's suffering to the realization "how terrible is the need of a woman by women in country towns" (175). Although she admits that women doctors "pay a price for our privilege" (123), she is sustained by her awareness that "the women all depend on me" (138). So the sense of usefulness becomes in itself a tool for empowerment. Power in the guise of usefulness is certainly the goal of Helen Brent when she proclaims, "I have a mission, a duty to perform" (40). Hers is the most encompassing calling: her "chief aim is to make all women find themselves" (104) for she is "determined to leave the world better" than she found it (31).

Nevertheless, despite these fine motivations and attributes, both male and a good many female protagonists within the fictions are shown as censorious of women doctors. Among the authors the pattern is one of a direct correla-tion between gender and attitude. The women writers present a far more positive image of the doctress than do the men. Meyer's Helen Brent is a veri-table superdoctress—beautiful, strong, calm, successful, and always in control of her professional (if not of her personal) life. She performs "difficult gyne-cological operations . . . that required nerve, coolness, daring, skill, a steady hand, and a delicate one" (15), and in her speech on her accession to the presi-dency of a women's medical college she vows to provide women with "the very best training," upholding "the very highest scientific standards" (20). Phelps's heroine, Atalanta Zay, too is independent, self-confident, and highly competent. Single-handedly she runs a rural practice in Maine, is "sent for all over the county" (86), goes out to night calls alone in her horse and buggy, handles minor surgery with "a firm and fearless touch" (47), and earns five thousand dollars a year, though she could make much more if she did not treat the poor for free. Jewett's Nan Prince is at a considerably earlier stage of her career than Helen Brent or Atalanta Zay, yet she already shows "a sort of self-dependence and . . . self-reliance" (103) together with an instinctive in-sight into people, and the "resource, bravery, and ability to think for one's self that make a physician worth anything" (138).

These commanding women physicians are a striking foil to Howells's Grace

Breen. An "inexperienced girl" (76), timid, hesitant, she is in constant need of reassurance and approval from her mother, who undermines her as consistently as does the narrator (who refers to her, for example, as that "girl"). At the beginning of the novel she has completed her training and is about to start practice; however, since she has only one patient, the title, *Dr. Breen's Practice,* sounds ironic. When faced with a critical medical situation Grace panics and calls in the elderly Dr. Mulbridge, who takes charge of the case while Grace, deferring to his superior judgment, reverts to the traditional womanly role of nurse. Self-deprecatory, lacking pride or a sense of self, the pathetic Dr. Breen seems so temperamentally unsuited to medicine as to be almost a cautionary figure. Midway between the reduction of Grace Breen by a male writer and the apotheosis of Helen Brent by a woman is James's portrayal of Mary Prance. She has well-developed self-esteem and a good deal of panache; however, she is hardly presented as attractive, even though she comes to rise in Basil's opinion. Yet the intelligent, learned, capable Dr. Prance is wholly overshadowed by the sexually alluring Verena, who captivates Basil but has not a thought of her own.

Dr. Prance, dissecting in her own home laboratory, is the most "scientific" of the doctresses in these five fictions. Her authoritative manner is reinforced by her somewhat mannish appearance and her brisk dismissal of "the sentimental" (33). She is set on competing with the gentlemen doctors, yet she can also be tender, maternal, and "redemptive," as is shown in her compassion for the dying Miss Birdseye. Just as committed to science and far more explicit in her pursuit of power is Helen Brent with her advanced operations, which put her in the vanguard of American gynecological surgery, pioneered by J. Marion Sims (1813–83). At the opposite end of the scale, Grace Breen, if and when she can muster the necessary self-confidence, is likely to prove maternal and maybe redemptive as she ministers to the women and children in her husband's factory town.

For their endeavors to conjoin the disparate styles of practice Dr. Zay and Nan Prince are the most interesting. Both have early on been empowered by supportive male role models: Nan by her guardian, Dr. Leslie, and Atalanta Zay by her father, who was a physician. As a child she liked "to be round his laboratories" (87), and though he died when she was only fifteen, he had made a deep impression on her, which has been intensified by his early death into an idealized memory. She believes that she "inherited" the "taste for science" (77) she discovered while at Vassar and that that has made medicine come more easily to her. The dissecting room was "a trial" (78) to her at first, she admits, but she experienced no difficulty in working alongside men, whom she found to be very courteous. But the really momentous impetus to become a doctor derives from her experiences with her mother. When she is asked why she decided "to make such a sacrifice of yourself? such a young bright life as yours" (75), she answers after some hesitation in a low voice: "It was owing to—my mother. She had a painful illness. There were only we two. I took care of her through it all. She spent that last summer here in Sherman,—it was cool here. She suffered so from the hot weather! My mother was greatly comforted, during a part of her illness, by the services of a woman doctor in Boston. There was one when we were in Paris too, who helped her. I said, When she is gone, I will do as much for some one else's mother" (76). From the outset, therefore, the male scientific example is partnered by a female maternal one in shaping her vision of medical practice. She sees the woman doctor as invested with the power to make a significant difference in the lives of other women. Here it is again very clear that doctresses equated power with usefulness.

That both these young women lost their parents while still young is important for their bold choice to go into medicine. As orphans they are freer from the directive constraints of close relatives and thus have greater liberty in pursuing their goals. Their education differs only in that Nan begins hers in apprenticeship to Dr. Leslie before going on to formal instruction in Boston and a postgraduate year in Zurich. Atalanta Zay, after training in New York, has also spent time in Zurich, as well as in Paris, seeking additional European credentials, as did many of the more eager and financially secure women doctors. Both ultimately go back to their native regions. Nan in *A Country Doctor* turns down offers of a position at a city hospital in favor of returning home to be a general practitioner specializing in pediatrics, aspiring to be Dr. Leslie's successor. She does so out of loyalty to both her mentor and the community where she grew up. The description of her return makes it clear that she will bring a large measure of the redemptive ideal of service to her patients to complement the science she has learned: "It was a great pleasure to belong to the dear old town, to come home to it with her new treasures, so much richer than she had gone away that beside medicine and bandages and lessons in general hygiene for the physical ailments of her patients, she could often be a tonic to the mind and the soul; and since she was trying to be good, go about doing good in Christ's name to the halt and maimed and blind in spiritual things" (252–53).

Dr. Zay likewise opts to practice in Maine, in an even more remote area than Nan. She prefers it to a town because it affords better opportunity to devote herself wholly to her professional obligations without the distraction of social demands. It is no coincidence that both *A Country Doctor* and *Dr. Zay* are set in New England. Together with New York, Boston was the prime center of medical education for women and consequently had a far higher concentration of female physicians than anywhere else: in 1880, 132 women were practicing in Boston alone, 14.9 percent of the city's medical force; by 1890 the figures had risen to 210 and 18.0 percent, respectively (in the rest of the country the corresponding percentages were 2.8 in 1880 and 4.4 in 1890).[47] It is also in keeping with historical facts that Dr. Zay is an adherent of homeopathy, which women doctors tended to espouse rather than the heroics of alleopathy.[48]

It is indeed in part Dr. Zay's allegiance to homeopathy that is instrumental in Waldo Yorke's decision to remain under her care, for homeopathy is the medical creed in which his mother believes. His trust in nurturing maternalism is thus transferred onto this first woman doctor he has ever encountered. He has little choice anyway since Dr. Zay is the only homeopathist within thirty miles of the place where Waldo, a Boston lawyer on business in Maine, has incurred a serious accident. The circumstances under which this particular doctor-patient relationship develops are perhaps unusual but certainly not beyond the bounds of credibility. Although both Dr. Zay and Nan Prince care primarily for women and children, neither of them is nonplussed by male patients, whom they acquire either as the result of accidents requiring immediate attention, as in the case of Waldo, or, occasionally, by virtue of their being the elderly spouses of their female patients. However, even Dr. Zay is forced to confess that never before had she treated a *young* man.

Her handling of Waldo is an example of her ability to unite the scientific and the redemptive in managing her power with the utmost tact. She gives expert care to the wound on his head, keeping watch at his bedside through the first critical night. He naturally takes her to be a nurse and repeatedly asks to speak to the doctor. Since the episode is presented from his point of view, the technique of suspense is cleverly deployed as the realization dawns on him that his gentle, competent attendant with the soft step and soothing voice *is* the doctor:

"Where *is* that doctor? I am too sick a man to be neglected. I must see the doctor."

"The doctor has been here," said the woman who was serving as nurse, "nearly all night."

"Ah! I have been unconscious, I know."

"Yes. But you have been cared for. I hope that you will be able to compose yourself. I trust you will feel no undue anxiety about your medical attendance. Everything shall be done, Mr. Yorke."

"I like your voice," said the patient, with delicious frankness. "I haven't heard one like it since I left home. I wish I were at home! It is natural that I should feel some anxiety about this country physician. I want to know the worst. I shall feel better after I have seen him."

"Perhaps you may," replied the nurse, after a slight hesitation. "I will go and see about it. Sleep if you can. I shall be back directly."

This quieted him, and he slept once more. When he waked, it was broadening, brightening, beautiful day. The nurse was standing behind him at the head of the bed. She said:—

"The doctor is here, Mr. Yorke, and will speak with you in a moment. The bandage on your head is to be changed first."

"Oh, very well. That is right. I am glad you have come, sir." The patient sighed contentedly. He submitted to the painful operation without further comment or complaint. He felt how much he was hurt, and how utterly he was at the mercy of this unseen, unknown being, who stood in the mysterious dawn there, fighting for his fainting life.

He handled one gently enough; firmly, too,—not a tremor; it did seem a practiced touch.

The color slowly struck and traversed the young man's ghastly face.

"Is *this* the doctor?"

"Be calm, sir,—yes."

"Is *that* the doctor's hand I feel upon my head at this moment?"

"Be quiet, Mr. Yorke—it is."

"But this is a a woman's hand!"

"I cannot help it, sir. I would if I could, just this minute, rather than to disappoint you so."

The startled color ebbed from the patient's face, dashing it white, leaving it gray. He looked very ill. He repeated faintly,—

"*A woman's hand!*"

"It is a good-sized hand, sir."

"I—Excuse me, madam."

"It is a strong hand, Mr. Yorke. It does not tremble. Do you see?"

"I see."

"It is not a rough hand, I hope. It will not inflict more pain than it must."

"I know."

"It will inflict all that it ought. It is not afraid. It has handled serious injuries before. Yours is not the first."

"*What shall I do?*" cried the sick man, with piteous bluntness.

(41–43)

The scene has, of course, a comic dimension as a variant on the stock fairy-tale recognition, where the frog turns out to be a prince. Here there is a kind of inversion as the prince (the doctor) turns out to be a frog (a woman).

Dr. Zay's surgical skill and sound judgment are kept very much in the fore-front. When Waldo suffers a complication, she knows exactly what to do, and does it briskly and with aplomb: "She drew her surgical case from her pocket, and selected an artery forceps. She opened the wound, and instructed Mrs. Butterwell how to hold the forceps while she ligated the artery. She bandaged the arm, and adjusted it to suit her upon a pillow. She had a firm and fearless touch. Her face betrayed no uneasiness; only the contraction of the brows inseparable from studious attention" (47). In his aftercare, too, her profession-alism is underscored and contrasted with his discomfort as she follows the rituals of the physician's visit:

This young lady required his age, his habits, family history, and other items not immediately connected in the patient's mind with a dislocated ankle.

"Now your pulse please," she said, when she had reached the end of her catechism. She took his wrist in a business-like way. The young man experienced a certain embarrassment. The physician gave evidence of none. She laid his hand down again, as if it had been a bottle or a bandage, told him she was greatly gratified with his marked improvement, prepared his powders, and, drawing the little rubber clasp over her medicine-case, gave him to understand by her motion and manner that she considered the consultation at an end. (51)

The balance of power has a special piquancy here through the reversal of the traditional gender roles. It is the man who has to be submissive as the patient and the woman who is in control as the doctor. Yet despite her impeccably professional conduct, Waldo cannot but see her as a "young lady."

As he moves beyond the crisis toward recovery, Dr. Zay's nurturing capacity reinforces her medical proficiency. The transition—and the fusion—is well illustrated at the moment when he begins to put weight onto the injured foot. After guiding him professionally through the appropriate movement, which is painful to him, "she melted like frost, and shone; she hovered over him; all the tenderness of the healer suffused her reticent face" (64–65). As in the recognition scene, here also there is an almost magic transformation implicit in the phrase "she melted like frost and shone." The coalescence of intelligence and warmth in her is directly articulated by Waldo's hostess, Mrs. Butterwell, who tells him: "There's more *woman* to our doctor than to the rest of us, just as there's more brains" (86). Subsequently the narratorial voice exalts her in hyperbolic terms as possessing "the mysterious odic force of the healer, which is above science, and beyond experience, and behind theory" (99). Dr. Zay is a new, late-nineteenth-century incarnation of the missionary to the bedside, female in gender and dually empowered by scientific knowledge and quasi-maternal tenderness.

This special blend of abilities pervades her relationships to her other patients too, although none is portrayed with the expansiveness of her rapport to Waldo, which is central to the plot. She deals with an outbreak of scarlet fever in the poor section of town with the same medical and human devotion she gives to her paying patients. In a more melodramatic incident, when a young man who has impregnated his girl tries to drown himself, she takes complete charge of both the physical and the psychological aspects of the crisis, not only reviving the would-be suicide but also prevailing upon him to marry the girl forthwith. With her "imperious voice," "firm hand" (139), dogged persever-ance at resuscitation, and calm persuasiveness, she exerts commanding power as her natural and rightful role.

Like Dr. Zay, Nan in *A Country Doctor* also often seems an idealized figure whose life story is a rewriting of that of the unhappy, abused orphan girl common in nineteenth-century fiction. Nan, by contrast, is well cared for and loved, becoming "a more and more useful little assistant" (94) as she goes on rounds with Dr. Leslie. The autobiographical element is quite strong here for Jewett was the daughter of a dedicated country doctor and was herself prevented by ill health from following in his footsteps. This early novel of hers is therefore a rewriting as wish fulfillment in more than one respect.

In observing Dr. Leslie, Nan absorbs alongside his practical methods and techniques his approach to patients, which is essentially a continuation of the older tradition of acting as missionary to the bedside and confidential friend. He appears to combine the scientific and the redemptive, although it is hard to assess the extent of his acquaintance with innovative medicine. The narra-tor expresses a distinct skepticism at the current "haphazard way of doctoring, in which the health of the patient was secondary to the promotion of new theories, and the younger scholar who could write a puzzlingly technical paper often outranked the old practitioner who conquered some malignant disorder single-handed" (140). But Dr. Leslie is exempt from such prejudices: he "was always trying to get at the truth, and nobody recognized more clearly the service which the reverent and truly progressive younger men were ren-dering to the profession. He added many new publications to his subscription list, and gleaned here and there those notes which he knew would be helpful" (140). He makes a trip to Boston to "visit some instrument-makers' shops and some bookstores" (113); what instruments and books he acquires is not stated. While Jewett is well informed and specific about the routines of country prac-tice, she is frequently vague and evasive about aspects of medical culture with which she had no personal familiarity. For instance, her handling of the train-ing Nan receives in Boston is conspicuous for its perfunctoriness.

Because *A Country Doctor,* in the manner of the Bildungsroman, focuses on Nan's discovery and pursuit of her vocation in her youth, there is less scope than in *Dr. Zay* to evince her interaction with patients. Only toward the end of the novel is she a fully qualified physician, but her healing power is shown before then. As a medical student, on an outing with friends she uses her knowledge of anatomy to manipulate a farmer's dislocated shoulder back into position. Stooping and unbuttoning her right boot, Nan plants her foot on the damaged shoulder and catches up the hand to give a quick pull; there is an unpleasant cluck as the bone goes back into the socket and a yell from the sufferer, who scrambles to his feet: "'I'll be hanged if she ain't set it,' he said, looking quite weak and very much astonished. 'You're the smartest young woman I ever see'" (198). Nan here displays the same self-assured, take-charge attitude as Dr. Zay, and again a male patient has to acknowledge a woman's medical skill. Her scientific competence in dealing with her patients' physical ailments is, as the narrator directly tells us (252–53), allied to a spiritual dimension, grounded in the religious imperative to do "good in Christ's name," so that she is also "a tonic to the mind and soul." Her nurturing understanding suffuses her tendance of the body in a holistic healing.

These novels about the doctress devote less space to the portrayal of the issue of power than do the narratives about male physicians discussed in the two previous chapters. None of the doctresses is shown using a stethoscope or a microscope or even a thermometer. Also remarkably absent are the class tensions that so determine and complicate the balance of power between doctor and patient in mid-nineteenth-century England. The doctresses and most of their patients are of roughly the same social level, although some of the rural patients in *Doctor Zay* and *A Country Doctor* are poor. It is tempting to argue that late-nineteenth-century American society was less obsessed with the subtleties of a class hierarchy than its British or European counterparts. More likely, however, the concern with gender is so overriding in these fictions as to relegate questions of class. Certainly the problems caused by gender are sufficiently pressing to overshadow the actual practice of medicine in favor of a concentration on the doctresses' personal and social predicaments.

Preeminent among these, corresponding to the professional choice between the scientific and the redemptive, was the dilemma in regard to marriage. Ironically, whereas marriage was considered a plus for a male physician as a stabilizing influence, for a doctress it was regarded as a drawback, a distraction from wholehearted attention to patients. At a time when marriage and motherhood were almost universally hailed as the only desirable way of life for women, the difficulty, perhaps impossibility, of reconciling the two was a paramount obstacle. Some, notably Jex-Blake, believed that marriage and medical practice were incompatible, for a married woman with a family would be "serving two masters";[49] she advocated a choice between marriage and a learned profession. Jacobi, on the other hand, while conceding that marriage, "which complicates everything else in the life of women, cannot fail to complicate their professional life,"[50] took her own marriage to Dr. Abraham Jacobi as the model for rejecting the notion that medicine exacts celibacy from women. When she wrote about marriage, asserting that medicine was not incompatible with marriage, she repeatedly used the word *adjustment*. Even more outspoken is the argument voiced in December 1886 by a contributor to *Alpha*, a journal edited by the physician Caroline Winslow: "A woman who has before her the broad avenues of usefulness, who has ambition and energy to develop her powers, will not be satisfied to tie herself down in the soul-cramping marriage. . . . woman's highest duty to herself and humanity demands her full development as a *Woman*, not as a *Wife* or *Mother.*" Like Jacobi and others in the United States, Elizabeth Garrett, who married J. G. Anderson in 1871, proved that marriage could be combined with medicine. Of the fifty women on the British Medical Register in 1886, thirty-two were single, ten married, five widowed, and one had begun to study medicine while married. In the United States, one-fifth to one-third of female physicians at that time did marry, often fellow doctors; some continued their practices, others chose not to do so.

In confronting the conflict between professionalism and marriage, the plots of these novels delineate a range of alternatives for women, some of which were startlingly audacious, particularly the notion that a woman might actually prefer a profession to marriage. The convention of marriage as the happy ending to the heroine's story is deeply ingrained in nineteenth-century literature. Jane Eyre's "Reader, I married him" could be uttered by the great majority of female protagonists. Ideally, as in Jane Austen's novels early in the century, the marriage is the right match between congruent partners. Romance is attenuated in mid-century realism when things no longer work out as easily or as well. Yet *Middlemarch* still pivots on a series of marriages: Dorothea and Casaubon, and eventually Will, Lydgate and Rosamond, Fred Vincy and Mary Garth, Celia and Sir James Chettam. Although the perplexities of the marital state are not suppressed, as in romance, its validity and desirability nevertheless remain unchallenged. Even Emma Bovary, who is so desperately unhappy with her husband, is unable to conceive of happiness for a woman other than through the agency of a man, some fantasy lover. Marriage was not only the norm for women; it was considered the absolute precondition for social respect and self-fulfillment. Failure to find a husband meant shame, degradation, possibly the humiliating necessity of having to earn one's living as a governess.

Within this social and literary tradition, the doctress novels attempt to mediate the clash between the conventional domestic role for women and the new paths explored by those who follow the calling to medicine. One obvious attempt to overcome this dichotomy was Blackwell's appropriation of maternity into medical practice. But there is no consistent correlation between nurturing medicine and marriage, on the one hand, and science and celibacy, on the other: Blackwell, the advocate of maternity, remained single, while the scientifically minded Jacobi married. Still, in the novels a broad pattern is discernible in the association of the predilection for science with singlehood and the inclination to redemptiveness with matrimony.

The most resolutely celibate among the fictive doctresses is Mary Prance in *The Bostonians*. Wedded, as it were, to scientific medicine, she is a confirmed spinster for whom marriage is not even an option.[51] Her mannish appearance and manner hint that she may be lesbian. Helen Brent too remains single, though perhaps not entirely by choice. She has been shabbily treated by her lawyer fiancé, Harold Skidmore, who breaks their engagement when she takes her medical degree and goes off to Germany. The prototype of the new liberated woman, she argues vehemently that women should no more be expected to give up their profession on marriage than men. Yet her life, full, rich, and busy as it is, is not complete. At the end of the novel, after Harold's wife has left him, he writes to Helen that "some day there will come knocking at your gates a broken Harold, as a suppliant" (196). This sentimental final twist is hardly convincing, but it does show the force of the convention of marriage as the preferred closure for the heroine, even if only as a prospect on the horizon.

Nan Prince's position is considerably more complicated. Though an adventurous tomboy in her childhood and later gripped by "the feeling of a reformer, a radical, and even a political agitator" (131), Nan is, it is emphasized, not "the sort of girl who tried to be mannish" (121). In Dr. Leslie she has a somewhat ambiguous model: he has for many years been a widower without a family, but his pleasure in bringing up Nan suggests his need for an emotional outlet beyond the care of his patients. Following his lone life, Nan rejects marriage when she turns down the rising young lawyer George Gerry. Because she finds him attractive, she goes through a phase of hesitant indecision, particularly during a sleepless night when "her old ambitions were torn away from her one by one, and in their place came the hardly-desired satisfaction of love and marriage, and home-making and housekeeping, the dear, womanly, sheltered fashions of life" (228). But in the clear light of day she understands that to marry would be to lose "the true direction of my life" and that her part is "to make many homes happy instead of one" (241). So marriage is to her a "temptation" (229) to be resisted because it would limit her potential for a wider usefulness. In making her choice, which is by no means easy for her, Nan is motivated by a commitment to service similar to the ideal of the redemptive missionary to the bedside. But as *A Country Doctor* shows, a woman's nurturing redemptiveness can be expressed in paths other than marriage.

Grace Breen, by contrast, beset by self-doubts about both her competence and her suitability to the profession, takes marriage as a way out, and probably also as a compensation for the early disappointment that led her into medicine. She rejects the proposal of the mature Dr. Mulbridge that they be "physicians in partnership" (322) as well as husband and wife. Her refusal becomes less puzzling in light of the terms he uses in addressing her. In his words, she has shown herself to be "faithful, docile, patient, intelligent beyond anything I have seen" (228), but, he assures her, "you could never succeed alone" (223). He is right about her intelligence, for she tells him bluntly that he is "a tyrant" who wants "a slave not a wife" (254). Meanwhile she has sought the advice of young Mr. Libby about Dr. Mulbridge's proposal, which gives her the opportunity to declare to him: "Don't you see that I love *you*?" (248). So Grace Breen-Libby moves to the factory town where her husband manages his father's mills and treats his workers' sick children. The pointed closing comment that "the conditions under which she now exercises her skill certainly amount to begging the whole question of woman's fitness for the career she had chosen" (271) is a harshly judgmental intrusion by the male narrator, still intent on denigrating Grace. Married and motherly, she alone among these fictive doctresses is weak and vacillating.

The complete opposite to Grace is the intrepid Atalanta Zay, the boldest of the women doctors portrayed in these fictions. She is strong-willed, self-assertive, and supremely confident of her ability to handle any professional situation. With her absorption in her flourishing practice, her dedication to helping women, and the gratitude and success she thereby earns, she appears the least likely to marry. But she ends by acceding to Waldo's persistent courtship, albeit on her own, perfectionist terms, in the conviction that the marriage can be *"divinely* happy" (248). She sorely tests Waldo, treating his love "like a fit of measles" (248) and sending him back to his law office in Boston to apply himself more diligently to his work. He returns after six months, the "new type of man" appropriate to the "new kind of woman," "a woman who diverged from her hereditary type" (244). The verve of the plot is heightened by the continued role reversal, for Waldo has been decidedly lackadaisical in his profession as a lawyer, barely earning five hundred dollars a year. He is made to undergo a kind of testing reeducation in order to become an acceptable spouse to Dr. Zay.

The ending of *Dr. Zay,* like that of *Jane Eyre,* patently veers into romance. "The miracle has happened!" Waldo ecstatically exclaims; "'We love each other,' he urged,—'we love each other!'" (243). Even at this climax, it is worth noting, he has to "urge" her, and still she hangs back: "'We think so,' she said sadly. '*You* think so'" (243). Only when she realizes that he does not want or expect her to give up medicine does she begin to soften. Then, as the tables of control are turned, the idiom smacks strongly of romance: "She stretched her hands out to him in mute appeal" (246), and he comforts her (and assumes authority over her): "'How tired you are!' he said, with infinite tenderness. 'I would have rested you, poor girl!'" (247). That last phrase is surprising and jarring, for never has the authoritative doctress behaved like the "poor girl" she seems to Waldo. While the phrase is protective, it is also demeaning. At least in his eyes the role reversal of the earlier stages of their relationship, when she was dominant, has to be undone in order to make the partnership acceptable to him. Whether she goes along with this remains ambiguous. Her loss of her voice at this point is in striking contrast to her previous self-possession; now she expresses herself in the language of gesture. "Before he had finished speaking, she glided up to him; her deep-colored dress and waving feminine motions gave her the look of some tall velvet rose, blown by the wind. She put both her hands in his, threw her head back, and looked at him. For that one moment she gave her soul the freedom of her eyes" (247–48). The comparison to a "tall velvet rose, blown by the wind" evokes

fragility as well as beauty. Her transformation from the briskly professional into
the softly feminine is clearly signified by the change in her garb from the
unobtrusive, neutral colors she favors on her rounds to the brilliance and soft-
ness of her dress on social occasions. *Dr. Zay* would have us believe that the
"strong-minded doctor" will coexist harmoniously with the "sweet woman"
(254) in the union with Waldo. But it cannot do so without recourse to a terminology that attests to a slippage into the realm of romance, which leaves
a shadow of doubt in the minds of today's readers. Will Dr. Zay be able to
acquiesce in the traditional wifely role of submissiveness within the home
and maintain her professional power outside?

   These novels, then, in addressing a controversial question of the day,
offer a variety of fear and wish projections through deflation or inflation.
Grace Breen can certainly be seen as a cautionary figure, a woman who has
strayed into a mistaken orbit. Likewise, Mary Prance, whose intellectual acuity hardly compensates for the forfeiture of her charm. Far more potent are
the idealized images represented by the other three, each of whom in her
own way attains an exemplary stature: Helen in her surgical and administra-
tive feats; Nan in her brave renunciation of marriage in order to seek fulfillment in service to others; and Dr. Zay in her bid to have it both ways. The
plausibility of these images is closely dependent on the literary quality of the
fictions in which they appear. Helen Brent, with her exclusive zeal for science
and her strident crusading, comes across as a cardboard character because
she is so grossly overdrawn. In the exaggeration of her exploits the line between
idealization and hyperbole has been crossed.[52] In *Dr. Zay* the perfect outcome
comes at the expense of a displacement into the genre of romance, which
modifies the credibility that can be invested in it. The most convincing is Nan
Prince because of the balance and moderation of the portrayal, especially
in the frank admission of the many struggles she has to face as she climbs the
"long hill" (134) that confronted a woman entering medicine at that time.

   These five American novels have their counterpart in five British fictions
that appeared at roughly the same time: Charles Reade's *Woman Hater* (1877),
G. G. Alexander's *Dr. Victoria. A Picture from the Period* (1881), the anonymously
published *Dr. Edith Romney* (1883), *Mona Maclean. Medical Student* (1893) by
"Graham Travers," the pseudonym of Margaret Georgiana Todd, Jex-Blake's
biographer, and Conan Doyle's short story "The Doctors of Hoyland," in his
collection *Round the Red Lamp* (1894). As in the United States, the sudden pop-

ularity of women physicians as fictive heroines was a concomitant of the battles raging in Great Britain most acutely from the late 1860s through the 1870s.[53] There are many parallels between the doctress fictions on the two sides of the Atlantic as the same themes are explored: surprise at the very idea of a woman's practicing medicine and even more at her competence, composure, and erudition; doubts about the propriety of such a course; the contrast with the conventional expectations of female conduct; self-justification and empowerment through usefulness in the form of service to fellow women; the schism between the scientific and the redemptive style of practice; and the ultimate quandary of marriage.

Like the American fictions, the British show doctresses at various stages in their careers, from differing gendered perspectives, and adopting a range of positions. Although there are no exact, one-to-one analogies between the British and the American figures, the similarities in the overall picture are quite apparent. Two out of the five British physicians opt for marriage, the same number as in the American narratives. Two, again as in the transatlantic cluster, are resolutely scientific, while the other three seek a compromise. Rhonda Gale in *A Woman-Hater,* who resembles Mary Prance in *The Bostonians* in her primary commitment to the scientific as well as in a certain mannishness, eventually wins approval for her tendance of young women. In "The Doctors of Hoyland" Dr. Verrinder Smith refuses a proposal of marriage and partnership from the town's doctor; like Dr. Zay with Waldo, she has attended expertly to the compound leg fracture he sustained in an accident and has earned his respect and affection. However, having just been accepted to do research at the Physiological Laboratory in Paris, she gives her suitor this blunt response: "There are many women with a capacity for marriage, but few with a taste for biology. I will remain true to my own line."[54] The sting of the woman's empowerment is to some extent defused by the tale's pervasive irony. Dr. Victoria also eschews marriage for reasons that are not clear from the overelaborate plot of the three-decker novel. Like Helen Brent, she is intrepid in performing audacious eye surgery on a young cousin, to whom she then extends maternal care, thereby ensuring the good outcome of the intervention. Edith Romney and Mona Maclean manage to bring all the disparate elements together: science and sympathy, practice and marriage. Both go through a phase of having to contend with severe difficulties, a sort of trial of strength from which they emerge triumphant. In the British novels the tendency to idealization and, with it, to romance predominates;[55] there is no equivalent to the ineffectual Grace Breen. Overcoming obstacles and setbacks, these determined doctresses win their way through to productive lives validated by their succor of women and children.

The doctress fictions have a dual significance. They are clearly the literary precipitate of a social phenomenon that excited and disturbed people as a particularized manifestation of the vexing "woman question." They are therefore to some extent indeed "personified arguments for or against a question."[56] But they are more than what this rather hostile critic implies, and on two grounds. First, several of them are very successful as popular novels that can still be read with considerable pleasure. The polemical aspects are well integrated, so that they do not overshadow interest in the plot and characters. They are by no means mere tracts for the exposition of certain ideas. Yet they also transcend the immediate controversy about women doctors by exposing the quandary that faced all doctors in the wake of the fundamental advances made in the course of the latter half of the nineteenth century. The problem was how to accommodate to the innovations: could physicians simply continue their traditional function as missionaries to the bedside, invoking such aids as the stethoscope, the microscope, anesthesia, x-rays, and so forth, as necessary? or did these developments entail a whole new style of medicine, and with it an altered balance of power? The tension between the redemptive and the scientific set up by Nathanael West encapsulates the crisis. The women doctors had to wrestle with this predicament in an acute form because their very suitability to medical practice was so strenuously queried as to intensify both their self-consciousness and their self-scrutiny. They had to try to blend the redemptive, maternally nurturing role into which they were socialized with the cool detachment of the scientific stance. Because of gender expectations, their task was more challenging than that faced by their male counterparts though basically no different. The doctress fictions afford insight into a profession in the process of transition from an older to a more modern format that not only accepted women but also recognized the need to relate to patients in a simultaneously redemptive and scientific manner.

5.

DISEASES AND DISEASED PEOPLE: THE NINETEENTH-CENTURY HOSPITAL

You should paint diseases rather than diseased people.
—ETIENNE JEAN GEORGET

No, NO, NOT TO THE HOSPITAL!"[1] Gervaise shouts in Zola's *L'Assommoir* (1877; trans. 1970) when her husband, a roofer, takes a bad fall and breaks his leg. Even though she is warned that it will be very expensive to look after him at home, she insists that he be transported to their apartment close by. The place is the working-class district of Paris, and the time shortly after the middle of the nineteenth century.

What are Gervaise's reasons for this horror of the hospital? It is significant that neither she nor the narrator sees the need to offer any kind of explanation, presumably on the assumption that readers of the period would immediately understand. The hospital was in fact widely perceived as "more threat than haven."[2] Because of the many trials of innovative drugs and treatments popular fear of experimentation was strong and not unjustified. In addition, the unhygienic conditions and the poor grasp of the mechanisms of contagion made hospitals a "seedbed of infection,"[3] where as many lives were claimed by cross-infections as by the diseases that had led to the hospitalization. To Gervaise the hospital is a place not to be restored to health but to die. The chilling description of the hospital as a "seminaria mortis" (seminary of death), coined by the eighteenth-century German scientist Gottfried Wilhelm Leibnitz,[4] still largely held true through much of the following century. The very terminology testifies to the menace: the typhus to which many medical patients succumbed was known as "hospital fever," and surgical patients fell victim to "hospital gangrene." Although the mortality rate in the Paris hospitals had been declining in the first half of the century from 1 out of 5.35 between 1805 and 1814 to 1 out of 11.03 in 1850,[5] it was still shockingly high.

So Gervaise has ample grounds for shunning the hospital and the diseases that it generated as a greater danger to her husband than his broken leg. Her fears are a component of popular culture, probably derived from gossip and cautionary tales to form an instinctive revulsion. Since Gervaise is neither educated nor articulate, she does not voice her anxieties except in that anguished outcry, "No, no, not to the hospital!" Yet well before her husband's accident her perception of the hospital is indirectly conveyed in a quite brilliant literary strategy. In the opening chapter of *L'Assommoir,* as she sits at the window waiting for her lover's return, "she looked to the right towards the Boulevard de Rochehcouart, where butchers in blood-stained aprons were standing about in groups in front of the slaughterhouses, and now and then the fresh breeze wafted an acrid stench of slaughtered animals. To the left her eyes ran along a stretch of the avenue and stopped almost opposite at the white mass of the Lariboisière hospital, then being built" (24). The Lariboisière Hospital, built in 1854 to supplement the Hôtel-Dieu, which had been partly destroyed in the great Paris fire of 1772, was regarded as a model of modern design; Florence Nightingale constantly referred to it in her *Notes on Hospitals* (1859). But to Gervaise it simply denotes the site of human death, corresponding to the slaughterhouse for animals. The point is forcefully reiterated in the closing words of the novel's first chapter as Gervaise is filled with dread at the prospect of living out her life "between a slaughterhouse and a hospital" (49).

Gervaise's attitude represents the norm for that period and points to the fundamental paradox besetting the nineteenth-century hospital. Though shunned by patients, it became "the backdrop of all medical thinking; all is applied in the hospital; all can be confirmed only there."[6] At the hospital the three key elements of the newly evolving scientific medicine—physical examination, autopsy, and statistics—could be fully deployed and developed. The hospital then began to occupy the position it now holds as the epicenter of advanced research and progressive practice. But however essential it was to physicians at the cutting edge, it did not bring positive benefits to a substantial number of patients until the late nineteenth century: "Only in the last hundred years have hospitals come to play an important role in the treatment of the sick," wrote Brian Abel-Smith in 1964.[7] To "promote higher standards of medical care, to undertake specialized treatments and operations" was only one and by no means the cardinal purpose of hospitals, which served equally "to maintain the suffering poor, to advance medical knowledge, to save doctors' time, to test whether patients were malingering, . . . to protect society, and to serve as doctors' workshops."[8] Likewise, "most Americans who sought the care of a doctor did not consider hospitalization," for "good treatment was home treatment"[9]—which confirms Gervaise's resolve to nurse her husband at home despite the depletion of her savings. Particularly in the early part of the century, when drugs and surgery could do little, patients were admitted for shelter, rest, warmth, and nourishment rather than for a specific course of treatment. Given the risk of cross-infection, the miserable conditions, and the restrictive rules, all who were able to do so avoided the hospital literally like, or as if it were, the plague.

The public prejudice against hospitalization was endorsed by the average physician too. As late as 1881 Cathell issued this advice:

> Be chary of ever sending people from their homes to hospitals, unless you are perfectly sure the management is humane and skillful. While hospitals are an unspeakable blessing to sick wanderers and to the homeless, they are less so to those who have friends and a place to call home. . . . To carry a weary or worn sick person from his home to a hospital, deprive him of his friends, neighbors, and companions, and all the little, endearing sympathies and solaces of domestic life, restrict his freedom by half-way imprisonment, and subject him to the risk of rugged indifference on the part of coarse nurses, and to austere, humdrum hospital rules—to bed, to meals, to everything at the sound of the bell; expose him possibly to public gaze, merely as an object of medical treatment, or for experiment with new remedies, or for the clinical advantage of medical students, clothe him hospital-fashion, and put him on diet prepared at regulation hours by stranger hands that know not his peculiarities or tastes, his likes and dislikes—if he be a person of domestic tastes and sensitive disposition, with a natural attachment to his home and its surroundings, such a change from home

treatment would be most hurtful and injudicious, and could scarcely fail to aggravate his disease.[10]

Cathell here sums up all the objections underlying Gervaise's protest. The hospital is to him a haven "to sick wanderers and the homeless," but those who have friends and a home should be cared for there so as to avoid the discomforts, indignities, and hazards of hospitalization. Cathell's advice, which does not even mention the risk of cross-infection, is directed at the financially able. Even though Gervaise is below that level of security, she insists on following middle- and upper-class custom in having her husband transported home.

The nineteenth-century repugnance toward hospitals can be better understood in light of their history. Institutions dedicated exclusively to the care of the sick grew out of the alms- and workhouses that were the last resort of the poor and the homeless. Among the unfortunates crowded into these dumping grounds were those unable to fend for themselves owing to sickness or injury and without either resources or family to tend them. So the almshouse, known too as the poorhouse, was the destination of the diseased before the establishment of infirmaries. In 1800 there were only two hospitals in the United States: the Pennsylvania Hospital in Philadelphia, founded in 1732, and the New York Hospital, inaugurated in 1771 and in operation since 1790. The oldest hospital in Europe, the Hôtel-Dieu in Paris, reputedly dates back to 660. The best-served city was London, with seven hospitals: St. Bartholomew's (established in 1123), St. Thomas's (1207), the Westminster (1719), Guy's (1721), St. George's (1733), the London (1740), and the Middlesex (1745). All these foundations had the same purpose, summarized in very similar phrases by medical historians: "a 'receptacle' for the dependent and indigent";[11] "to maintain the suffering poor";[12] to give shelter to "the poor and those without roots in the community";[13] to provide "a refuge for the penniless sick."[14] In every instance the motive is a social rather than a medical one, an act of mercy to meet the most basic needs of the impoverished sick. Living—or, frequently, dying—conditions, described by Guy Williams in *The Age of Agony* (89–103) for the eighteenth century, were disgusting and appalling in the extreme and had not changed substantially by the early nineteenth century.[15] At best, "this refuge was neither very restful nor very clean,

but at least, within its crowded, malodorous and noisy wards, the impoverished could get food, a bed, and physic."[16] Yet often they had to share a bed.

These institutions, whatever their internal organization, were supported
by charitable donations. This was another major reason why they were so
vehemently spurned by anyone with the slightest pretension to the respectable social status to which Gervaise still aspires at the point in *L'Assommoir* when her husband falls. For apart from the physical risks and discomforts
involved in going into hospital, there was also a psychological factor that
played a decisive role. To accede to hospitalization amounted de facto to a
confession of failure, to an incapacity financially and socially to muster care
for oneself. It meant not merely a surrender of freedom but an avowal of
neediness that brought shame and opprobrium. Gervaise's stand is undoubtedly animated almost as much by pride as by concern for her husband's
welfare. The force of her feelings can be gauged from the fact that this is
the only occasion when she really asserts herself, for she is an essentially yielding personality. That it was social not medical necessity that called for hospitalization through most of the nineteenth century is primary among the
whole concatenation of considerations that shaped the intense resistance.
Even fairly late in the century, home care remained the norm and the desideratum. Victims of street accidents in Boston, for instance, were transported
to their homes, and to the hospital only if there was no other suitable accommodation. Surgery too was performed at home, the makeshift setup on
the kitchen table being preferable and almost certainly more salubrious than
the hospital. The moral aspect of hospitalization surfaced also in the social
manipulation in which hospital authorities felt not just at liberty but under
a veritable obligation to engage. Rules to curb all forms of licentiousness,
notably drinking and gambling, were stringently enforced in the belief that
the institution had the right, indeed the duty, to control and reform patients'
lives. The self-righteously judgmental dichotomy of "worthy" and "unworthy"
poor, pervasive in the nineteenth century, underpinned the hospital's sense
of mission to correct the morals of its inmates. Perhaps the very scantiness
of the physical improvement the hospital could hope to effect contributed to
the emphasis on spiritual melioration.

The recurrence of such words as *poor, pauper, penniless, dependent,* and *indigent* is a clear pointer to the class system that governed hospital use. All recent

studies of the socioeconomic status of hospital patients document the overwhelming preponderance of the lower working class throughout the century. The one extant volume of case records for the London Fever Hospital
for 1824–25 lists 130 consecutive female admissions: "Not surprisingly, most
of the women in employment were servants, though several nurses also became patients. Eight of the women were transferred from workhouses."[17] Of
the 10,414 inmates classified in the census of London hospitals in 1861 all but
157 were wage earners, employed in industry, domestic service, or agriculture.[18] Warner's detailed profiles of the Massachusetts General Hospital between 1823 and 1885 and of the Commercial Hospital of Cincinnati between
1838 and 1851 produce the same findings.[19] This study is particularly telling because of the exceptionally complete case records on which it is based. In both
hospitals the patients' occupational standing was considerably lower than that
of the corresponding general population. At the Massachusetts General Hospital the male patients were most commonly blue-collar laborers or sailors.
Similarly, at the Commercial Hospital of Cincinnati between one-half and
two-thirds of the sample from the 1830s through the 1860s were unskilled
laborers and boatmen. While the average length of stay amounted to several
weeks and not infrequently to some months, the relatively large number of
patients discharged during the first week reflects the high incidence of patients
admitted solely for drunkenness or exhaustion.

    This heavy overrepresentation of the lower classes corroborates the tradi-
tional association of hospitals with almshouses. Even in the 1870s, "hospitals
were perceived as the kind of place that all but the desperate would want to
avoid."[20] Class is thus a further factor in Gervaise's adamant opposition to
her husband's hospitalization; a skilled laundress, she cherishes the ambition
to open her own business at the time of her husband's accident. Her sense of
self-respect rebels against the very idea of accepting charity and being grouped
with the type of people who entered these institutions. According to Charles
Rosenberg, "lingering unwillingness of the prosperous and respectable to be
treated in a hospital" persisted into the closing decade of the century.[21] Indeed,
it was actually considered reprehensible for those who were not needy to use
hospitals. In 1853 the British Medical Journal ran a series of articles excoriating
"gentlemen's servants, clerks and well-to-do tradespeople with their wives
and children [who] absolutely encumber the waiting-rooms of the London
hospitals."[22]

    The waiting rooms here referred to are those of outpatient departments, but even they were considered the reserve—in a sense, the prerogative—of the needy. This is vividly illustrated in the scene witnessed by the medical student Philip in Somerset Maugham's *Of Human Bondage* (1915) when he is on duty in the outpatient clinic:

> They came in one by one and walked up to the table at which sat Dr. Tyrell. They were old men and young men and middle-aged men, mostly of the labouring class, dock labourers, draymen, factory hands, barmen; but some, neatly dressed, were of a station which was obviously superior, shop-assistants, clerks, and the like. Dr. Tyrell looked at these with suspicion. Sometimes they put on shabby clothes in order to pretend they were poor; but he had a keen eye to prevent what he regarded as fraud and sometimes refused to see people who, he thought, could well pay for medical attendance. Women were the worst offenders and they managed the thing more clumsily. They would wear a cloak and skirt which were almost in rags, and neglect to take the rings off their fingers.
>
> "If you can afford to wear jewellery you can afford a doctor. A hospital is a charitable institution," said Dr. Tyrell. (397)

The time of this episode is approximately the late 1880s. Although similar complaints of "abuse" were still being voiced around 1900, a system of graduated payments had already been introduced. It was initiated at the specialized hospitals that developed out of the outpatient departments devoted to particular fields, which began in London with, for instance, an ophthalmic clinic at St. Thomas's in 1871. By the 1880s departments of dermatology, otolaryngology, gynecology, dentistry, and electrotherapy had multiplied and were being consolidated at a rapidly accelerated rate into specialist hospitals.[23] In pursuit of expert treatment some better-off patients who would not have gone to a general hospital but who could not afford the customary guinea (one pound and one shilling) for a private consultation with a specialist were attracted to these new institutions, where they were charged according to their means. Despite their contributions to their care, these patients had none of the control over their doctors exercised by affluent paying patients in the mid–nineteenth century, such as Lady Arabella and Sir Roger in *Doctor Thorne*, who could and did switch medical attendants at will. The middle-class patients at the new specialist hospitals, though they needed the subsidization

of their fees, sought the expertise available only there. So the growing specialization of medical care directly enhanced doctors' power by limiting patients' choices. Some of the small British provincial "cottage" hospitals also
began collecting graduated amounts from patients in the latter part of the
century. The difference between the patient's payment and the total cost was
often defrayed by subscribers.

In return for their donations, regular subscribers had the privilege of a
certain number of "letters" per year giving them the right to nominate beneficiaries. The allocation was generally in proportion to the level of the subscription, with some earmarked for admission to the hospital and others
restricted to outpatient treatment. Prospective patients had to make the
rounds of listed subscribers in order to plead for a "ticket." Those with an influential patron stood a better chance of being admitted than those who
lacked influence, as the poor did. This method became less rigid only toward
the very end of the century.

The tribulations and humiliations that the letter system entailed for patients
are fully exposed in George Moore's *Esther Waters* (1894) as the servant girl
searches for a bed to deliver her illegitimate baby. Since she is not yet in labor,
she cannot be admitted as an emergency patient and is told to procure a letter. She is charged a shilling for access to the book with subscribers' names
and addresses, but unable to read, she does her best to memorize a few as
they are recited to her. Then begins her round in search of the elusive document. An elderly lady rejects her, saying "she did not wish to judge any one,
but it was her invariable practice to give letters only to married women" (110).
At houses where the mistress or master is out she is snubbed by footmen,
who either discourage her from waiting or insist that she divulge her business.
When she finally finds a kindly donor disposed to help her, he has already dis-
tributed all his tickets for the year and can only offer to send her to a friend,
a large subscriber. Emotionally and physically exhausted from her quest, Esther gives up. Equally devastating is the experience of the textile mill workers
in Elizabeth Gaskell's *Mary Barton* (1848), who petition their employer for a
letter on behalf of one of their fellow workers who has been struck with
fever. In one of the novel's most searing and poignant scenes the gaunt, pale
weavers are ushered into the mill owner's home just as he is polishing off a
sumptuous breakfast midmorning. He responds to their urgent begging non-
chalantly: "I doubt if I've an inpatient order to spare at present; but I'll give

you an outpatient's, and welcome" (64). The prospective patient dies in his damp, dark hovel—as he would likely have done in the hospital anyway.

As the locus of death, the hospital fulfilled an important function in the development of medicine by supplying the corpses necessary for the exploration of anatomical pathology. According to Foucault, "The corpse became the brightest moment in the figures of truth."[24] Paris, which had had a Dissection School since 1797, took the lead, and as humoral pathology was replaced by anatomical pathology postmortems became routine on those who died in hospitals in order first to identify the lesions that had caused death and ultimately to learn from them how to diagnose the signs of disease in the living. After the British Anatomy Act of 1832 physicians at the London Fever Hospital performed autopsies on two-thirds of their fatal cases,[25] while during the 1850s some 250 postmortem examinations were carried out annually at Guy's.[26] As a result, "intellectually ambitious young physicians began to seek out the autopsy room and not the library as the principal theater in which to earn their intellectual laurels."[27] The prevalence of autopsy performed on those who died in hospitals added an extra dimension to the fear and revulsion already felt: anxiety that one's body would be appropriated for dissection. Those whose remains were not claimed by relatives for burial were indeed quarry for research. Stories of desecration after death greatly intensified popular suspicion of the hospital.

Fear of body snatching is one of the central themes of the four chapters in Eugène Sue's Les Mystères de Paris (1844; The Mysteries of Paris, n.d.) that are set in a hospital.[28] This four-volume potboiler, with its involuted, melodramatic plot, enjoyed immense popularity during its serialization in the Journal des Débats between June 1842 and October 1843. In its heyday it was "one of the most important events in French life."[29] It was adapted for the theater in 1844 and again in 1889. As the scion of a distinguished dynasty that comprised more than four generations, between 1699 and 1865, including fourteen surgeons, five professors, five members of the Academy, and five holders of the Legion of Honor, Sue was able to draw on intimate knowledge of the medical scene. Although he himself resisted the pressure to become a doctor, he was for a while apprenticed to his father at the Hôpital de la maison militaire du roi (The King's Military Hospital) and subsequently spent a year each at hospitals in Spain and Toulon. In a lengthy footnote (missing in the English version) prefatory to volume 4, chapter 12, "The Hospital," Sue makes a kind of apologia for what follows. The illustrious work of his father, grandfather, great-uncle, and great-grandfather, whose name he has the honor to bear, prohibits him, he maintains, from making the slightest attack or heedless allusion to doctors. This disclaimer serves merely to heighten the gravity of Sue's indictment of the fictional Dr. Griffon as he parades through his ward with his obsequious entourage of assistants and students.

The impact of this scene is intensified by the suspense created through the delay of Dr. Griffon's appearance, which occurs only some two-thirds of the way into the episode. It is anticipated in a series of three frames, each opening out of the preceding one. The first, a continuation of the prefatory remarks, consists of authorial footnotes directed against the evils of hospitals, here again deemed "the last refuge of the poor" (4:132n). This phrase is part of a lengthy quotation from an article of 19 January 1836 in the journal *Constitutionnel* that accuses hospitals of aggravating their patients' ills and asserts that "cures are now carried out in the way that punishments used to be" (4:133n). The quotation, intended to support Sue's position adds in effect, as a footnote to a footnote, another frame to the initial one. The great majority of this authorial material is concentrated in the opening few pages; only an occasional observation is inserted later.

The second, more straightforward frame establishes the contract between the author-narrator and the reader, who is twice invited to enter the hospital and watch the happenings under the narrator's guidance. This is the gateway to the main narrative, which begins with a description of the setting: "Nothing is more melancholy than the somber sight of the vast hospital ward into which we will now introduce the reader" (4:132). All the adjectives as well as the details of the smells and sounds dwell on the noxiousness of this environment. A vignette of action forms the climax and the conclusion of the reader's initiation into the world of the hospital: the arrival of a priest who performs a ceremony at a bedside while a nun prays alongside. "Then silence reigned again. One of the sick had just died" (4:134). These lapidary sentences, which present death as an everyday occurrence, are characteristic of the laconic starkness that puts the reader into direct confrontation with the sights, sounds, and happenings in this hospital. This effective sparseness is made possible by the relegation of authorial commentary to the footnotes. The rationale for the multiple frames becomes apparent in the dramatic economy of the exposition of the fictional happenings.

The focus then shifts onto three women patients in the ward. As their beds are close together (though one is dying of tuberculosis), they begin to whisper to each other, and soon they are exchanging tales of the misadventures that have reduced them to hospitalization. All three have been plunged into their present "ruined" destitution by their betrayal and abandonment by men on whom they had relied. Interspersed in their recountings of the past are expressions of concern about the future, especially their terror at the prospect of being "dissected, . . . cut up into pieces" (4:138). This is a repeated motif of their conversation as they recall other patients who had been tormented by the same apprehension and scheme how to save one another from this horrifying fate by arranging to have the body claimed. Even the poorest of them has laid aside a small sum for burial. It is striking how their distress circles around not their present gruesome conditions nor their imminent death but precisely the issue of dissection. They express no religious scruples, simply an instinctive revulsion against the prospect of the violation of their remains.

Finally, the instigator of the evil enters to make his rounds. Dr. Griffon is described in two kinds of terminology: that of warfare and that of science. In contrast to the dejected patients, he is "as ingenuously satisfied and triumphant as a general after a victory very *costly* in soldiers' lives" (4:129). He is thus immediately cast as an insensitive, egocentric killer. To him the hospital is "the theater of my glory" (4:145) where he commands a considerable "body of staff" (4:146). This military language is overlaid with references to his scientific prowess; four times he is called "this prince of science" and his followers are his "scientific cortege" (4:146). "Cortege" is ambivalent in its dual resonance, evoking in its celebratory sense the retinue of a distinguished person and carrying in its darker association echoes of a funeral procession. His ruthless indifference in the name of devotion to science is revealed in his proud declaration that "here we begin on the living experiments and studies that we complete in the amphitheater on the cadaver" (4:147). The corpse in the dissecting room is here made the fulcrum of the hospital, whose raison d'être is the advancement of knowledge, not healing.

This scenario is borne out by Dr. Griffon's tour of the ward. The patients are no more than numbers to him, objects of research. Told that "number 1" had died at 4:00 A.M., he expresses surprise that it had not happened earlier, as he had predicted, and then he graciously bestows this superb specimen on one of his assistants, who immediately inscribes his initials onto the body to signal his possession of it. As Dr. Griffon moves from bed to bed in the ward he scrutinizes each patient with a penetrating gaze, sometimes asking brief questions about symptoms he is expecting. He never, however, inquires of a patient how she feels; there is no interaction between doctor and patient, only a brusque interrogation to satisfy the physician's curiosity. He does not perceive the sick as human beings, only as embodiments of various pathologies. He laughs at the women's reluctance to strip naked before a throng of spectators and reminds them that cooperation is the condition for their admission to the hospital. He hardly glances at several cases who offer "nothing interesting or compelling" (4:149) but delights in those who present something unusual, notably "a new subject" (4:154) who has a rare disease he has been longing to observe. Dr. Griffon is, it is twice noted, "most jolly" (4:151, 154) as he surveys the creatures who are the fodder for his scientific experiments. His name is well chosen: a griffon (griffin) is in ornithology a bird of prey, a type of vulture, and in mythology an animal with the body of a lion and an eagle's head and wings. This doctor devours, and what is more, he does so with undisguised pleasure for the sake of science.

Dr. Griffon's ward round is portrayed in dramatic style, almost totally in dialogue between him and the members of his entourage. This lively immediacy contrasts with the earlier parts of the episode, which are mediated by the narratorial voice and punctuated by authorial footnotes. The voices missing during the doctor's visit are those of the patients. They are explicitly forbidden to speak in his presence except in direct response to his queries. Their silencing underscores the extent to which they are reduced to insensate objects, sacrifices on the altar of science, "ample material for observation" (4:145), as Dr. Griffon boasts. This is an enactment of the "medicine of observation" fostered by the Paris hospitals, based on a veritable philosophy of observation.[30] The shortcoming, namely, that there was too much reading and too little observation, was corrected by mid-century as the site of instruction was transferred from university lecture halls to the bedside of institutionalized patients. But observation and experimentation exacted their toll too, as Dr. Griffon's conduct reveals. He regards his ward as a testing ground for trying out on the poor medications that he may later prescribe for his rich private patients.

This episode in Les Mystères de Paris must prompt the question of exaggeration. How credible is Dr. Griffon in his overwhelming zeal for research that obliterates all humanity? His symbolic name in itself already arouses some suspicion. Yet Sue insists on the literal veracity of his portrayal, categorically stating in a footnote that "this is in no way exaggerated" (4:131n) and arguing that the figure of Dr. Griffon can be granted "without too much hyperbole" (4:130). How much hyperbole is involved here? Is he a monster, a madman "of unprecedented savagery" (4:157), or an example of those "respectable" (4:127) doctors whose heads have been turned by the potential of science? The ambiguity should perhaps be read as an expression of Sue's own ambivalence toward the medical profession, a mixture of the admiration he records in his prefatory remarks and censure of current grave abuses in hospitals. But even after a certain dramatic intensification is discounted, the situation depicted in these hospital chapters of *Les Mystères de Paris* is a fundamentally accurate rendering of the then prevailing etiquette of power in charity hospitals. The doctor could exercise an unchecked tyranny over the destitute sick who had accepted his suzerainty in return for shelter and what passed for care. Once they entered into the bondage of the institution, the poor abdicated rights over their own bodies in life and in death. The contract amounted in effect to a total surrender on the patients' part and an unlimited empowerment of the physician. These are the conditions that motivate Gervaise's adamant stand against her husband's hospitalization.

That Sue's image of Dr. Griffon's treatment of his patients is more than an unfounded parody is borne out by the testimony of extraneous witnesses. Many American physicians in Paris for further study "reported disapprovingly of having observed in their French mentors the sort of indifference and brutality toward patients that Sue portrayed in Dr. Griffon."[31] The tendency to abstraction led some Parisian clinicians to envisage the sick as specimens of pathology divorced from human context.[32] In the huge Allgemeines Krankenhaus (General Hospital) in Vienna too Dr. Patrick A. O'Connell, of Boston, noted that patients were used "as if the principal purpose of their being in the hospital was to illustrate the lectures."[33] Nor are complaints from patients lacking: "The doctors visit you incessantly, and . . . you feel as if you were not exactly an ailing human being but merely a 'case' that was being read as one reads a novel which is interesting enough, no doubt, but which is expected to develop a much more interesting phase, to wit, the catastrophe, at almost any moment."[34]

These criticisms reflect a heightening clash of opinion about the definition of the hospital: was its primary purpose to care for the sick or to be a great scientific research laboratory? Medical historians are in agreement on the fundamental change in the practice of medicine wrought by the developments in the nineteenth century: "The rise of 'hospital medicine' involved a dramatic transformation in both the *location* of medicine and its *content*."[35] Removed from "the family, the natural locus of disease," the patient becomes an example to be classified as "beneath the eye of the doctor, diseases would be grouped into orders, genera, species, in a rationalized domain."[36] Parisian hospitals "shaped an academic style of clinical activity oriented not toward the care of particular patients, but toward the accumulation of knowledge based on the treatment (and possibly autopsy) of numerous patients with similar ills."[37]

The spread of the statistical method was an important impetus to the progressive reification of the patient. So was the introduction of such instruments as the microscope and, toward the end of the century, x-rays, which resulted in the physical separation of the doctor from the patient in the diagnosis of disease. This alteration in the doctor-patient relationship was acknowledged by some physicians, and not without a certain note of regret: "our eyes and our minds are rather apt . . . to dwell too much on our detailed notes and manifold instrumental aids, and too little on the patient, his personal peculiarities, and the ultimate nature of his ailments."[38] The attention and respect commanded by the findings produced by the new technology, which led from the bedside to the laboratory, were among a variety of factors that coalesced to increase the emotional distance between doctor and patient. The localization of disease and the consequent specialization resulted in improved diagnosis and treatment but also led to a fragmentation of care, the opposite to the holistic understanding of patients in their social context that was the salient strength of the missionary to the bedside. In place of the continuity and comprehensiveness that Mr. Gibson, Dr. Thorne, and Mr. Lydgate bring to their patients, the hospital physician is bound by the very definition of the situation to handle an episodic crisis in a case torn out of its natural surroundings. The artificiality of the encapsulated hospital incident inevitably results in the treatment of diseases rather than of diseased people. And the focus on the disease naturally augmented the doctor's power and reduced that of the patient.

The hospital, as *Les Mystères de Paris* shows, fulfilled another important function through teaching. "Walking the wards" was initially a casual and voluntary part of medical education that enabled students to gain practical experience by actually seeing cases of various diseases. With the move away from theoretical medicine to practical physical examination, growing emphasis was placed on the necessity of firsthand knowledge. In the early prescriptions for the reform of medicine young doctors were urged to seek education not from books but at the bedside. By the 1870s what had been innovative advice had become the cardinal rule, namely, that from the day a young man decided to be a doctor he had to visit the hospital. So the hospital, which in the eighteenth century had been founded by laymen to provide for the poor, was promoted in the nineteenth century by physicians to serve medical students and their teachers. The hospital became a classroom in which the patients were the subjects (or objects) of study. Since the students paid for their instruction, teaching was a source of income as well as an investment for the future, when pupils could be expected to refer their own patients to their mentors for remunerative consultations.

The hospital's role in teaching and in research effected a change in its status in the last third of the century. As the center for medical education and advanced practice, it was transformed from a shelter for the destitute sick into the arena for students' training and doctors' experimentation. In the United States the proliferation of medical schools, whose number rose from 75 in 1850 to 160 in 1900, was accompanied by a proportionate increase in hospitals, from 178 in 1872 to more than 4,000 by 1910.[39] Expansion was parallel though less spectacular in London, where there was a 41.4 percent increase in teaching hospitals between 1855 and 1889.[40] A pattern of reciprocal accommodation resulted from physicians' need for access to hospitals and hospitals' need for patients. In London, for instance, St. Bartholomew's Hospital closed its fever wards in 1885 at the insistence of its governing board, yielding to the doctors' demand for more teaching space.[41] In the hospital's new teaching capacity, the outpatient department, or "dispensary," assumed a crucial role in screening, selecting, and procuring patients. By a process of triage from a large pool of prospective patients those with interesting diseases were admitted to hospital. This system could be mutually beneficial insofar as the sickest were given care and the doctors acquired the cases they wanted for teaching purposes. On the other hand, it was also open to abuses such as those depicted in Les Mystères de Paris if doctors were unscrupulously motivated by their own agendas more than by solicitude for their patients. The whole question of inclusions and exclusions grew more problematic as general hospitals refused incurables and chronic cases in favor of the acutely sick.

The centrality of teaching in the major hospitals also altered the balance of power as it became triangulated through the presence of students. At its worst this could result in exploitation, as in *Les Mystères de Paris* when the patient is treated as a nameless number who is in the hospital to further the doctors' research and the pupils' education. The hospital population, consisting as it did of the poor and sick, was utterly stripped of any power, with the patient assigned "a passive and uncritical role in the consultative relationship, his main function being to endure and wait. . . . The special qualities of the individual case were swallowed up in vast statistical surveys."[42] The repression of the individual's personality was implemented by the regimentation imposed by the rigid, impersonal hospital routines that superseded moralistic paternalism as the hospital itself came under the domination of science. Mind and body, integrated in early-nineteenth-century bedside medicine in the home, were sharply separated in hospital medicine as part of the growing trend toward specialization. The body was treated as a self-contained, almost mechanical entity, while mental and emotional disorders became the purview of "alienists."

Another form of dichotomization permeated the power structure as the outcome of the prevalent hierarchical social order, which created a great distance between penurious hospital patients and their middle-class physicians. Two different styles of medicine came into being side by side, or rather on opposite sides of the great financial and social divide between the haves and the have-nots. Cathell, who writes for the private family practitioner, makes no bones about the differences between the treatment to be meted out to the desired "wealthy and pampered," however trying they might be as patients, and "hospital and dispensary patients, soldiers, sailors, and the poor," who he claims are "much easier to attend than the higher classes."[43]

> With hospital patients, sailors, soldiers, paupers, etc., there are but two classes—the really sick, suffering from affections of a well-marked type, and malingerers. Hence, exclusive hospital education and practice are apt to lead to a rough-and-ready habit of treating every patient as if very sick, or else as having little or nothing the

matter with him. These crude or possibly overactive methods may answer in public institutions, but they will not suit squeamish people with nerves tuned to a high key, so often seen in private practice, with indefinite or frivolous ailments for which the physician trained only in a hospital could hardly fail to feel and manifest contempt. Hospital practice is so different from private that but few members of our profession shine conspicuously as practitioners in both spheres. . . . The two fields are essentially different, and lead the mind in different directions. (51–52)

This gives a telling insight into the late-nineteenth-century double-tiered medical system, with paying patients looked after at home and entitled to consideration despite their maybe "frivolous ailments" and silly whims and the poor remaindered, as it were, in hospitals, where roughness toward recipients of charity was regarded as permissible, even justifiable.

The brusqueness that was the normal tone in hospitals is evident in *Esther Waters* when Esther is admitted as an emergency case already in labor. The mere fact that she has to go into the hospital for her confinement is indicative of her lowly standing: "Any woman who was willing to give birth in a public hospital . . . was either desperately poor or a prostitute."[44] The reluctance to use hospitals for lying-in was mutual to patients and trustees, and for the same reason: fear of childbed fever. A large proportion of those who resorted to hospital were, like Esther, unmarried and without a home. There is no suggestion in *Esther Waters* of the blatant cruelty in *Les Mystères de Paris,* merely gross insensitivity and tactlessness on the part of most of the midwives and students who attend her. The gentleness of one midwife and one young student redresses the balance, averting the unmitigated negativity characteristic of Sue. Another major difference between the two hospital scenes lies in the focalization. In *Les Mystères de Paris* it is the narrator-author who filters and relates what happens. In *Esther Waters,* by contrast, the perspective is that of the patient giving birth; consequently the images are a fragmentary collage of her impressions as she drifts into a light sleep or is wrenched by pain. By this means, at the very least the patient's humanity is recognized.

Nevertheless, the experience is full of horror for Esther. She is as frightened on arrival by the steel instruments and basins she sees laid out on a round table as by the screams she hears. She is disturbed, too, by the students' loud laughter, their frivolous chatter about plays and novels, their sudden stampede to the window to see a passing band, and the crunching of the candy they are eating. These homely details, registered through Esther's eyes and ears, effectively make Moore's point without any of the voiced authorial comment so prominent in *Les Mystères de Paris*. The situation is explained to Esther as she tries to run away because the young men strike her as "all beasts!" "'Come, come, no nonsense!' said the nurse, 'you can't have what you like; they are here to learn'" (115). Eventually, after she has overheard a nurse talk about an unsuccessful operation that ended with the patient's death and snatches of argument about her progress, which is not as smooth as had been anticipated, a doctor arrives who ushers in "silence and scientific collectedness" (117). Esther has little awareness of him for he administers chloroform, which makes her lose sight of the circle of faces. But she does register that he speaks "in a low whisper" (117), a welcome relief from the students' rowdiness. When she comes round, "the doctors and nurses were still standing round her, but there was no longer any expression of eager interest on their faces" (117). She is not an interesting case. Once again the patient is depicted as wholly at the mercy of medical attendants, who may give good care, as the doctor does, but who are mostly inconsiderate and egocentric. The division of power is quite simple: all to the physician, none whatsoever to the patient.

A complement to *Esther Waters* is Somerset Maugham's *Of Human Bondage*, which takes place in a London hospital at approximately the same time. But here the angle of vision is that of the medical student Philip, who after trying several other career paths has finally decided to follow in his father's footsteps as a doctor. The second half of the novel traces his progress through the stages of his education and into his first position as a locum in a town on the south coast. At "St. Luke's" hospital he combines theoretical lectures with practice in bandaging, learning auscultation, use of the stethoscope, and dispensing in preparation for his rotation through the main departments: outpatient, medicine, surgery, and midwifery. A qualified physician himself, Maugham is able to give an accurate and persuasive picture of hospital work. The melodrama characteristic of *Les Mystères de Paris* is completely absent here, or rather it is displaced onto Philip's troubled relationship with the fickle Mildred. In fact, his training at the hospital is the firm anchor of his life as he finds his true identity and develops self-confidence through his mastery of his profession.

At the beginning, in the outpatient department, Philip works with Dr. Tyrell, "a successful man, with a large consulting practice, and a knight-hood in prospect" (395). Dr. Tyrell is so popular with students that they com-pete to be his "clerk." But toward patients his "healthy man's jovial condescension" and his "patronizing air" are inappropriate, though not ill-in-tentioned: "He made the patient feel like a boy confronted by a jolly school-master; his illness was an absurd piece of naughtiness which amused rather than irritated" (395). The comparison of the patient to a naughty schoolboy and of the doctor to a jolly schoolmaster vividly conveys the uneven balance of power. Dr. Tyrell is by no means sinister or evil like Dr. Griffon in Sue's novel; however, as a healthy man without imagination, he is lacking any shred of empathy for the sick. Patients are assigned to a clerk, who has to question and examine them and then present summary findings and a ten-tative diagnosis to Dr. Tyrell. As in *Les Mystères de Paris*, patients serve as in-structional material, displayed and inspected for the edification of the small crowd of students who follow the doctor on his rounds. Yet although patients clearly are being used, the ritual is carried out with a dispassionate neutral-ity that is not offensive:

> If there was anything interesting to hear students applied their stethoscope: you could see a man with two or three to the chest, and perhaps two to his back, while others waited impatiently to listen. The patient stood among them a little embarrassed, but not altogether displeased to find himself the centre of attention: he lis-tened confusedly while Dr. Tyrell discoursed glibly on the case. Two or three students listened again to recognize the murmur or the crepitation which the physician described, and then the man was told to put on his clothes. (398)

This scene effectively illustrates that "the change in medical knowledge" was "based essentially on the fact that the doctor came close to the patient, . . . began to perceive what was immediately behind the visible surface."[45] The possible findings are subsequently discussed at greater length by Dr. Tyrell with the students in order to formulate a method of treatment. Occasionally

there is a certain frivolity at patients' expense but no cruelty. In fact, one patient is described as "not altogether displeased to find himself the centre of
attention." However, he has power only to the extent of *his* usefulness to the
hospital for teaching purposes. This is an interesting inversion of the position
of the doctresses, whose justification lay in *their* usefulness to patients. The
system in *Of Human Bondage* is designed for the instruction of the clerks; any
benefit to patients is quite secondary and incidental. Teaching and learning
take precedence over healing. The patients' subjugation and the humiliation inflicted on them is obliquely suggested by the word "herded" (398) applied to the next batch, the old women, who are ushered in as if they were
animals.

But Maugham's novel also admits an exception in Philip, who replicates
the one young student in *Esther Waters* who shows some concern for her well-
being. "It seemed to Philip that he alone of the clerks saw the dramatic interest of those afternoons. To the others men and women were only cases,
good if they were complicated, tiresome if obvious; . . . But to Philip there
was much more. He found an interest in just looking at them, in the shape
of their heads and their hands, in the look of their eyes and the length of their
noses. You saw in that room human nature taken by surprise, and often the
mask of custom was torn off rudely, showing you the soul all raw" (399–400).
The cases, interesting, hopeless, or just humdrum, are here recuperated
through Philip's vision into human beings with souls. His imaginative insight
is perhaps carried over from his earlier calling as an artist; even though his ex-
pressive abilities proved inadequate, he has an artistic sensibility. In addition, he himself knows suffering from his physical disability of a clubfoot.
This too differentiates him from the vigorously healthy Dr. Tyrell and gives
him greater understanding of those destined to be patients.

It is no surprise that Philip develops a very good rapport with patients
when he works with them one-to-one, without the intrusive intermediacy of
a supervising physician. Although he takes due care "to preserve the distance
between the hospital patient and the staff" (422), he becomes "a favourite
with the patients" (481) for professional and personal reasons. Apart from his
"gentle, sensitive hands which did not hurt them" (481), he has the equally
valuable quality of a good humor that is not merely an assumed bedside manner but stems from his deep sense of both their vulnerability and their sto-
icism in bearing their lot. The exclusively scientific attitude toward patients

in *Les Mystères de Paris* is tempered in *Of Human Bondage* by a redemptive humanity. The difference in context surely also affects doctors' perceptions of their patients: as a pupil in a London hospital at the turn of the century, Philip is not under the same pressure to do research that dominated the Paris hospital in mid-century. Hospital patients are still tools but not pawns.

In one cardinal facet, however, the balance of power is alike in these two narratives. It is the physician who controls the interaction with patients by initiating the questions that accompany the physical examination. Often these questions are quite pointed, aimed at ascertaining the presence or absence of particular symptoms that could differentially confirm or rule out any of a variety of possible diagnoses the physician is considering. This mode of approaching patients is a concomitant of disease specificity, which recognizes clusters of signs typical of one syndrome or another. The doctor therefore has to take the lead after allowing patients an opening statement of the chief complaint. This style of directed interrogation differs from the free narration patients gave of their illness as they saw it at the time of humoral medicine. Mr. Gibson in *Wives and Daughters* and Trollope's Dr. Thorne proceed by listening open-endedly and drawing their conclusions from the patient's account and from observable signs such as pulse rate and skin color. The intercalation of disease specificity thus induces a signal shift in the balance of the doctor-patient encounter. The command over a growing corpus of arcane knowledge that is not accessible to lay people bolsters the physician's authority (and mystique). The emergence of specialties and subsequently of subspecialties further fosters this trend through the formation of a professional elite of experts in one area or another.[46] The distance between hospital patients and staff, rooted in social and pecuniary discrepancies, is reinforced by the cognitive incommensurability.

By the latter half of the nineteenth century the disparity between doctor and patient spread also to the affluent middle and upper classes. Whereas in the early part of the century communication between doctor and patient had been predicated on shared assumptions, this consensus was sharply disrupted as the doctor became less dependent on patients for information about their condition and turned more to objective measurements derived extraneously from the new technologies. The students in *Of Human Bondage* use their stethoscopes to hear murmurs and crepitations without speaking to the patient at all. The attenuation of the "two-way channel" between doctor and patient is ascribed by Jewson to "the emergence of Hospital Medicine [which] severed the link between the concepts of medical theory and the naive experiences of sufferers from disease."[47] This is perhaps an overstatement, for the change was gradual and at first only partial when medical theory was still rather limited. The severance was indeed most abrupt and most apparent in the hospital, where it was compounded by the social and educational hiatus between inmates and staff. But it extended beyond the infirmary as an erosion of the patient's idiosyncratic voice in the face of the authoritativeness of the doctor's idiom, buttressed by science and technology. What Jewson calls in broad strokes in his 1976 article "The Disappearance of the Sick Man from Medical Cosmology" has been redefined in communicative terms by Mary Fissell as "the disappearance of the patient's narrative and the invention of hospital medicine." Fissell argues that early in the eighteenth century "the patient's and the doctor's words are one" (99) as patients constitute a narrative from the physical manifestations of their illness that the doctor accepts because doctor and client are "on near-equal hermeneutic footing" (92). In the context of increasing medical autonomy "the patient's narrative of illness was made utterly redundant. Hospital medicine came to focus on signs and symptoms, which provided doctors with a disease-oriented diagnosis conducive to the demands of hospital practice and reflective of its social structure" (93).

The change of balance, whose beginnings Fissell already discerns in the eighteenth century, assumes far greater force in the nineteenth in the wake of the scientific and technological advances that gave the physician diagnostic and therapeutic means extrinsic to the patient's narrative. In 1880 Jacobi impressed on women medical students "that what the patient has to tell you constitutes precisely the least important part of what you must learn about him in order to be able to understand his case, and to do him any good" because only the physician can "understand the pathological significance of one symptom as compared to that of another."[48] These are the words of the advocate of the scientific approach, which clearly leads to the supremacy of the physician's observational and evaluative powers over the patient's naive, personal experience of illness. So the importance of the patient's narrative decreases, though it can never be wholly eliminated because it forms the point of departure for the physician's examination and questions. What is more, its worth is in direct proportion to the individual narrator's reliability, so that it pales beside the objective evidence of the stethoscope, the microscope, and the other "scopes" devised in the nineteenth century that allow physicians to form their own assessment based on direct confrontation with the disease rather than through the intermediacy of the diseased person. Although these instruments too demand skill, dexterity, and discernment on the operator's part,[49] thus entailing certain hazards of their own, they can nevertheless be expected to yield more accurate findings than the patient's subjective sensations.

The weakening of the patient's voice may in part account for the puzzling dearth of literary portrayals of hospital medicine in the nineteenth century compared with the profusion of works that show variants on the doctor as missionary to the bedside. It is surely no coincidence that the two novels that deal most fully with the hospital, *Les Mystères de Paris* and *Of Human Bondage,* were written by men who had themselves served on hospital staffs. The patients, overwhelmingly poor and possibly, like Esther Waters, illiterate, were unlikely to convert their experiences into fiction. Here too the element of class again comes strongly to the fore, for nineteenth-century novelists and their readers by and large belonged to the middle class, who would shun the hospital as a disgrace attendant on penury. It is significant that Gervaise in *L'Assommoir,* when she has descended to the most abject straits near the end of her life, passively lets her husband be admitted to the St. Anne hospital for delirium tremens after he has been picked up off the street during one of his frequent alcoholic sprees. Broken in health and spirit by hunger, liquor, and abuse, she has sunk to that level of the population that had no choice but to resort to hospitals. It is curious, however, that the hospital is missing from the two ambitious nineteenth-century French social panoramas, Balzac's *La Comédie humaine* and Zola's *Les Rougon-Macquart.* Balzac focuses on the middle classes, especially on their efforts to rise in the opportunistic world of capitalism. For them to patronize a hospital would be an unthinkable degradation. In *Le Père Goriot* as the old man lies on his deathbed in a garret, reduced to pauperism by his predatory daughters, he is tended as well as possible by his two young fellow boarders, a medical and a law student, who never consider consigning him to hospital. Even more striking is the virtual absence of the hospital from the *Rougon-Macquart* cycle, which deliberately set out to survey social institutions. The railroads, government administration, agriculture, department stores, the mines, the church, prostitution, the stock exchange, the army, art, and the Parisian markets are all featured, but medicine, in the final novel of the sequence, *Le Docteur Pascal,* is represented in the persona of a private practitioner-researcher without hospital affiliation.

This gap is all the more surprising in light of the transformation of the hospital in the course of the nineteenth century from the "receptacle of all miseries" to the "cradle of new medicine."[50] More crucial for this change than either the elaboration of investigative instruments or the understanding of disease specificity were two other developments. The most dramatic was the discovery of anesthesia: a public demonstration of the efficacy of ether in dental surgery was given by William T. G. Morton in Boston on 16 October 1846.[51] Dentists could reap immediate financial gain by offering painless treatment, which vastly increased their practice. A year later, on 10 November 1847, James Simpson presented his paper on chloroform to the Medico-Chirurgical Society of Edinburgh.[52] The first appendectomy was performed by Henry Hancock in London in 1848.[53] Even more critical to the transformation of the hospital was the adoption of antisepsis through the use of carbolic acid, evolved in the 1860s by Joseph Lister (1827–1912). While surgery could be performed without pain by the 1850s, it remained an extremely risky venture because of the very high mortality rates from postoperative infections. Sepsis was considered an inevitable concomitant of cutting, and death resulted in 24–60 percent of the cases, depending on the hospital.[54] Wards were filthy, with the same bowl of water and sponge used to clean all the wounds in a ward. Lister disproved the old theory that it was oxygen that caused suppuration, and through his exceptional skill with the microscope (which his father had perfected in 1829) he became convinced that germs introduced in the course of the surgical act were the culprit. His postoperative mortality rates for amputations, then the most common surgical procedure, fell from one death in every two and one-half cases to one in every six and two-thirds.[55] Asepsis, the scrupulous sterilizing of everything that will touch the area of the operation, superseded antisepsis, the disinfection of the wound site, in the 1880s. Antisepsis and then asepsis "rejuvenated surgery entirely and transformed surgical wards, after centuries of hospital gangrene, into places which one could hope to enter with the hope of leaving alive."[56] The heavy casualties in the American Civil War added further impetus to the growth of hospitals.[57] From about 1870 onward hospital admissions began to soar as medicine became more active and intrusive, especially through the new possibilities for surgery. Between 1861 and 1891 expansion was so rapid in London that the need for proper planning became a matter of urgency.[58] Also in the 1870s, twenty-four-hour staffing with trained nurses able to give skilled care was introduced. Scientific knowledge fostered social change, reshaping a welfare institution into a place of potential healing.

The cumulative conjunction of asepsis and anesthesia, which made lifesaving interventions possible, was an incentive for even those who had homes to undergo surgery in the now safer and better- equipped environment of the hospital. The introduction of x-rays in 1895–96 brought an added motivation for hospital use since the early machines were too cumbersome for a practitioner's office. In response to the needs of the new type of patients hospitals changed in many ways. Separate pavilions were constructed to improve ventilation and to minimize the risk of cross-infection as well as to segregate charity from paying patients, who were cossetted in settings similar to those of a luxury hotel, accommodated in suites, their meals served on linens, china, and silver in an attempt to replicate the lifestyle to which they were accustomed. But much dissent ensued over pay and part-pay beds, especially over the establishment of a middle tier for those who could afford to pay part of the cost.[59] By the end of the century more members of the middle classes were seeking care away from home when they were ill, and not solely for surgery. Physicians saw the advantages of hospitalization in facilitating closer supervision of the patient, preventing the spread of disease, and actually exerting a therapeutic effect through removal of the patient from the tensions of home surroundings. The rise of the hospital undoubtedly intensified the doctor's power in many ways and substantially eroded that of the patient.

Still, Gervaise's cry "No, no, not to the hospital!" is echoed in Mrs. Vidler's equally firm declaration in A. J. Cronin's *Citadel* (1937): "No, sir, I won't have my Harry in a hospital!" (307). The place is London, the time the late 1920s, but the sentiments are remarkably similar. Pride plays a greater part for Mrs. Vidler than fear of infection; the hospital is no longer seen as the locus of death, yet it continues to be regarded as a humiliation by the Vidlers, "respectable, hard-working tradespeople" (306) who keep a shop in Paddington Street "named, rather magnificently, 'Renovations, Ltd.'—one half devoted to boot repairs and the other to the cleaning and pressing of wearing apparel" (306). With this business of their own, the Vidlers are of a somewhat higher social level than Gervaise and her husband, who are employees. So when her

husband needs surgery Mrs. Vidler is adamant: "I won't have Harry go beg-
gin' for subscribers' letters, and standin' in queues, and goin' into a public
ward like he was a pauper" (307). The old association of the public hospital
with poverty persists into the early twentieth century.

That this aversion is more than mere prejudice is borne out by Cronin's
description of the Victoria Chest Hospital, "one of the oldest and most famous hospitals in London" (263). "The Victoria Hospital was unquestionably
old. . . . Upon the gloomy, dilapidated façade was a great placard in red and
white, which seemed obvious and redundant: VICTORIA HOSPITAL IS FALLING
DOWN. . . . The untiled walls were painted a peculiar shade of dark chocolate,
the uneven passages, though scrupulously clean, were so ill-ventilated that
they sweated, and throughout all the rooms there hung the musty odour of
sheer old age" (263). Not surprisingly, the young tubercular woman admitted
there fails to thrive and is eventually moved to a private clinic in the country,
where the pure air and calm are conducive to her recovery. Despite its fame,
this hospital is not beneficial to the patient.

Mrs. Vidler's resolve, however, does not work out well. Wanting the very
best for her husband, she specifies that it must be in "a private home" (307).
The terminology is potentially confusing here, for in British English a private
home, or, as it is more commonly called, a nursing home, is something very
different from the long-term custodial place for the aged and infirm to which
these terms refer in America. Nursing homes, of which there were at least
fifty in London in 1900 and a good many more later, were generally small,
for-profit establishments with facilities for surgical and noninfectious medical
cases. Some were owned by surgeons and physicians who filled them with
their own patients; more often they were started and run by women with
or without nursing qualifications. The hospitals did not exactly endorse these
competitors, but they welcomed the removal of paying patients for fear
that their presence might have an adverse effect on fundraising activities.
Conditions in nursing homes ranged from reasonably satisfactory to almost
sordid: "In some of them no trained nurses were employed, the food was
meagre and badly cooked and the accommodation inconvenient, noisy and
dirty."[60] Complaints from patients and their relatives about the low standard
of care and the exorbitant charges in some homes were printed from 1900
onwards in the *British Medical Journal* and *The Hospital*.[61] In fact, Harry Vidler
is rather fortunate in the Brunsland Nursing Home in Brunsland Square: "It

was a clean, old-fashioned home not far from Chesborough Terrace, one of many in the district where the fees were moderate and the equipment scanty. . . . Like every other home which Andrew had entered in London, it had never been intended for its present purpose. There was no lift, and the operating theatre had once been a conservatory. But Miss Buxton, the proprietress, was a qualified Sister and a hard working woman. Whatever its defects, the Brunsland was spotlessly aseptic—and even to the furthest corner of its shining linoleum floors" (308).

It is not the nursing home that kills Harry Vidler but a surgeon so grossly incompetent as to verge on the criminal. He has no hospital appointment, yet there is nothing to stop him from operating in a nursing home. Although all the medical personnel present in the operating theater realize that the surgeon's ignorance has cost the patient his life, Mrs. Vidler has no suspicions whatsoever, accepting at face value the surgeon's mendacious excuses. When the family doctor, Andrew Manson, who had made all the arrangements, later broaches his own sense of guilt for what happened, she brushes aside his attempted confession of complicity in having worked with so crude a surgeon. Manson has defaulted on his obligation to assess the surgeon's competence critically and to steer his patient toward a more skilled operator. A physician's failure to exercise power wisely, *The Citadel* shows, can be disastrous to the patient even in the absence of ill intentions. The physician's greatly enhanced empowerment also entails greater responsibility in the decision-making process, including the scrupulous avoidance of negligence. Ironically, Mrs. Vidler's trust in her longtime physician is so deeply ingrained that she cannot at all register that he is trying to own up to his share of the blame for the debacle. She finds pathetic consolation in her certainty that "my Harry had the best that money could give him" (353). In this instance at least the hospital, with its accredited staff, would have been a better choice despite the perceived taint of social disrepute. On the other hand, for Mary Boland with her tuberculosis the Victoria Hospital spelled a slow death. Cronin, himself a physician turned novelist, uncovers in *The Citadel* many facets of the defectiveness of the medical system in Britain in the 1920s, including the decrepit state of the hospitals and the scandal of uncontrolled nursing homes.

Caveat emptor is Gervaise's and Mrs. Vidler's stance in regard to hospitalization. But when the buyers in question are diseased people and their families, common sense and even instinctive criteria may have to yield to the imperatives of the disease itself. Whatever its drawbacks, by the end of the nineteenth century the hospital had become an indispensable necessity from both the doctor's and the patient's point of view for the practice of scientific medicine, which was "not a matter of the same game, somewhat improved, but of a quite different game."[62] This "different game" transformed the balance of power by making the patient more and more dependent on the doctor's expertise.

6.

THE QUESTIONABLE SANCTUARY: THE RESEARCH LABORATORY

The true sanctuary of medical science is a laboratory.
—CLAUDE BERNARD

THE CONCEPT OF THE LABORATORY as "the true sanctuary of medical science" was formulated by Claude Bernard (1813–78), the most illustrious French representative of experimental medicine. He himself carried out important research on the function of the pancreas in digestion and on the relationship between the body's central and sympathetic nervous systems. He is still best known for his *Introduction à l'étude de la médecine expérimentale* (1865; *Introduction to the Study of Experimental Medicine*, 1927), which sponsored a new view of medicine as a science governed essentially by observation, experimentation, and comparative analysis. It is in consonance with this vision that the laboratory is cast as "the true sanctuary," in contrast to hospitals, which Bernard saw only "as the entrance to scientific medicine, . . . the first field of observation which a physician enters."[1] Bernard's monograph made an impact beyond the world of science and medicine through its fervent adoption by Emile Zola, the leader of the naturalist writers. Zola's treatise *Le Roman expérimental* (1880; *The Experimental Novel*, 1963) is openly modeled on Bernard's methodology in that it attempts, with limited success, to transpose the system of experimentation based on observation into literature so as to turn the novel into a social document.

Bernard's idealistic view of the laboratory is projected in his use of the evocative word *sanctuary,* which denotes a holy place, a shrine, the most sacred part of a place of worship. Its distinct religious aura recalls *missionary* and *redemptive*, those other terms chosen by nineteenth-century medical men to characterize their professional activity. Bernard's exaltation of the laboratory as "the true sanctuary" fuses the spiritual with the scientific. The tension between the redemptive and the scientific of which Nathaniel West spoke (incidentally, some twelve years later) does not exist for Bernard, who subsumes the redemptive into the scientific. Bernard's belief that it is in the laboratory that "true medical science" will be achieved invests it with a quasi-utopian force. According to Bernard, the laboratory is the means to fulfill medicine's redemptive mission to the human species. His championship of the laboratory suggests "that the transition to laboratory medicine was a revolution at least as great [for the history of medicine] as the transition to hospital medicine which preceded it."[2]

The crux of this second revolution, and the reason for the centrality of the laboratory, lies in the convergence of science and medicine. Bernard always writes of not just medicine but of medical science. Without denigrating the role of clinical observation in the hospital or sickroom, he argues forcefully that it is no more than a preliminary stage: the ultimate basis of scientific medicine must be the laboratory because there the explanation of morbid phenomena and their divergence from normal states can be explored. "The laboratory . . . must therefore be the culminating site of the scientific physician's studies" (110). The laboratory, and it alone, could produce the rigorous taxonomy of diseases that had to precede the elaboration of therapeutics. And it was precisely its disengagement from the idiosyncrasies of individual patients that was the source of its strength. The evidence culled from patients, though by no means negligible, could nonetheless never attain the authoritative universal validity to be derived from laboratory observation and experimentation. Clinical medicine, and with it the patient, take second place in this enthronement of the laboratory.

By infusing the ideology of science into medicine Bernard's arguments laid the theoretical foundation for the supremacy of the laboratory. His stance was remarkably prescient, for in the mid-1860s few of the major breakthroughs that resulted from laboratory experimentation had yet been achieved, although important beginnings had been made. Chemistry had been modernized by the advent of quantitative analysis and the expression of results in mathematical form. *Cellular Pathology* (1858), by Rudolf Virchow

(1821–1902), is a significant landmark for its understanding of disease as a disorder not of form but of function and its argument that physicians must turn to pathological physiology rather than pathological anatomy in order to solve the fundamental riddle of sickness. In 1865, the year of Bernard's monograph, Louis Pasteur (1822–95) identified the microorganisms that were attacking the silkworm and ruining the industry, and in 1871 he was able to do the same for beer.[3] But it was only in 1877 that he extended his studies to diseases of higher animals and human beings, not only identifying the disease-producing microorganisms but also working toward the preparation of preventive vaccines. His most spectacular success, vaccination against rabies, came in 1885. Germ theory, the realization that certain diseases are caused by contagion through living animalculae, previously disputed, was definitively proven by Pasteur's work. The fact that he was actually a chemist, not a medical man, undoubtedly raised the prestige of the laboratory and fostered an understanding of the importance of the sciences for medicine.

The other great late-nineteenth-century bacteriologist was the German Robert Koch (1843–1910), who began his career as a country doctor and achieved his first triumph in 1876 with his studies of the etiology of anthrax.[4] By developing new methods of fixing and staining he was able in 1879 to identify the bacteria causing wound fever, thereby paving the way for the control of sepsis. It was also Koch who established the criteria for the acceptability of research data in bacteriology.[5] His further prodigious discoveries included the tuberculosis bacillus in 1879, the cholera bacillus in 1883, as well as the organisms responsible for cattle plague in South Africa in 1897 and for the plague in India in 1898. Among the signal advances made by others in the last quarter of the nineteenth century was the identification of the bacilli of typhoid fever by Karl Eberth and Georg Gaffky in 1880, of diphtheria by Edwin Klebs and Friedrich Loeffler in 1883, of tetanus by Arthur Nikolaier and the German-trained Japanese Shibanuro Kitasato in 1884, and of bubonic plague by Kitasato in 1894.[6]

These fundamental steps toward the conquest of some of the most lethal diseases were bound to lead to a heightened awareness of the role of the laboratory in medicine. American physicians, who had gone to the lecture halls of Edinburgh in the early nineteenth century and to the Paris hospitals in mid-century, gravitated to German laboratories in the final third of the century. By the 1870s a few of the better American hospitals had set aside small areas for laboratory work, and in this and the following decade the appointment of a pathologist to hospital staffs became increasingly common. Progress was slow, however; even in the early 1890s facilities were often quite inadequate.

Such hospital laboratories did not, however, correspond to Bernard's ideal. The term *laboratory*, derived from the medieval Latin *laboratorium*, meaning simply "workshop," assumed a range of denotations stemming from its original signification of a room or building equipped for scientific experimentation, research, and testing. The private facility, such as Dr. Jekyll's in *Dr. Jekyll and Mr. Hyde*, Lydgate's in *Middlemarch*, or Dr. Rougon Pascal's in Zola's *Docteur Pascal*, became ever rarer with the growing complexity of the necessary equipment. Laboratories where diagnostic tests could be carried out at the physician's behest as a crucial adjunct to clinical practice were incorporated into hospitals in the late nineteenth century. As those who could rely on a laboratory acquired a new elitist status, freestanding private laboratories were established in the 1890s that were accessible to all physicians.[7] Parallel to, but different from, these laboratories with a directed function were purely research institutions, which were divorced from the immediate needs of medical practice but were expected in the long run to be able to convert their theoretical investigations into therapeutic applications. It is this latter type of laboratory that met Bernard's definition as "the true sanctuary of medical science" and that is the subject of this chapter.

The research laboratory as a distinctive entity was developed in the last third of the nineteenth century partly in connection with the growing attention to public health. The first general institute devoted to all aspects of research in public hygiene was founded in Munich in 1879 under Max von Pettenkofer (1818–1901).[8] Germany remained in the forefront of laboratory medicine with no fewer than eleven institutes constructed at German universities between 1870 and 1890. But the most famous in Europe were the Pasteur Institute, established in Paris in 1888, and the Koch Institute, established in Berlin in 1891. These two were entirely heterogeneous in organization: the Pasteur Institute, funded by philanthropic donations as well as professional and state contributions, was set in an out-of-town environment; it had a multiplicity of scientists who worked together with a remarkable team spirit. The state-supported Koch Institute, in contrast, was squeezed into an urban location where there was a shortage of space; it was confined to those with medical qualifications and, perhaps because of its rigid hierarchical structure, beset by embittered tensions.[9] The early 1890s were the heyday for the inauguration of research institutes: the Institute for Experimental Medicine in St. Petersburg in 1892, the British Institute of Preventive Medicine in London in 1893, and the Serotherapeutic Institute in Vienna in 1894. It was also in 1892 that the first American laboratories of hygiene opened at the University of Pennsylvania and in New York City as part of its health department, and in 1894 the Johns Hopkins University dedicated its William Pepper Laboratory.[10] In addition, commercially motivated research laboratories began to appear, though not until the early twentieth century, when the money-making potential of science was becoming evident. An important example of such a self-supporting laboratory is that of Sir Almoth Wright in London; it grew out of a poky basement room, where Wright was intent on finding a weed-killer for bacterial farming in 1902, to the rather grand enterprise occupying two storeys in a spacious modern building where Alexander Fleming stumbled on penicillin in 1928.[11]

Despite this increase in the number and scope of laboratories, public response was mixed, tending toward skepticism. On the one hand, the existence of a rabies vaccine had an enormous and very positive effect; on the other hand, the social impact of the laboratory was limited because therapeutics mostly lagged considerably behind diagnosis. Before 1900 only diphtheria antitoxin afforded the possibility of decisive intervention in the course of an acute nonsurgical ailment. But diphtheria antitoxin and the rabies vaccine were exceptions. The introduction of serological tests for typhoid (1897) and syphilis (1906), though impressive as scientific achievements, were more relevant to prevention than to cure. In the 1860s and for several decades thereafter it seemed that the laboratory was able to fathom causes rather than to produce treatments. Whereas microscopy and analytical chemistry had early diagnostic applications, therapeutic spin-offs of laboratory science were few until the very end of the century. Dissatisfaction with the outcome of laboratory research was vented in the German slogan "Wir wollen heilen, und nicht klassifizieren" [We want healing, not classification].[12] As the gap between knowledge and therapeutics widened, there was considerable frustration at the shortcomings of bacteriology in translating its findings into practical means for helping the sick. A salient example of the problem was the disappointment following the premature announcement in 1890 that Koch's tuberculin offered a cure for tuberculosis, not merely the diagnostic tool it turned out to be. The disenchantment with laboratory science was rendered no less keen by the fact that it was shortsighted and misguided. It overlooked, for instance, the large number of specific drugs synthesized in the laboratory at an accelerated rate from the early 1860s onwards, including such staples as barbituric acid (1863), digitalis (1869), salicylic acid (1874), and phenacetin (1887).[13]

The failure of the laboratory's power to cure is revealed in Zola's *Docteur Pascal,* which is set in the south of France in the early 1870s. Rougon Pascal, trained as a physician in Paris, where he came under the influence of Bernard, like Lydgate aspires to combine clinical practice with research. Thanks to his independent income he can afford to practice medicine part-time and devote most of his energy to his research. Already in his late fifties at the novel's opening in 1872, Pascal visits patients only on Thursdays. He no longer even maintains an office; instead, he has turned his own quarters upstairs into "a sort of laboratory,"[14] which remains secluded, "like a sanctuary" (5:939). Zola's term "tabernacle," while not replicating Bernard's "sanctuary," places Pascal's work in the same pseudosacred context. His research is indeed a secularized religion to him, as he spends entire days in his laboratory, experimenting with mortar and pestle and test tubes.

Dr. Pascal aims to perfect a new remedy, nothing short of a cure-all: "he believed he had discovered a universal panacea, the elixir of life destined to combat human debility, the only real cause of all ills, a genuine scientific fountain of Youth which, by giving strength, health, and willpower, would recreate a wholly new and superior human breed" (5:940). Pascal's search for a universal panacea has both mythical and topical elements. On the mythical level it derives from the chimerical wish for a single, simple, quasi-magical antidote to all ills. His research has been described as obsessive, devolving from alchemy, rather than objective and disinterested, as science is expected to be.[15] Its filiation from alchemy is important for its arrogation of mysterious, almost supernatural powers; on the other hand, obsessiveness was by no means alien to scientific research, as is illustrated by the life stories of many nineteenth-century scientists who persisted despite successive setbacks. On the more immediate historical level, Pascal's endeavor is in keeping with the widespread vogue at that time of various secret remedies, for which enormous claims were made.[16] The public's gullibility in regard to such elixirs was supported by bona fide advances in chemistry and by the consequent difficulty lay people had in distinguishing the spurious from the genuine. Pascal's quest for an all-encompassing rejuvenating remedy, like Lydgate's pursuit of primitive tissue, is a fantasy-driven enlargement of contemporary possibilities. However, the attribution to Pascal in 1873 of Jules Chéron's 1893 ideas and practices makes his research an anachronism, thereby propelling it in the direction of romance.

Although Pascal himself maintains his belief in the potential of laboratory research ultimately to make significant improvements in human life despite his own current shortfall, blighted hopes such as those portrayed in Zola's novel created a distrusting ambivalence toward the laboratory, not least because they were echoed by real-life disillusionments. If to Bernard it was "the true sanctuary," to many it seemed a highly questionable institution that resulted in more disappointment than reward. The intervention of the laboratory thus shaped the perception of medicine as possessing a harmful as well as a redemptive capacity. The discrepancy between Pascal's hyperbolic hopes and his paltry results casts a highly dubious light on laboratory research, nullifying the very powers it claims. The limitations rather than the successes of medical research are shown in Le Docteur Pascal: one of Pascal's patients dies of an embolism following his injections, and none of them shows more than temporary improvement. The variety of diseases to which he applies the elixir of life testifies to his faith in its blanket efficacy: one patient has ataxia and paralysis secondary to syphilis, another is a homicidal maniac, a third is suffering from a bout of depression. Overcoming his devastation at his failure, Pascal begins to grasp that such therapeutic effects as he has achieved are primarily psychological; once he realizes that the elixir is a placebo, he takes to injecting simply water, which proves no less salutary. In this instance the laboratory's product is at best useless, at worst noxious. So in competition with Bernard's utopian concept of the laboratory as the true sanctuary of scientific medicine a dystopian suspicion forms that it is a sort of diabolical kitchen.

Nowhere is this as apparent as in Robert Louis Stevenson's Strange Case of Dr. Jekyll and Mr. Hyde (1886). The term "case" in the title draws the story simultaneously into both the medical realm and that of detective fiction. The central figure, Henry Jekyll, is at the outset presented as a most eminently respectable physician through the enumeration of his scientific degrees and

honors: "M.D., D.C.L., LL.D., F.R.S." (9). Yet just as much as his evil double,
Mr. Hyde, he is made an object of mystery. Since he is already dead before
the beginning of the narrative, readers have only mediated access to him
through the eyes and testimony of those surrounding him. So a distancing is
effected through a series of interlocking frames: the intercalated letters, en-
closures, and accounts open up a multiplicity of perspectives, which deepen
the perplexity. All the foreground action is among those who are trying to
grapple with the case, which is not solved until the closing section, "Henry
Jekyll's Full Statement of the Case" (48–62), an autobiographical confession
of the lurid fate that had befallen and destroyed him.

The key to the mystery lies in the laboratory below Dr. Jekyll's cabinet.
Originally it had been a dissecting room, for Dr. Jekyll had bought the house
from the heirs of a celebrated surgeon, but "his own tastes being rather
chemical than anatomical" (22), he had adapted it to his own purposes. The
sinister charge carried earlier in the century by the locus of autopsies is
now transferred onto the laboratory. As a visitor, the lawyer Mr. Utterson,
passes through the laboratory he senses its vaguely menacing character:
"he eyed the dingy windowless structure with curiosity, and gazed round
with a distasteful sense of strangeness as he crossed the theatre, once crowded
with eager students and now lying gaunt and silent, the tables laden with
chemical apparatus, the floor strewn with crates and littered with packing
straw, and the light falling dimly through the foggy cupola" (22). The eeri-
ness of this ramshackle space is set off against the normality of Dr. Jekyll's
cabinet with its fire, lighted lamp, and business table. It can hardly be called
cozy, for the windows are dusty and the fog seems to be creeping in, but its
discomforts are domestic in nature, not uncanny as in the laboratory. The
two rooms represent the dualism that is the theme of the tale and that surfaces in many little details. For instance, Mr. Utterson is "amazed to find a
copy of a pious work for which Jekyll had several times expressed great esteem, annotated, in his own hand, with startling blasphemies" (40). On the
lawyer's second visit to Dr. Jekyll's home the cabinet appears almost cheerful,
with a singing kettle and things laid out for tea beside the good fire in the
glow of the lamplight, "the quietest room, you would have said, and, but
for the glazed presses full of chemicals, the most commonplace that night in
London" (39). Here, in the presence of the chemicals, the agents of catastrophe are named, if not yet identified.

For Dr. Jekyll's criminal other, it transpires, "mostly comes and goes by the laboratory" (15). The "really damnable" (6), "deformed" (7) Mr Hyde is presented as the laboratory's product: "a masked thing like a monkey" that jumps down "from among the chemicals" (37). The incarnation of the lower elements in Dr. Jekyll's soul, he has been released through the drug compounded by the doctor. Dr. Jekyll's scientific curiosity drives him on to pursue an experiment that he knows to be perilous: "the temptation of a discovery so singular and profound at last overcame the suggestion of alarm" (50). It is to a "temptation," to the seduction of a course of action recognized as unwise or even wrong, that Dr. Jekyll yields and eventually succumbs. For a time, as "the record of a series of experiments" shows (44), he succeeds in containing the forces he has released, turning himself at will into Mr. Hyde and back again into his public persona. The process of transformation itself is described by Jekyll as an experience at once agonizing and "from its very novelty, incredibly sweet" (50). Although Hyde's depravity as he veers "towards the monstrous" leaves Jekyll "at times aghast," he is able to maintain "his good qualities unimpaired" (53). But finally things get out of control as Hyde's preponderancy grows, and with it Jekyll's sickliness, until the draught wholly loses its effect to restore Jekyll to his own shape. In a clever denouement, Jekyll concludes that it was an "unknown impurity" in his first batch of chemicals that had imparted efficacy to the drug.

That word "impurity" on the penultimate page is pivotal to the story. It is something contaminated and unchaste that has unleashed the vicious Hyde. This could be taken as to some extent an exculpation of scientific experimentation. Earlier Jekyll had insisted that "the drug had no discriminating action; it was neither diabolical nor divine" (51–52). Science itself, this implies, is intrinsically neutral, but even in the hands of a well-meaning person it can lead to dire consequences. Far from being readily amenable to regulation, scientific experimentation can run amuck, wreaking havoc in totally unforeseeable ways. *The Strange Case of Dr. Jekyll and Mr. Hyde,* like the folktale of the sorcerer's apprentice, shows how deceptively tenuous is the human capacity to regain authority over the mechanisms of the universe once they have been unleashed. Since moral judgment is absent from Stevenson's story, it is not just a cautionary fable. Readers' response is prefigured in the puzzled, stunned horror of Mr. Utterson and others associated with Dr. Jekyll as they gradually uncover what has happened. In this example of the uncanny, as in

Mary Shelley's *Frankenstein* (1818), the vileness originates not in some super-natural witches' kitchen but in a scientific laboratory. Its negative potential is cogently demonstrated in the scientist's loss of control over his experiment. He is disempowered and indeed destroyed by the very agencies through which he had hoped to expand man's mastery of the body by the mind.

An even more threatening role is ascribed to the laboratory in Aldous Hux-ley's *Brave New World* (1932). The Central London Hatchery and Conditioning Centre, whose motto is Community, Identity, Stability, is devoted to the perfection of the species by selective breeding of the fittest and ablest, delib-erately harnessing Darwinian principles to human reproduction in feats of genetic engineering. Its nucleus is the Fertilizing Room: "The enormous room on the ground floor faced towards the north. Cold for all the summer beyond the panes, for all the tropical heat of the room itself, a harsh thin light glared through the windows, hungrily seeking some draped figure, some pal-lid shape of academic goose-flesh, but finding only the glass and nickel and bleakly shining porcelain of the laboratory. Wintriness responded to wintri-ness. The overalls of the workers were white, their hands gloved with a pale corpse-coloured rubber. The light was frozen, dead, a ghost" (15). The con-trast between the intended life-producing purpose of this room and its ac-tual deadening effect emerges from all the descriptive notations: the dominant wintriness in the cold, the northern exposure, the "harsh thin light," the per-vasive whiteness, the "pale corpse-coloured rubber," the "bleakly shining porcelain of a laboratory," the light "frozen, dead, a ghost." Another, more glaring contrast is latent in the unvoiced subtext of the disparity between the warm spontaneity of natural procreation and the icy calculation of this cali-brated process. The word "hatchery," generally applied to animals, points to the dehumanization inflicted by this system. Huxley's novel is, like Orwell's *1984* (1949), a mordant satire, a fantasy dystopia of the future. Significantly, the agent and the site of the evil, as in *Dr. Jekyll and Mr. Hyde,* is a laboratory that has been perverted to nefarious ends in the name of designed progress. In both these works the activity in the laboratory backfires to create not a melioration of the human condition but a terrifying travesty. The laboratory may be a kind of enclosed sanctuary, but it is malevolent in its ensorcelment of those who come into its orbit.

The unmitigated negativity of *Dr. Jekyll and Mr. Hyde* and *Brave New World* is not replicated in either of the two main literary works about the research laboratory, Sinclair Lewis's *Arrowsmith* and A. J. Cronin's *Citadel*. However, both are decidedly critical in the cutting satire directed against research institutes. Since there is an interesting pattern of similarities and differences between these two novels, I will analyze them comparatively by juxtaposition.

The structure of both works is that of picaresque narrative, as the adventures of the main protagonists are depicted in an episodic series of incidents. In each one the pivotal character is a physician, Martin Arrowsmith in Lewis's novel and Andrew Manson in Cronin's. The shared, though inverted, initials of their names suggest a certain consanguinity. The place and time of the action are fairly far apart: *Arrowsmith* is set in the United States between 1897 and the early 1920s, *The Citadel* in Great Britain between about 1921 and the mid-1930s. The temporal scope of *Arrowsmith* is longer because it starts in Arrowsmith's adolescence, when he begins to be attracted to medicine, and follows him through medical school, general practice in the Midwest, a stint in public health in Nautilus, a position as pathologist at a fancy clinic in Chicago, and eventually on to a research institute in New York. *The Citadel* opens somewhat later in Manson's career with his first two positions as an assistant in general practice in Welsh mining villages, follows him through his move to London, his employment for a time in a research laboratory, and his subsequent return to private practice. The varied environments in which Arrowsmith and Manson work give the opportunity for a wide-ranging overview of the prevailing conditions and problems in medicine at their respective historical and geographical junctures. *Arrowsmith* has indeed been seen as "the recapitulation in one man's life of the development of medicine in the United States,"[17] while *The Citadel* fulfills the same function in regard to British medicine. Their emphasis is somewhat different, as the titles suggest: in *Arrowsmith* the focus is more on the individual's choices, whereas in *The Citadel* it is on interaction with the established system. Yet the two heroes are quite alike in character: enthusiastic outsiders who become rebels in their challenge to professional norms.

Both novels are based on close personal knowledge of medical etiquette. Lewis's grandfather, father, and uncle were all family doctors, and his brother Claude was a highly respected surgeon in St. Cloud, Minnesota. Doc Vickerson's small town office in Elk Mills and Arrowsmith's own practice in Wheatsylvania are modeled largely on the country practice of Lewis's father, with a certain dramatic heightening, for instance, of Vickerson's disorderliness.

Lewis was able to glean information about medical school as well as technical details from his brother. In addition, he sought the expert advice of the bacteriologist Paul de Kruif, who was fresh from the Rockefeller Institute of Medical Research, where he had been an associate of the biologist Jacques Loeb. After their meeting in 1922 Lewis and de Kruif spent hours in laboratories and traveled together to the island of Santa Lucia. De Kruif instructed Lewis on medical and scientific matters, including the usage in laboratories and the construction of complete professional histories for Arrowsmith and his teacher, Gottlieb. Lewis thus assured the soundness of the medicoscientific data.[18] Cronin had no need of such assistance since he himself had taken the M.B., Ch.B. (the normal British medical degree) with honors in Glasgow in 1919, and the advanced M.D., also with honors, in London in 1925. He practiced in the bleak coalmining region in South Wales until 1930, when he began to write his first novel, *Hatter's Castle* (1931), while convalescing from gastric ulcers. From then on he earned his living as a writer, enjoying great celebrity, especially with his television series about Dr. Finlay. The career of Andrew Manson obviously draws on Cronin's own early experiences.

A paramount theme of both novels is the transition from an older style of medicine to one that integrates scientific methods into practice. At the opening of *Arrowsmith*, Doc Vickerson's chaotic office, in all its "wild raggedness," is described as "the incarnation . . . the soul and the symbol" of his amateurish, slovenly habits as medical equipment jostles the debris of his daily existence: "The most unsanitary corner was devoted to the cast-iron sink, which was oftener used for washing eggy breakfast plates than for sterilizing instruments. On its ledge were a broken test-tube, a broken fish-hook, an unlabeled and forgotten bottle of pills, a nail-bristling heel, a frayed cigar-butt, and a rusty lancet stuck in a potato" (7). The rusty lancet stuck in a potato is an unforgettable emblem of unscientific practice. What Vickerson's patients think of him and his habits is not divulged; the appellation "Doc" suggests an affectionate familiarity, and probably there was no other practitioner within reach. But for all his backwardness and negligence, one of the two pieces of advice that Vickerson gives to the young Arrowsmith is to "get your basic science," the other being not to be "a booze-hoister like me" (8). Arrowsmith's own first office, when he sets up in Wheatsylvania, is hardly the acme of modern technology: the reception room is furnished with seedy chairs from the attic; an ancient bookcase, newly lined with pink fringed paper, becomes an instrument cabinet; a lumpy couch, covered in white oil-cloth, serves as a temporary examining chair; two cubicles at the back are turned into a consultation room and a laboratory. Arrowsmith cuts out racks for the glassware and turns a discarded kerosene stove into a hot-air oven for sterilizing glassware (149). Improvisational though it is on account of Arrowsmith's lack of capital, it is a signal advance on Vickerson's place. Yet Arrowsmith promises his wife that he will not "go monkeying with any scientific research" (149) instead of devoting his energy to earning a decent living. The little laboratory is represented here not as an adjunct to Arrowsmith's medical practice but as a danger, a lure away from the down-to-earth concern with patients and income.

The growing importance of office equipment, as medicine wants at least to appear more scientific, is brought out in the advertising brochure Arrowsmith receives from the New Idea Instrument and Furniture Company. It contains, Arrowsmith notes, "a quantity of poetic prose" and an "inspiring promise" (147):

> Don't you WANT to be a high-class practitioner? Here's the Open Door.
> The Bindlerdorf Outfit is not only useful but also exquisitely beautiful, adorns and gives class to any office. We guarantee that by the installation of a Bindlerdorf Outfit and a New Idea Panaceatic Electro-Therapeutic Cabinet (see details on pp. 34 and 97) you can increase your income from a thousand to ten thousand annually and please patients more than by the most painstaking plugging. (148)

This is clearly the voice of the satirist who had critiqued small-town social mores in *Main Street* (1920) and exposed big business in *Babbitt* (1922). Medicine too tends to be regarded as business in *Arrowsmith,* and not just by the New Idea Instrument and Furniture Company. Its (pseudo)scientific equipment is touted not as a supportive accessory to diagnostics or therapeutics but as essentially a means to increase income. Concern with income had been a commanding motif in Cathell's *Book On the Physician Himself* a good forty years before Arrowsmith's debut as a practitioner. But, significantly, the late-nineteenth-century dispenser of advice, though very intent on the furnishing of the office and the impression it will make, mentions hardly any equipment, and none beyond the basic microscope and test tubes. What has been called "the laboratory revolution" had in the meanwhile changed patient expectations. Esoterically named and probably peculiar-looking machinery is now deemed likely to impress patients and therefore to raise revenues. So equipment, irrespective of its usefulness, becomes a tool of empowerment for the doctor.

In *The Citadel* the office of Dr. Page, the disabled old physician in Blaenelly whose assistant Manson becomes straight out of medical school, is barely described, for almost all the work is done on rounds in the miners' houses. The surgery, as it is called in British terminology, lined with blue and green bottles on dusty shelves, serves mainly as a dispensary. Blaenelly, as Manson is soon told, has "no hospital, no ambulance, no X rays, no anything. If you want to operate you use the kitchen table. You wash up afterwards at the scullery bosh" (12–13). Manson's informant is the brilliant maverick Dr. Philip Denny, assistant to another local doctor. Denny contends "that all over Britain there were thousands of incompetent doctors distinguished for nothing but their sheer stupidity and an acquired capacity for bluffing their patients" (25). Manson begins to believe him after encountering Dr. Bramwell, who has "a grand manner, and some attitudes worthy of a great healer" (27), together with uncut hair sweeping over the back of his soiled collar, dirty fingers, and an overall air of seediness. The positive personal qualities, including even the clean, neat appearance so recommended by Cathell, recede here before "a grand manner" that suffices to satisfy the impoverished, uneducated clientele of miners. From the vantage of his loftier social and financial position Dr. Bramwell indulges in a personal and professional negligence that expresses indifference or even contempt for those under his care. Because he fails to diagnose appendicitis, a young patient dies. The relative degree of power he so readily commands appears to have induced degeneration in him.

Faced with a crisis caused by negligence in public health, Manson and Denny take matters into their own hands quite literally during a severe outbreak of enteric fever in a part of town served by a leaking sewer. Denny, who owns a fine Zeiss microscope, has spotted "the rod-shaped clusters of bacteria" (19) on the slides he has made, and Manson too recognizes them immediately. The local medical officer, "a lazy, evasive, incompetent, pious swine" (19), according to Denny, refuses again and again to take any action. So the two young physicians sneak out one night and blow up the sewer, the only way they can force construction of a new one. The black humor of this episode is more mellow than Lewis's satire, but like the difference between Vickerson's office and Arrowsmith's, it testifies to the generational conflict across the divide of scientific medicine. Its discoveries enable doctors by the early twentieth century to prevent and treat some diseases better than their nineteenth-century predecessors could; however, especially in remote areas and among working-class patients older practitioners are shown as indolent in putting the new capacities of scientific medicine into effect.

At Aberalaw, Manson's next post, conditions are somewhat better for there is a community hospital, although the town's senior physician keeps it as his exclusive preserve. Most of the members of the group practice are only a little better than Dr. Bramwell; one of them is very deaf, and another a fervent evangelist. Even the best of them, Dr. Urquart, "was old, rather automatic, and absolutely without inspiration" (131). The "good old type of family doctor," shrewd, painstaking, experienced, he "had not opened a medical book for twenty years and was almost dangerously out of date" (132). The generational disparity is very evident between these elderly men's dated styles of practice and that of the young Turk, Manson, who would "like to see more scientific methods used" (126). By means of the microscope Denny had given him, which Manson sets up in a room in his house designated as the laboratory, he does brilliantly original research on miners' lung disease resulting from dust inhalation, developing a technique for a complete clinical survey and tabulating the data. Although he sees himself as "no laboratory worker" (178), his is definitely a scientifically oriented brand of medicine far ahead of the primitive methods of his fellow assistants.

In dealing with silicosis *The Citadel* takes on a topical issue of its time. In the late 1920s and particularly during the Great Depression into the 1930s a liability crisis had developed in the political debate about miners' entitlement to disability pensions. The sandblasting pneumatic tools and other recently introduced mechanical devices had dramatically increased workers' exposure to silica dust, but compensation boards were slow and reluctant to admit liability.[19] The role of clinical laboratory research such as Manson carries out was absolutely crucial in establishing diagnostic and compensatory criteria. The laboratory, in the wider sense of scientific research, does in this part of *The Citadel* have a positive function as a sanctuary for Manson himself, relief from the harsh physical strain of his rounds on foot over hilly terrain in often rough weather, and above all for the miners whom it will benefit in the long run.

Manson's dogged lone quest has its parallel in Arrowsmith's experience in public health in Nautilus, where he is expected to be "epidemiologist, bacteriologist, and manager of the office clerks, the nurses, and the lay inspectors of dairies and sanitation" (183). His chief, Dr. Almus Pickerbaugh, whose "scientific knowledge was rather thinner than that of the visiting nurses" (202), is intent on "selling the idea of Better Health" (188) through the marketing ploy of rhyming limericks. His antics turn his self-proclaimed allegiance to "the up-to-date and scientific manner" (189) into a grotesque parody of the kind of medicine he purports to practice. Pronouncing himself "a laboratory man" (233), Arrowsmith finds refuge from Pickerbaugh's extravaganzas in a sustained series of experiments that will be published as a paper in the *Journal of Infectious Diseases*. To Arrowsmith, as to Manson, the laboratory is a sanctuary where he can validate himself. His persistence through the vicissitudes of his long and at times fruitless research is contrasted to the approach of Pickerbaugh, who "had published scientific papers—often. He had published them in the *Midwest Medical Quarterly*, of which he was one of the fourteen editors. He had discovered the germ of epilepsy and the germ of cancer—two entirely different germs of cancer. Usually it took him a fortnight to make the discovery, write the report, and have it accepted. Martin lacked this admirable facility" (248). Through irony of overstatement Lewis here conveys how laboratory research can be perverted not only into a phony activity in the hands of a consummate manipulator such as Pickerbaugh but also into a pathway to power. For the showman rapidly advances into a political career as "The First Scientist Ever Elected to Congress" (244), as the local newspaper announces. His weeks dedicated to "Better Babies," "Banish the Booze," "Tougher Teeth," "Stop the Spitter" (214), and so forth, his highly publicized Health Fair, and his slogan, "Just elect him for a term/And all through the nation he'll swat the germ" (244), prove big hits. The hollowness of his self-promotion is uncovered when his slackness in dealing with the real threats to public health in Nautilus becomes apparent. He is too preoccupied with his social climbing and his blatant hucksterism to give much heed to his pedestrian professional obligations, which he leaves to Arrowsmith. Pickerbaugh unscrupulously exploits the promise associated with scientific medicine for his own purely egocentric ends.

The portrait of Pickerbaugh has been described as a "painfully funny cari-cature."[20] Its comic exaggeration into the preposterous defuses the gravity of the public health officer's misuse of his power. Arrowsmith is dismayed by "the slimy trail of the dollar which he beheld in Pickerbaugh's most ardent eloquence" (218). His perception is confirmed by the future prospect that Pickerbaugh holds out to him of a "very lucrative practice" with "high-class" patients (204), whom he can meet by joining the country club and playing golf. Pickerbaugh thus functions in the novel as a foil to Arrowsmith's gen-uine, often frustrating questing in the laboratory. He is too absurdly over-drawn to be a sinister figure like Mr. Hyde or the engineer in *Brave New World*. Yet he is a menace to the community he is supposed to be serving because he deludes himself, and others, into mistaking his tawdry stratagems for public health endeavors. By violating professional etiquette, not to mention ethics, he achieves signal success in a society that is beguiled by his chicanery.

Manson and Arrowsmith are both rewarded for their research by recogni-tion and prestigious appointments at organized institutes. Manson is awarded the M.D. (a high and rare degree in Great Britain) and given the position of full-time medical officer at the C.M.M.F.B., the Coal Mines and Metaliferrous Fatigue Board. This sonorous name belongs to a government-sponsored in-stitute in London that has decided to open up the whole question of dust inhalation with a view to preparing a report to the Parliamentary Committee. Manson's work in the Welsh mining villages makes him exceptionally well qualified to pursue such an investigation. Excited at the prospect of ample time and proper facilities, he arrives in mid-August full of eagerness to get started. However, he has to accommodate to the lethargic pace of a govern-ment agency. Nothing can be done until the board convenes in mid-Septem-ber. Meanwhile Manson is to familiarize himself with the files (which he does in a single morning), drink endless cups of tea, read the *Times,* and go out to lengthy lunches. His colleague, a promising young bacteriologist, greets him with: "So you've come to join the forgotten men. . . . I'm, Doctor Hope. At least I used to think I was Hope. Now I am definitely Hope deferred." As for his work, he confesses: "Some of the time I sit and think. But most of the time I sit" (199). The entire environment is geared to leisurely comfort rather than work. Manson's office is "a warmly carpeted, restful sunny room with a superb view of the river" where "a large bluebottle is making 'drowsy' noises against the windowpane" (196). Working hours are ten to four, and the most "useful chap" in the department is a sedate, uniformed commissionaire who "makes delicious hot buttered toast" (196). These casual, concrete details about the C.M.M.F.B. amount to a telling indictment of its inertia, made the more effective by Cronin's ironic understatement.

The tragicomic pretense continues when the board finally meets. Its members are a mix of superannuated relics who have lost touch with current problems and careerists who pander obsequiously to their still influential seniors. The grandiloquence of the rhetoric sets off the pettiness of the sponsored projects. So enthusiastic support is expressed for the new medical officer's "all-important study of dust inhalation," which is to be brought to "its ultimate and scientific conclusion" (203) under the aegis of the C.M.M.F.B. If Manson's hopes are raised by these auspicious speeches, they are rudely shattered by the bathetic triviality of the task he is required to do first because it is a "pressing matter" (203): the inspection of first-aid equipment at all mines, with particular attention to standardizing "the size and weave of bandages, the length, material, and type of splints" (204). The sheer imbecility of this assignment as well as its utter inappropriateness to Manson's abilities adds up, beneath the ludicrous surface, to a bitter deflation of organized research. Taken aback yet trying to be cooperative, Manson tours the mines, cataloguing bandages "with alarming conscientiousness" (206), and as if in revenge submits a report crammed with "statistics by the tubful, pages of tables, charts, and divisional graphs showing how the bandage curve rose as the splint curve fell" (207). After this mockery of research is commended as "highly scientific" with "excellent graphing" (207), the futile discussion of bandage sizes makes Manson lose his temper. The misuse of scientific methodology for an inane objective and the resultant thwarting of what should have been his real work provoke Manson's resignation. To be cast as "a bandage counter-for life" (206) is the cipher of his impatience, irritation, and disillusionment. This laboratory—and there is one tucked away in a remote corner of the building—is a sanctuary only in a bad sense, a backwater of prevarication.

The abuse of power and the gross infraction of etiquette at this institution are epitomized in the incident with which this segment of Manson's career and of The Citadel ends. Book 3 closes with the announcement that "silicosis was, in that year, scheduled as an industrial disease" on the basis of medical evidence provided by Dr. Maurice Gadsby, the slimiest operator on the board, who is "acclaimed by the Press as a Humanitarian and a Great Physician" (210). That Manson's work bears fruit only as a result of a de facto theft by a well-connected insider is a sharp barb at the hollowness and deceit of the research establishment. What is most striking is the inverse outcome between the momentous findings of Manson's work in Aberalaw, unfunded, part-time, and improvised, and the paltriness of the task he is made to do as a full-time, government-sponsored researcher.

Arrowsmith also ends by giving up organized research, but his path is more circuitous and his story more complex. His article in the *Journal of Infectious Diseases* earns him an invitation to join the McGurk Institute in New York, a privately funded foundation after the manner of the Rockefeller Institute for Medical Research, which had been established in 1901. The McGurk cultivates the image of being "the soundest and freest organization for pure scientific research in the country" (137), dedicated solely to the advancement of basic research by men without obligations other than to their experiments. That it is "probably the only organization for scientific research in the world which is housed in an office building" (265), on the twenty-ninth and thirtieth stories of the McGurk Building, is an early hint of its covert commercialism, of which Arrowsmith is unaware for quite a while. Significantly, the institute's social amenities, from its "forbiddingly polite" reception room with "its white paneling and Chippendale chairs" (265) to its "real wonder" (271), its grandiose dining hall, are its most prominently mentioned facilities. Arrowsmith's laboratory is "smallish but efficient, the bench exactly the right height, a proper sink with pedal taps" (268). With its "decent, clean rows of test-tubes" (269), it strikes him so emphatically as a sanctuary for research that he is moved to formulate the prayer of the scientist: "God give me unclouded eyes and freedom from haste. God give me a quiet and relentless anger against all pretense and all pretentious work and all work left slack and unfinished. God give me a restlessness whereby I may neither sleep nor accept praise till my observed results equal my calculated results or in pious glee I discover and assault my error" (269). The religious aura surrounding medicine is here evoked once more. Arrowsmith's primary desire is to give service to humankind by applying his intellectual powers wisely, honestly, and selflessly. His ethos is the opposite of Pickerbaugh's.

For a time Arrowsmith's enthusiastic immersion in his experiments keeps him oblivious of the more questionable aspects of the McGurk Institute.

Readers are disabused sooner than he is, so that dramatic irony permeates this part of the novel. The ceremonious Scientific Dinners, which the researchers are obliged to attend, are obviously designed to impress important visitors. Altogether a great deal of effort in invested in window dressing to assure favorable publicity and to gratify donors. The institute's speciousness is implied by the comic-strip names of its directing personnel: Dr. A. DeWitt Tubbs, Dr. Rippleton Holabird, and its major benefactor, Capitola McGurk, who treats the institute as if it were a toy and its scientists "her husband's pensioners" (281). The position of its director, Dr. A. DeWitt Tubbs, as mediator between science and commerce is denoted by his office, which is "except for a laboratory bench at one end, most rigidly business-like" (272). The financial strings attached to allegedly pure science become apparent when accuracy is relegated to second place behind expediency. This verges on corruption as the scientists are urged to produce speedy, flashy results with immediate practical applications. In projecting these expectations the institute's administration is probably trying to meet the hopes of the time. By the 1920s scientific research, which had earlier "called up an ambiguous response" in American culture, had "increasingly become an object of inordinate respect, for men of science were truly 'miracle men.'"[21] Nevertheless, the avidity to cater to market forces leads to pressure to publish prematurely and so actually creates an atmosphere inimical to genuine research. Despite its front of respectability as a serious institute for advanced research, the aims of the McGurk are curiously reminiscent of Pickerbaugh's. Though more sophisticated in its means, this group also seeks to harness the power of scientific medicine for self-aggrandizement.

The institute's dominant though covert agenda is strenuously opposed by two scientists each of whom plays an influential role in Arrowsmith's life. The younger is Terry Wickett, M.D., Ph.D., "a first-rate chemist" (275) and a skeptical nonconformist who corresponds to Philip Denny in *The Citadel*. It is Wickett who enlightens the incredulous Arrowsmith about much of the institute's pretentious shamming. For instance, he reveals that the famous "finest centrifuge," the speediest in the country, is in practice useless: "The only trouble is, it always blows out fuses, and it spatters the bugs so that you need a gas-mask if you're going to use it" (275). As a useless showpiece the centrifuge is the symbol of both the institute's ostentatiousness and its ineffectiveness. Wickett contemptuously resists all the posturing; he even walks out on Capitola McGurk as she drools over "the poor little guinea pigs and darling rabbicks" (283). His intransigence, condemned by the administration as rude and uncouth, is an expression of his uncompromising adherence to absolute rectitude in scientific research. Wickett's integrity, like his anger, stems from his understanding of the responsibility that must go with his power and privileges as a scientist. While he does not comply with the social etiquette of polite conduct, he does honor the more arduous etiquette of medical power. His example makes Arrowsmith begin "to wonder about the perfection of his sanctuary" (284).

Arrowsmith is made to wonder even more by the controversial position in the institute's schemes of Max Gottlieb, the German bacteriologist who had first kindled his interest in scientific research during his student days. Gottlieb had preceded him to the McGurk, so that he takes the senior scientist's presence there as a warranty of the institute's authenticity without realizing the extent to which Gottlieb himself has been bamboozled and exploited. To the aging man the McGurk seems a sanctuary after his unhappy struggles to find an appropriate forum for his work. The centrality of this figure is indicated by the title Lewis originally considered, *The Shadow of Max Gottlieb*. The novel does indeed trace the shadow Gottlieb casts over Arrowsmith as his mentor and ideal; its crucial action is the younger man's eventual emancipation from that shadow through an independent decision that contravenes Gottlieb's scientific principles while satisfying Arrowsmith's own humanistic tendencies. In the conflict between the two ethical systems *Arrowsmith* not only reaches its climax but also raises most acutely the issue of the function and purpose of laboratory research in the context of medical healing.

Gottlieb is the incarnation of absolute troth to the ideal of pure scientific research. His history is carefully delineated so as to make his extremism credible. Born in 1850, he had taken his medical degree at Heidelberg, where he had been drawn to biology in the wake of Koch's discoveries. At forty, infuriated by discrimination against Jews and by Germany's growing militarism, he had come to the United States. In thirty years he has published a mere twenty-five papers, "all exquisitely finished, all easily reduplicated and checked by the doubtfulest critics" (120–21). His lifestyle is simple to the point of asceticism, but on his desk lie "letters, long, intimate, and respectful, from the great ones of France, Germany, Italy, Denmark and from scientists [in] Great Britain" (122). Heedless of financial reward, facile publicity, or social eminence, he is "an authentic scientist": "He had never dined with a duchess, never received a prize, never been interviewed, never produced anything which the public could understand, nor experienced anything since his schoolboy amours which nice people could regard as romantic" (121). Gottlieb conceives great scientists as members of a priesthood to whom the laboratory is a sanctuary in its literal religious meaning. His total commitment to "Pure Science" is summarized in the comment that "he would rather have people die by the right therapy than be cured by the wrong" (120). Such relentless fanaticism is the dark underside of his inexorable allegiance to research; he disregards present, individual suffering in a manner that seems inhumane for the sake of his ideal, which is to obtain long-term, incontrovertible proof of the validity of the experiment. His austere, inflexible scientific etiquette dictates his stance: his only interest is in the deployment of intellectual power, almost as an end in itself. This ethos is the crucial frame for the moral choice that later faces Arrowsmith.

Gottlieb appears sporadically throughout the novel as Arrowsmith's guide, mentor, and conscience. It is he who teaches him the basic principles of scientific experimentation, such as the necessity for maintaining an untreated "control" (42) in every experiment, and who reassures him when he is beset by doubts about his ability to be a scientist. The acerbic Gottlieb also formulates the distinction between the mentality of the researcher and that of the run-of-the-mill physician: "There are two kinds of M.D.'s—those to whom c.c. means cubic centimeter and those to whom it means compound cathartic. The second kind are more prosperous" (36). This apparently cynical comment characterizes the two types of power attainable by a physician: cognitive and financial. That Gottlieb considers the two alternatives mutually exclusive and evidently despises the second is in fulfillment of his function in *Arrowsmith* as a sublime fool in a world dominated by moneygrubbers. His lasting innocence represents for Arrowsmith throughout his career a potent model of idealism against which to measure his own course.

The bustling, at times frenetic activity at the McGurk is in direct contrast to the inertia at *The Citadel*'s C.M.M.F.B. Politicking is rampant, an incessant jostling for power, privileges, and recognition that becomes particularly intense when a new director is to be chosen. Arrowsmith, though he comes to realize that the McGurk is not the "kind of scientific Elysium" he had naively imagined it to be,[22] steers clear as far as possible of the factions and intrigues to devote himself to his work. True to his "natural aptitude for cloistered investigation," he is even ready to give up "three or four hours of wholesome sleep each night" (286) to learn, under Terry Wickett's tutelage, the advanced mathematics he needs to know. His long hours sequestered in the laboratory are clothed, as Rosenberg has put it, "with a spiritual, an inherently transcendent quality" that recalls the missionary nature of medicine.[23] The institute's power ploys and internal strife do not prevent Arrowsmith from creating for himself a true sanctuary for scientific medicine. Like Gottlieb, he is able to maintain his uprightness through a dedication to his work so wholehearted as to afford effective protection from interference by extraneous forces.

Arrowsmith's discovery of an antitoxin for the plague, like Manson's work on silicosis in *The Citadel,* has a topical dimension. The choice of the plague as the immediate challenge is most apposite, for in the plague "the final diagnosis—the identification—is impossible without a laboratory."[24] The laboratory holds sole authority for distinguishing between the three types of plague: the bubonic, spread directly by rat fleas, the even more lethal septicaemic, and the pneumonic, which can spread by infected droplets in the breath. In prelaboratory times diagnosis was effected symptomatically, that is, by the presence of buboes, while the specific causal agent was unknown. The elaboration of identifying tests in the microbiological laboratory was therefore a crucial advance. This transformation in the understanding of the plague was achieved during an epidemic in Hong Kong in the summer of 1894 when the Japanese bacteriologist Shibasaburo Kitasato, a student of Koch's, and Alexandre Yersin, a Swiss microbiologist out of the Pasteur school, discovered the plague bacillus.[25] In recounting the history of this breakthrough, Cunningham repeatedly emphasizes "the essential role of the laboratory."[26] The mechanism whereby the body could acquire immunity against infection was fiercely debated. In 1917 a new theory was proposed by the French-Canadian bacteriologist Félix d'Hérelle (1873–1949), who suggested that a living ultramicroscopic filter-passing virus was responsible for causing lysis (breaking down) of the infective bacteria, thus giving the body immunity against a particular bacterium. He called this virus "bacteriophage," meaning "bacteria eater," signifying a virus that feeds on living bacteria as a parasite and breaks them down.[27]

This is the medicohistorical context for Arrowsmith's research on "phage."

Opinion was sharply divided whether it could have a therapeutic as well as
a prophylactic effect. Arrowsmith is strongly urged by the McGurk's director
to make the transition from "fundamental research" to "practical healing":
"Enough of this mere frittering and vanity. Let's really *cure* somebody!" (316).
The prospect of the kudos and, even more, the financial yield of sensational
medical discoveries is the motivating factor in the pressures brought to bear
on Arrowsmith. Scientific integrity, modeled on Gottlieb, makes him resistant
to undue haste; results have to be repeated, checked, and verified until their
validity is beyond doubt before publication and human testing are warranted.
In an intercalation of historical fact Lewis has D'Hérelle beat Arrowsmith by
a hair's breath with his published report on phage. Arrowsmith's regret at the
forfeiture of the glory (and income) he might have reaped is tempered by the
inner satisfaction of having stuck to his principles as a scientist. This incident
is of importance in the development of the plot as a prefiguration of Arrowsmith's subsequent actions; it shows that he is in fact a most scrupulous
scientist who does not lightly depart from the correct etiquette.

Arrowsmith's opportunity to test the efficacy of his phage comes fortu-
itously in an epidemic of plague on a tropical island. His intention is to conduct a carefully controlled experiment by comparing a cohort of vaccinated
individuals with a parallel group of the unvaccinated. "Martin swore by
Jacques Loeb that he would observe test conditions; he would determine forever the value of phage by the contrast between patients treated and untreated and so, perhaps, end all plague forever; he would harden his heart and
keep clear his eyes" (333). Before he leaves for the island he is very categoric
in insisting on the need for "real test cases" so that his experiment will not be
"mucked up" (334). He refutes "with close-reasoned fury" the argument that
"in this crisis mere experimentation was heartless" (335); the scientist has to
make short-term sacrifices for the sake of long-term gains. He finds it much
harder to maintain his position after actually experiencing the devastation
of the plague: "He had seen the suffering of the plague and he had (though
he still resisted) been tempted to forget experimentation, to give up the possible saving of millions for the immediate saving of thousands" (358). But he
swears "that he would not yield to a compassion which in the end would
make all compassion futile" (359). At this point the shadow cast by Max Gottlieb is very strong as Arrowsmith recalls his mentor's teaching when he refuses phage to half the islanders: "'I'm getting to be good and stern, with all

you people after me. Regular Gottlieb. Nothing can make me do it, not if they tried to lynch me,' he boasted" (375). To those working alongside him he seems, though "quite a decent young man, . . . a fanatic" (361). Even after his closest coworker has succumbed to the plague, he continues to resist the demand that he give the phage to everyone, boasting: "I'm not a sentimentalist; I'm a scientist!" (365).

In light of these reiterated boasts and declarations Arrowsmith's sudden and complete volte-face following his wife's death from the infection is a surprising plot development. "Oh, damn experimentation!" he now exclaims as he orders phage to be dispensed to everyone who asks for it (376). In a moment of distress, when death touches him personally, not just professionally, he throws away the chance to carry through his controlled experiment and thereby betrays the principles Gottlieb had inculcated into him. True, he had previously fleetingly queried the basis for Gottlieb's severity: "It came to him that Gottlieb, in his secluded innocence, had not realized what it meant to gain leave to experiment amid the hysteria of an epidemic" (359). This lays the foundation for his emancipatory rebellion. It would be satisfying, and flattering to Arrowsmith, to be able to argue that he is motivated by the very compassion he had earlier condemned. There are some indications to support such a view. His "prayer of the scientist" (269) as he takes possession of his laboratory, in its fervent appeal to an unknowable deity, contravenes science's fundamental rationalism. Also his avowal that "he loved humanity as he loved the decent, clean rows of test-tubes" (269) testifies to a dualism alien to Gottlieb. If such a hypothesis could be upheld, his renunciation of experimentation in favor of succoring the suffering masses could be read as a grand romance act that would cast Arrowsmith as the rescuing knight in shining armor and the phage as a magic potion.

But such an interpretation cannot be sustained. The unglamorous fact is that Arrowsmith "went to pieces" (376), and what is more, he drinks quite heavily. Prior to issuing the order for the universal use of phage he gulps down several glasses of raw rum, which may well have clouded his judgment. "His falterings are often of his own making, and when he botches the chance to make a definitive test of the value of his bacteriophage, the cause is his own choice made on the basis of humane emotional considerations instead of the purely intellectual integrity he had hoped to attain."[28] Here "falterings," "botched," and "had hoped to attain" are negative expressions redo-

lent of failure, while "the purely intellectual integrity" is the ideal for which
he strives. However, the "humane emotional considerations" that sway Arrowsmith's choice at this point cannot be branded as simply a fault in his character. His choice denotes both a shortcoming and a virtue: a shortcoming
in him as a research scientist and a virtue in him as a human being. For it is
precisely Arrowsmith's infraction of the dour etiquette of pure science that
makes him a warm and attractive figure.

This episode forcefully poses the question whether the pursuit of scientific knowledge should override all other considerations, as Gottlieb believes.
Ultimately what is at stake here is the relationship of laboratory medicine
to bedside medicine, or, as it has so aptly been designated, "the bedside-bench
ambivalence."[29] Is there a radical distinction between the culture of laboratory
research and that of clinical practice in hospital, office, or home? The division
of intellectual labor in the laboratory is based, it has been argued, not upon
particular organs or diseases, as in clinical practice, but upon conceptual de-
marcations derived from scientific disciplines. Thus, in the words of N. D.
Jewson, "the problems encountered in medical practice rapidly declined as
a legitimate point of departure for the discourse of medical investigators."[30]
Jewson calls the laboratory "an insulated intellectual cocoon" (238) with ex-
acting and exclusive specifications for membership and a technical jargon that
serves as a ritual mode of differentiation between the initiated and outsiders.
Detachment is a determining trait of the researcher's psychological profile,
together with a clearcut monodimensional rapport with peers in place of the
physician's multidimensional, at times difficult interaction with sick people.

The tension between research and practice, delineated by Jewson for the
period 1770–1870, became more strained toward the end of the nineteenth
century as the laboratory gained importance. Traditional physicians resented
the veneration for scientific findings because they felt it implied a disdain
for clinical acumen. "The appeal of the laboratory and its transcendent claims
seemed to many clinicians a dangerous will-o'-the-whisp."[31] Such suspicion
of the laboratory is very explicit in *Dr. Jekyll and Mr. Hyde.* And earlier the populace of Middlemarch is leery of Lydgate on account of his reputation for
experimentation. The dichotomization of researcher and practitioner is present in *Arrowsmith* too: "Martin himself attended the sick man [Sondelius],
trying to remember that once he had been a doctor who understood ice-bags
and consolation" (365). The distinction is between the clinician's attention

to an individual's present physical and psychological needs and the researcher's focus on the possibility of saving millions in the future.

This divergence of aim entails a sweeping alteration in the etiquette of
power. The researcher's thrust toward universalism means that differences
between patients have to be minimized for the sake of delineating the typical characteristics of an objectified disease. The individual patient has to become "merely a point on a curve";[32] to put it even more crassly, "it made
relatively little difference whether that [disease] process was going on in an
Irish immigrant or a laboratory dog."[33] It did, of course, matter to the extent
of the disparity between human and canine physiology and pathology, but
the point is well taken that the patient is to the researcher a generic entity,
as it were. Since "the occupational activity of medical investigators hence-
forth took the form of the extension of certified knowledge rather than the
servicing of clients," the sick person was conceptualized "as a material thing
to be analysed." Consequently, "laboratory medicine, by focusing attention
on the fundamental particles of organic matter, went still further in eradicating the person of the patient from medical discourse."[34]

Such attenuation of interest in the individual as he becomes a case is amus-
ingly illustrated in Conan Doyle's story "The Third Generation" when Dr. Ho-
race Selby suddenly tells a patient consulting him in his office: "'Curiously
enough, I am writing a monograph upon the subject. It is singular that you
should have been able to furnish so well-marked a case!' He had so forgotten
the patient in his symptom, that he assumed an almost congratulatory air towards its possessor. He reverted to human sympathy again, as his patient asked
for particulars."[35] The doctor here, normally humane, sees the patient mo-
mentarily as "able to furnish" research data. His pain is forgotten in the doctor's pleasure at coming upon further useful evidence. This incident also gives
a glimpse of the way the late-nineteenth-century doctor establishes his authority by knowledge and allegiance to science more than by behavior ("ice-
bags and consolation"). On the patient's side too a modification takes place
when confidence in the physician stems indirectly from belief in his mastery of
the sciences. But a possible conflict begins to emerge here, for patients, probably without realizing it, come to have dual expectations: ideally, they want the
new scientific expertise to be conjoined with traditional comforting. The discord is intensified by patients' awareness of a reduction in heed to their idiosyncrasies in favor of a standardized armamentarium of procedures and drugs.

That Arrowsmith has to move literally out of the orbit of the laboratory in order to remember that he was once a missionary to the bedside is a telling confirmation of the researcher's abstraction from the patient. Manson differs from Arrowsmith in this respect: he is, and remains, primarily a clinician whose research grows out of his practical work with his patients. He realizes "that he was no laboratory worker, that the best, the most valuable part of his work was that first phase of clinical research" (178). He certainly respects and productively draws on scientific methods, "conducting a systematic examination of every anthracite worker on his list" (129), taking "the pit workers and surfacemen as controls" (159) until he has perfected his technique and is able to present his results according to the accepted protocol: "He drew up a series of tables indicating the ratio-incidence of pulmonary disease, amongst the various grades of anthracite workers" (176). The ultimate basis of his research, however, resides not in the laboratory's test tubes and samples but in his clinical brilliance in following up on his observations and measurements in a lengthy series of patients. Manson converts practice into research, pragmatically deducing a theory from his bedside findings. The miners recognize that "he can do the real stuff, like, when it's wanted" even though he is "a bookish chap" (158) whose medical interests transcend the daily round. His rather hasty rejection of organized research, while partially justified by the way he is treated at the C.M.M.F.B., may be an expression of his underlying preference for the practical over the theoretical.

So Manson returns to practice. In London he goes through a phase of materialism as he lets himself be implicated ever more deeply in the glittering whirl of high-society medicine, where lucrative honoraria are easily garnered for medical care so sleazy as to verge on the scandalous. But after a series of shattering reversals, including the death of a patient through a surgeon's gross ignorance and the loss of his wife in a street accident, Manson breaks loose from the vanities of this corrupt existence to found a community health center in a Midlands town in partnership with Dr. Hope and Dr. Denny. With this fresh start *The Citadel* ends quite positively as Manson reverts to the role of missionary to the bedside. He has come to learn that his true power as a doctor springs from the care of patients; whether he will ever engage in research is left open to conjecture. However, he will assuredly draw on the resources of modern scientific medicine in caring for his patients. The laboratory is a false sanctuary to him, deflecting him from his true vocation. But *The Citadel* does not project a blanket condemnation of the laboratory as quintessentially nefarious in the way that *Dr. Jekyll and Mr. Hyde* and *Brave New World* do. Instead, criticism is sharply focused on one particular type of government-sponsored laboratory without impugning the worth of medical experimentation per se. Yet the implication is that the genuinely positive contributions are made by the exceptional lone researcher, not by the lumbering state organization.

Like Manson, Arrowsmith turns his back on institutionalized research but not on the laboratory itself, for in contrast to his British counterpart, he feels it to be his natural medium. As in *The Citadel,* there is a strong suggestion that the best research is conducted aside from the questionable sanctuary of the organized establishment. With considerable panache Arrowsmith flees the McGurk Institute and his opulent socialite second wife to follow Terry Wickett into the remote northern woods, where Wickett has set up an improvised laboratory in a shack. This sensationalist closure has been greeted with a good deal of skepticism: one critic called it "a little fantastic . . . and quite unpersuasive,"[36] and another deemed "the Shangri-La of a two-man research lab in the Vermont mountains scarcely a convincing denouement."[37] The flight into the wilderness enacts the romance motif of repudiation of society in favor of a supposedly simple existence in the country, but it brushes aside such realities as funding and appropriate working conditions. This extravagant protest, while more striking than the modest ending of *The Citadel,* is ultimately less hopeful. For it goes beyond endorsing individual over group effort; it also seems to infer that disinterested medical research is hardly feasible in the commercially driven everyday world and that isolation is the price for probity. The backwoods laboratory to which Arrowsmith and Wickett withdraw is certainly a sanctuary for them; however, is their gesture a retreat, a self-assertion, or a mixture of the two? Can this setting, with all its hardships and deficiencies, prove propitious for the rigorous and often complicated processes of twentieth-century medical research?

The laboratory thus assumes in late-nineteenth- and early-twentieth-century literature a far more problematic guise than Claude Bernard could have imagined. His sanctification of the laboratory is countered by its aggressive demonization in *Dr. Jekyll and Mr. Hyde* and *Brave New World.* Mostly, however, medical research is portrayed as characterized by ambivalences: between idealization and vilification, between stringency and meretriciousness, between the lone effort and the organized institute, between fidelity to science's slow, deliberative processes of controlled testing and the desire for instantaneous application of life-saving discoveries, between the allure of basic research with its long-term hopes of momentous progress and the shorter-term gratification of caring for and healing the sick. Such ambivalence also pervades the image of the researchers in the tension between suspicion of their weird, perhaps dangerous pursuits and admiration for their potential power to ease humanity's suffering. Bernard's term "sanctuary" in fact has the capacity to accommodate these disparate conceptions. Although he certainly invested the word with a solely positive meaning, it can also carry other, more dubious connotations. For a sanctuary, a safe place, is also by definition a cloistered space at a remove from the mainstream of daily activity. Its seclusion is a prerequisite for its status as a sanctuary, yet it inevitably has the effect of distancing those within its walls. This applies equally to the laboratory, which is both "the true sanctuary of scientific medicine" and a system that separates doctor from patient. Although it is essential as a sanctum for research, it can nevertheless become questionable if it degenerates into the corrupt instrument of power exposed in these novels.

7.

EYEING THE INSTITUTION: THE TWENTIETH-CENTURY HOSPITAL

———————————————————————————

Doctored, they say of drinks that have been tampered with, of cats that have been castrated.—MARGARET ATWOOD, *Bodily Harm*

———————————————————————————

THE INSTITUTIONAL EYE TENDS to become focused on the lung, and it forgets that the lung is only one member of the body."[1] This critique of the hyperspecialization, fragmentation, and consequent disregard for the whole person of the patient was voiced, not within the past ten years, but as long ago as 1927 by Frances W. Peabody, M.D., in a lecture to students at the Harvard Medical School entitled "The Care of Patients." By then patient care had been sufficiently downgraded to warrant discussion as part of an attempt to revive the skills and attitudes that in earlier periods had been regarded as vital to the physician's positive interaction with patients. With the professionalization of nursing into a highly trained occupation and the development of a succession of new therapies and procedures, caring for the patient became assigned to nurses, while the doctors' task was curing. This dichotomization of care and cure is one of the hallmarks—and bugbears—of medicine today.

By the 1920s many of the problems that bedevil the contemporary hospital had already crystallized. The transformation of the hospital from a refuge for the indigent sick into "the temple of science"[2] had as its concomitant its promotion to the central role in medical education, therapeutics, and research: "if the hospital had become medicalized by the 1920s, it must be emphasized that the medical profession had by the same time become hospitalized."[3] The hospital had also attained acceptance as an essential community institution patronized by patients of all social levels. As the custom of referring difficult cases for diagnosis and treatment grew the hospital came to be seen as the best place for surgery and for treatment of any serious acute ailment. The necessity for hospital admission was no longer predicated on the social criterion of poverty but on the presence of a medical condition requiring sophisticated attention. However, even as "the inmate was becoming a patient,—the patient [became] a diagnosis."[4] For with the elaboration of rigid routines for the sake of efficiency, the hospital tended to lose sight of patients as individuals. Their reduction to physiological, biochemical, and pathological entities is indicated by their frequent anonymity through the habit of substituting the nomenclature of their disease for their personal name.

It is this narrowing of focus and depersonalization that is the object of Peabody's strictures on the methods of the "institutional eye." In an eloquent passage he contrasts the missionary to the bedside with the hospital physician:

> When the general practitioner goes into the home of a patient, he may know the whole background of the family life from past experience; but even when he comes as a stranger he has every opportunity to find out what manner of man his patient is, and what kind of circumstances make his life. . . . What is spoken of as a "clinical picture" is not just a photograph of a sick man in bed; it is an impressionistic painting of the patient surrounded by his home, his work, his relations, his friends, his joys, sorrows, hopes and fears. Now, all of this background of sickness which bears so strongly on the symptomatology is liable to be lost sight of in the hospital: I say "liable to" because it is not by any means always lost sight of, and because I believe that by making a constant and conscious effort one can almost always bring it out into its proper perspective.[5]

The mild nostalgia inherent in this scenario does not detract from Peabody's argument; it is less a critique of the hospital per se than a plea for the incorporation of the valuable aspects of the old style of home-based bedside medicine into the new hospital mode. Indeed, he sees no incompatibility between the two as he asserts: "The treatment of a disease may be entirely impersonal; the case of a patient must be totally personal" (877). Peabody's statement represents an affirmation of the duality of medicine. To revert to the idiom of the nineteenth century: although the scientific ("impersonal") approach is unquestionably the dominant one in this century, the redemptive ("personal") side should not be eradicated.

In the seventy years since Peabody's speech medicine has made unprecedented scientific and technological advances, which have intensified rather than decreased the problem he identified in 1927. The late-twentieth-century hospital has been described as at once "the triumph of modern medical science" and the embodiment of "the most unfortunate features of modern medicine."[6] Public belief in scientific medicine and its curative benefits has fostered increasing trust in the expert authority of the hospital's physicians. Yet this magnification of medical supremacy has not only resulted at times in a shortfall of excessive expectations on the part of patients but also substantively changed the balance of power by making patients totally dependent on their doctors' knowledge, a level and type of knowledge far beyond the grasp of even well-educated people. The early- to mid-nineteenth-century model of consultative cooperation between doctor and patient has been confuted by the many recent innovations in medicine. On the one hand, these are undoubtedly to the patient's therapeutic advantage; on the other hand, they open up a chasm between the medically trained and laypersons that results in a fundamental imbalance of power. The institution of "informed consent," which dates from 1960,[7] is intended to give patients some understanding of what is about to be done to them; however, its ulterior motivation is to protect medical personnel from charges of malpractice in case of mishap by spelling out the potential risks. The very need for such a ritual indicates the covert tensions between doctor and patient and the possibility of their mounting into oppositional clashes in lawsuits.

So the "reign of technology" has had, besides obvious gains, less apparent "losses to the sick patient, to the physician as clinician, and to society." The preponderance of the machine has the effect of blunting both the verbal and the affective aspects of the doctor-patient exchange as purely subjective elements in favor of the preferred objective data: "modern medicine has now evolved to a point where diagnostic judgments based on 'subjective' evidence—the patient's sensations and the physician's own observations of the patient—are being supplanted by judgments based on 'objective' evidence, provided by laboratory procedures and by mechanical and electronic devices."[8] The consequences of this shift for clinical practice are discussed in a textbook whose title reiterates Peabody's phrase, *The Care of Patients*. According to this book, because the "scientific basis for medical practice has placed an unfortunate emotional barrier between some doctors and their patients, . . . meticulous listening, empathic understanding, and compassionate concern for the patient have grown ever more important."[9] As more potent interventions have expanded the range of cure the emphasis on mere care has continued to diminish. So much so that a separate institution, the hospice, has recently been established for those patients who are beyond curative intervention and who need comforting attention.

To counter the mechanism bred by reliance on technology, deliberate efforts have been made to rehumanize hospital medicine. In 1983 Derek Bok, then president of Harvard, devoted his annual report to a survey of the system of medical education at that university and made recommendations for far-reaching changes. Nineteen eighty-three was also the year when the American Board of Internal Medicine issued its "Report of the Subcommittee on Evaluation of Humanistic Qualities in the Internist," a cogent reminder of the importance of qualities other than scientific expertise in the healing relationship between physician and patient. This was followed in 1985 by the same board's "Guide to Awareness and Evaluation," designed to help program directors evaluate and teach candidates in regard to "integrity, respect, and compassion."[10] A program to foster precisely such qualities has been outlined by Rita Charon, a practicing physician and a graduate student in English at Columbia, who underscores empathy as "one of the most challenging and important tasks of medical students. They must learn to empathize without losing their objective stance."[11] To achieve this desired combination, she encourages students to acknowledge their fears, anxieties, frustration, and anger through verbalization; to heed patients' experience, often overlooked in the central drama of health professionals' activity; and to widen their imaginative horizons by both reading and creative writing.

Such attempts to reinject more humanity into American medicine can be seen as part of the thrust to restore an image that has been progressively bruised in the course of the past quarter-century. The vicissitudes of Americans' attitude toward the medical profession are traced by Starr in *The Social Transformation of American Medicine*. After the wariness that prevailed in the early to mid–nineteenth century, devotion to medical authority grew in the twentieth century with the impressive increases in medicine's curative capacity. But "medicine, like many other institutions, suffered a stunning loss of confidence in the 1970s" (379), which Starr attributes to a multiplicity of factors including the challenge emanating from the women's movement and the abuses uncovered in malpractice suits. Symptomatic of this suspiciousness was a sensationalist book, *Medical Nemesis: The Expropriation of Health Care,* published in 1976 by the radical social critic Ivan Illich, who claimed that medical care actually caused more disease than it cured and that people would be healthier if they liberated themselves from dependence on the entire malignant apparatus of modern medicine. The doctor-patient relationship took a dangerously adversarial turn as each side came to feel that it had to protect itself from the other: the doctors from vindictive lawsuits initiated by patients disappointed by their outcomes, the patients from medical personnel perceived as uncaring to the point of negligence and corrupted by greed. In a curious paradox, the immense increase in the physician's power was accompanied not by a corresponding growth of trust but instead by a wariness prompted by misgivings that could amount to fear.

This "desanctifying of the medical profession" following "Americans' gradual disillusionment with technology and paternalism in general" has come to the fore in television serials and films as well as in narratives.[12] For in contrast to the avoidance of the hospital through most of the nineteenth century, in the past forty years it has become a favored setting for works in various media that purport to play out "real-life" dramas. This shift from shunning to what seems like fascination is in part connected to the hospital's changing social position. Once the despised refuge of the down-and-out, it is now a constituent of every community, familiar yet still enveloped in a mystique that evokes a curiosity compounded of trepidation and excitement. With its own rules, hierarchies, and usages, it forms an esoteric world within a world, the site, in Charles Rosenberg's words, of "the most fundamental and unchanging of human experiences—birth, death, and pain." He adds, "It is no accident that both black comedy and soap opera should have found the hospital a natural setting."[13]

Many recent novels and films present decidedly negative images of physicians. The organ snatchers in Robin Cook's *Coma* (1977) are the most lurid and memorable of a string of malfeasant doctors at the center of the enormously popular thrillers by this graduate of Columbia Medical School. The brilliant surgeon Dr. Thomas Kingsley in *Godplayer* (1984), who murders for the sheer pleasure of his power; Dr. Trent Harding, the anesthesiologist in *Harmful Intent* (1990), who frames a colleague to cover his own crimes; and the mafiosolike web surrounding Dr. Norman Wingate in the in vitro fertilization business in *Vital Signs* (1991) are further examples of gross abuse of medical power out of greed, jealousy, or psychopathology. The debased, perverted doctor is common in films too: the venial Dr. Chris Nichols in *The Fugitive* (1992), who does not hesitate even to murder his colleague's wife because she has discovered that he has falsified his experimental data by switching tissue in order to gain approval of a defective drug in which he has a large financial stake; the demented, drug-addicted twin gynecological surgeons in *Dead Ringers* (1988); the homicidal gasher in *Dr. Giggles* (1992); the negligent anesthesiologist Dr. Tower in *The Verdict* (1982); Dr. Welbeck in *The Hospital* (1971), so deeply engrossed in the management of his proliferating investments that he repeatedly botches surgery; the corrupt administrator of a VA hospital in *Article 99* (1992), who diverts supplies, depriving the patients of necessary equipment; the skeptical, resistant neurologists in *Lorenzo's Oil* (1992), who obstinately block trials of a seemingly promising treatment for a rare fatal disease out of a misguided sense of professional solidarity. What all these figures have in common is a megalomaniacal sense of their own power as exceeding the limits of social and even legal bounds.

These inventive contemporary variations on the theme of the harmful doctor are descended from a long tradition of attacks on the medical profession in literature. But they differ in an important way from their predecessors, which targeted the ineffectiveness and frequently the quackery and pretentiousness of the medical fraternity. The mordant tragicomic satire of medicine in the plays of Molière (1622–73), himself a sick man who actually died on stage, typifies the earlier approach.[14] In the late-twentieth-century instances that I have just cited it is not merely incompetence that is exposed but a moral vileness that undermines the very foundation of the healing vocation by putting self-interest, at times of a pecuniary nature, above service to others. It is as if medical power has an autointoxicating effect on some practitioners. The *New York Times* article on these lapsed physicians, subtitled "A Steep Slide," contrasts the medical delinquents so prevalent in television and film nowadays with their forerunners—Dr. Marcus Welby, Dr. Ben Casey, and Dr. Kildare on the small screen, and on the larger one *Dr. Ehrlich's Magic Bullet*

(1940), about the discoverer of a drug against syphilis, and D. W. Griffith's short *Country Doctor* (1911), which shows a doctor leaving the bedside of his sick son to answer a call from a patient.[15] To this company should be added the newly updated revival of the British series about the Scottish Dr. Finlay and his partners. All these conform to the old heroic model of the doctor as essentially noble, generous, and self-sacrificing. This is as much an idealization, a wishful projection, as the currently fashionable demonization is a grossly inflated expression of apprehension. The endless altruism of doctors always at their patients' beck and call and never sending a bill has to be recognized as an exaggeration in the same way as the unscrupulousness of the self-promoters. What must not be overlooked is the corrective presence among the bad doctors of honest, benevolent counterparts who stake their careers and even their lives to redeem the damage wrought by their culpable colleagues: Dr. Roger Kimble in *The Fugitive*, who is finally exonerated of charges of murder and in clearing his own name uncovers the real criminals; the idealistic young surgical team in *Article 99*, who run the very serious risk of dismissal and disbarment when they steal from their own hospital stores the supplies needed by their patients; the intrepid, imaginative Dr. Marissa Blumenthal in Cook's *Vital Signs*, who fathoms the bizarre crookedness of the infertility clinic; the resourceful Dr. Cassie Kingsley in *Godplayer*, who survives her husband's murderous ploys by ingenuity and enterprise; the determined Dr. Jeffrey Rhodes in *Harmful Intent*, who, like Dr. Kimble, restores his reputation by tracking down the vicious miscreant; the chief of medicine in *The Hospital*, who refuses to be tempted away from his responsibilities. The latest television serials too, such as *Dr. Quinn, Medicine Woman, Chicago Hope*, and *ER*, redress the balance by a return to a far more benign image that admits individual foibles but on the whole stresses integrity.

A blend of "desanctifying" with rehumanization occurs in the film *The Doctor* (1992) through the role reversal a hardened surgeon has to undergo when he becomes a patient in the hospital where he has worked. The drastic change of perspective very quickly makes him painfully aware of the patient's dilemma in having to deal with cavalier physicians as well as with a life-threatening disease. He submits to a sobering transformation as he is subjected without mercy to the callous handling of patients that he himself had previously condoned. The neat plot ends with a humorous twist when he makes his students become patients for seventy-two hours to expose them all to the tests, humiliations, and helplessness imposed by hospital protocol in hopes of raising their consciousness regarding the proper exercise of the power they themselves will soon have. This ironic wit counteracts the slightly sentimental closure as Dr. McKee's aloof pride in his technical virtuosity is tempered by a measure of sensitivity.

The undeviating imperatives of the hospital's power structure are also shown in Diane Johnson's novel *Health and Happiness* (1990) as they affect a spectrum of patients with illnesses of varying severity. All are without differentiation processed, as it were, by standardized routines. Without exception they are completely disempowered as soon as they come under the sway of the hospital's mechanisms. The aged, moribund Mrs. Tate is "being tortured" (289) by futile interventions that have ravaged her body as much as her disease has. Similarly, Randall Lincoln, who has advanced sickle cell anemia, is heroically resuscitated, kept alive through weeks of coma by sophisticated equipment at extraordinary cost (239), to be displayed at a fundraising event as an exemplar of the hospital's success, while in actuality he is a pathetic, doomed travesty of a human being. These hopeless cases are a foil to the novel's two central characters, both of whose minor ailments are grotesquely overtreated. Ivy Tarro, who turns out to have a clogged mammary gland from breast-feeding, nearly succumbs to the effects of a wholly inappropriate toxic drug infused in response to a misdiagnosis. And when Mimi, a hospital volunteer, is struck by an agonizing pain in her back, she is taken (because her doctor is away) to the emergency room, where she is "rendered virtually immobile all day, strapped, led, wheeled, carted" like "an anonymous log" by people who "were firm, kind, and paid no attention" (259). X-rays, an electrocardiogram, ultrasound, and blood enzyme tests reveal nothing, and she is scheduled for an angiogram when it is noticed that she has "a terrible bruise" (263) on her back. Johnson, who dedicates the book to her physician husband and to "many other friends who are doctors, with affection and apologies," has a sharp eye for the defects in the hospital system and steers with considerable skill between the tragic and the comic. But the sentimental strain of romance between Dr. Philip Watts, a senior professor of medicine, and his patient, Ivy, is an incongruous intrusion that undermines the novel's realism and detracts from serious consideration of its implicit issues.

This flaw is even more pronounced in a narrative that has attained notoriety in the medical community, *The House of God* (1978). Published under the pseudonym Samuel Shem, it is a first-person, quasi-autobiographical rendition of the experiences of the internship year. Since the author is himself a physician, the account has a basis of authenticated inside familiarity with hospital practices. But the characters and happenings are so grossly exaggerated as to amount to a mockery. The parody is most fully exemplified in the "Laws of the House of God" (420), which are impressed upon the interns: one of them, for instance, mandates: "At a cardiac arrest, the first procedure is to take your own pulse," while another rules: "The delivery of medical care is to do as much nothing as possible." The consistent message is physicians' prior obligation to care for their own welfare instead of being exploited, exasperated, and exhausted by patients' insatiable demands. This representation of patients as predatory aggressors against whom doctors must protect themselves as best they can is a cynical reversal of medical etiquette. Although many of the incidents are hilarious, all too often the humor becomes farcical and salacious. The interns' main objective, apart from self-preservation, is sex with the nurses. As a picture of the late-twentieth-century hospital *The House of God* moves beyond satire to slapstick comedy, where buffoonery dislodges plausibility. Yet does not physicians' overt anger at this image of hospital life perhaps suggest a tiny core of veracity to the parody?

The House of God and *Health and Happiness* both dwell on that staple of popular hospital culture, the romance between members of the staff or between physician and patient. This motif is peremptorily dismissed by Robert Klitzman in *A Year-Long Night* (1989) as a feature of "Hospital TV" (109) and a rarity in real institutions because of the extreme fatigue and time pressures under which doctors often work. Klitzman's book is one of three autobiographical accounts of medical education that appeared in a cluster in the later 1980s: Perri Klass's *Not Entirely Benign Procedure* (1987) and Melvin Konner's *Becoming A Doctor* (1987) are the other two. All of them deal with the rites of initiation into the profession through their hospital service, and all express concern about the dehumanizing impact of this process on budding young doctors. The etiquette of power inculcated in the 1980s is seen as having a deleterious effect on medical practice, especially on the interaction with patients.

These works are particularly valuable for the insight they afford into the contemporary hospital through the eyes of writers who are simultaneously outsiders and insiders. As newcomers to medicine, they still possess a freshness of perception that enables them to see with great clarity the qualities and

deficiencies of the accepted etiquette. At the same time, however, they cannot remain detached because they themselves are being assimilated into the
profession. So they record the rituals of entry, focusing on the inner and outer
difficulties they encounter as they are socialized into the proper behaviors.
All of them come to acquire a better understanding of the rationale motivating the conduct of doctors toward their patients, yet despite their acquiescence
in the prevailing professional ethos, they continue, to varying degrees, to
question and to resist those aspects that strike them as reprehensible. Their
double status as novices being turned into competent practitioners grants
them a unique perspective from which to appraise current hospital medicine.
That this dualistic vision is the mainspring and prerequisite for their writing
is most categorically enunciated by Klass: "I have to see and hear things not
only as a doctor, who would take most hospital sights, most medical locutions,
completely for granted, but also as a nondoctor" (16). And the exemption of
these autobiographical narratives from the necessity of constructing the neat
plot expected in a fiction reduces the likelihood of the sort of idealization
or demonization common in popular novels and films.

   Although these three accounts are fundamentally similar, they differ in
several respects. The writers concentrate on diverse segments of their apprenticeship and organize their narratives in disparate ways. Konner centers
his on the third year in medical school because he regards it as crucial since
it is "the first of total clinical immersion" (xii), when the student is fully involved in daily work with patients. He moves in a strictly linear progression
through his rotations in the emergency ward, anesthesiology, surgery, neu-
rosurgery and neurology, psychiatry, pediatrics, obstetrics, gynecology,
pathology, and medicine. The symmetry of his design is completed by a chapter entitled "The Fourth Year" and a conclusion, corresponding in reverse
order to the opening introduction and the chapter entitled "Basic Clinical
Skills." Klitzman opts for a later stage, the internship year, when the newly
minted M.D. crosses another major threshold by assuming at least partial responsibility for diagnosis and treatment. Accordingly, each of his chapters
turns on a single case even as he too rotates through medicine, emergency
room, neurology, and pediatrics. As in *Becoming A Doctor*, the disposition in *A
Year-Long Night* is chronological, following the academic year from July to
June, although the sequence here is more loosely picaresque and more dramatic in its greater concentration on the fate of patients than on the learning

experience. In contrast to the compact time frame of the year chosen by Konner and Klitzman, Klass's is expansive, covering all her four years as a medical student episodically in a mixture of the chronological and the topical. She is more issue- than case-oriented, partly because she takes in the entire span of medical school and partly owing to the fact that her book originated as discrete pieces for a weekly column in the *New York Times* and occasional articles for journals.

Both Klass's and Konner's viewpoints are decisively shaped by their personal circumstances. Klitzman, however, remains reticent about his identity beyond his professional persona. He divulges nothing about his history or situation, not even his age or appearance. The result of this discretion is a narratorial "I" that is shadowy to the verge of disembodiment. Only at Thanksgiving is he seen in relation to family members, and even then it is above all in his new capacity as a medical man. But what seems at first a somewhat disconcerting lacuna in fact underscores the main point of *A Year-Long Night*: the absorption in the microcosm of the institution so complete as to result in the virtual obliteration of the world outside and the temporary submergence of the self. When he finally comes off his last thirty-six-hour shift he experiences a surprise that is like a rebirth. "My mind was drained, and I felt weak. My legs barely held up my body. I walked into the white sunlight outside and gazed at people strolling up and down the sidewalk, looking healthy and free from IV poles. Familiar yellow taxicabs hurtled down the street uncaring. I had forgotten that the world still existed outside. I was surprised to see it, fresh, again" (222). The renewal of ordinary life in the bright natural light is a metaphoric spring after the year-long winter of darkness and anguish that the internship denotes for him.

Konner and Klass, by contrast, openly address the ways in which their personal lives impinged on their training and directly contributed to the shaping of their vision. Konner was in his early thirties when he embarked on medical training, with a Ph.D. in anthropology, a major book, and a successful teaching career to his credit. He has a good measure of intellectual self-confidence and a secure family base in his wife and two small children and, beyond that, the wider circle of parents, uncles, and aunts. Although he maintains that his age, his "atypical turn of mind," and his "stage of life" make him "not ideal for medical school" (28), it is arguably those very traits that make him an ideal *writer* about medical school. He cites his familiarity with anthropological methods, which he feels to be in his bones, as his greatest asset in his analytical record of his initial encounters with clinical medicine: "I am an anthropologist trained to study odd and complex social worlds through the marvelous prism of participant observation" (xiv). Konner is fully conscious of, even self-conscious about, this capacity to be at once participant and observer: "I *was* in and out of it at one and the same time" (xvii), he remarks as he finds himself frequently "watching doctors instead of trying my damnedest to become like them" (xvi–xvii). Besides a certain maturity, he has a professional eye that enables him to interpret the ritualistic behaviors he registers. The circumstances of his personal life as a husband, father, son, and nephew are also introduced fairly often, notably as he weighs the pros and cons of his position compared with the relative freedom of his younger fellow students. While his status as a father intensifies his pleasure in obstetrics and his attraction to pediatric endocrinology, it is ultimately his professional gaze as an anthropologist that is the foremost characteristic of the narrator of *Becoming A Doctor*.

In *A Not Entirely Benign Procedure* the family issues that are a backdrop to Konner's training stand in the forefront. Klass had done some graduate work in zoology and spent a year abroad, but the determining factor in her life is the baby she has during her second year in medical school. As a result she has constantly to juggle her time in order to arrange care and feeding schedules between her own obligations and those of her graduate student husband. Like Konner, she sees her embedment in family as both an advantage and a drawback: after long stretches on duty she imagines coming home to a quiet, calm apartment instead of to a noisy six-month-old, but she also realizes how restorative it is to go back to such a sound family life. Klass's role as mother more immediately affects her medical existence than does Konner's as a father. She feels outrage at the lack of instruction about normal pregnancy in favor of concentration solely on potential pathological complications (48–51). In a comical but revealing episode ("Baby Poop," 177–83) she makes the mistake of offering to change the diaper of an infant who is the object of a neurological consultation. The doctors prefer to endure an unpleasant smell for forty minutes rather than to stoop to the indignity of a nurse's work. Klass learns a lesson about the separation she is expected to make between her professional and her private persona, yet she continues to insist on the import on her medical education of her sensibility as a woman and a mother.

The differing emphases of these works are conveyed in their titles. Konner's *Becoming A Doctor* is the most direct and straightforward, while his subtitle, "A Journey of Initiation in Medical School," points to his anthropological perspective. Klass's *Not Entirely Benign Procedure* is much more artful. As an inverted mimicry of medical parlance, it is an irony of understatement that immediately implies a critical, somewhat mocking stance. Even more evocative is Klitzman's *Year-Long Night*, a metaphorical title that is glossed in the subtitle, "Tales of a Medical Internship." The phrase "year-long night," borrowed from William Morris's *Earthly Paradise*, forms one of Klitzman's epigraphs. The other, from Walt Whitman's *Hospital Days*, speaks of "the whole interest of the land, north and south [as] one vast central hospital." Taken together, Klitzman's title and epigraphs project somberness, sorrow, weariness, the perception of the internship as a long dark tunnel, almost an earthly hell. The image is upheld throughout the narrative: toward the middle of the year he says, "I had ceased to believe I'd see the light of day again" (99). The sustained metaphor from the title serves as a substitute frame for Klitzman's "tales" in place of the cognitive reflections characteristic of Konner and Klass. Klitzman's method is more distinctively literary as he uses a poetic motif rather than the personal element as the unifying thread.

The presence of metaphor as well as such other marks of literariness as patterns of repetition and contrast raises a question that needs to be considered as a preliminary to analysis of the way these writers eye the institution and its power structure: to what extent have the personal, autobiographical experiences been metamorphized into fiction? Clearly, autobiography can offer only a version of a truth because it is filtered through the eyes of the self-beholding author. What is the nature of the interface between the autobiographical and the fictive in these three works, and above all, how does it modify their credibility?

All three writers draw directly on their immediate memories of initiation into the profession. They show varying levels of awareness of a possible tension between the demands of truthfulness, of individual, perhaps idiosyncratic input, and of vivid reportage. Konner, who gives the most thought to this issue, explains in his preface his deliberate choice to steer his narrative between the social-science mode, "cast in appropriate psychologese" (xiii), and "what they call in Hollywood a 'punched-up' docudrama" (xiv). He decides to resort to generic names in an "effort to protect the privacy of the patients, physicians and other persons who appear in this book, as well as the confidentiality of the proceedings or relations described" (ix); so his is the Galen Memorial Hospital of the Flexner School of Medicine. Apart from this screen, however, he is remarkably forthright, especially in regard to his own reactions and feelings. He makes a fine point about the interplay between objectivity and subjectivity: "I have attempted to give an objective account of what I experienced, but I have not pretended that it is an objective account of what happened; on the contrary, I have tried to describe all events in the light of a full and frank subjectivity: my subjectivity as an anthropologist; as an educator; as a husband and father in his middle thirties; and as a medical student and future physician" (360). Klitzman opts for an entirely different approach: though of the three he is the most inclined to both metaphor and the dramatizing dialogue normative in a novel, he is at the same time largely self-effacing. He tries to extend objectivity by acting as a sort of registering and recording conduit with a minimum of cognitive reflection. By deemphasizing the personal aspects of his internship he underscores their universality as typical of that phase of medical education. Despite his often intense emotional involvement, he chooses to concentrate on his responses as a professional rather than as a particularized human being. Klass is at the opposite pole to Klitzman in her tendency to self-dramatization. In the section "A Weekend in the Life" (249–74) she shifts openly into fictionalization in chronicling two days in the life of an alter ego called "Elizabeth which is, in fact, my middle name" and "who is more than a little like me" (251). Though this "story" is an exception in *A Not Entirely Benign Procedure,* it is indicative of the method whereby Klass moves out of her self in order to watch her own performance. The outer experience is a platform for the elaboration of her inner reactions. This is very apparent in her presentation of her role in the attempt to resuscitate a patient (147–52), where she envisages herself as an actor in a drama. In a corresponding crisis Konner sees himself as a bystanding observer (102). It is precisely his intermediate position as a semi-participating spectator and his explicit admission of the imbrication of the subjective in the objective that makes him the most thoughtful and balanced witness of the hospital scene.

In the arduous process of education and socialization the interaction with patients is central in enabling students to learn both the appropriate medical treatments and the appropriate etiquette. All the apprentices at first feel acute apprehension stemming from their fear of actually inflicting harm on a patient through lack of manual dexterity or as a result of an oversight but also from a deeper anxiety about their own adequacy to their chosen profession. *Terrifying* and *terrified* are adjectives Klass uses again and again to describe her reactions to the ever new challenges she has to face. "The clinical years, especially the third year, are in some ways a very harsh experience. It is frightening to feel yourself very ignorant in a setting where sick people are depending on you for care. It is terrifying to learn on patients how to start an IV. You worry about making a mistake. You worry about hurting someone" (57). The "you" form that Klass uses here is a way of drawing readers into her experiences by appealing to their capacity to identify with her. One antidote to the terror for Klass is the comfort of food, but it cannot counteract the worst of the fears that come with the transition from medical student to doctor, the "terror of responsibility" (149)—and power. Hands-on procedures such as setting up intravenous lines, drawing arterial blood, doing lumbar punctures, or performing minor surgical repairs, initially done under supervision and with advice ("talked through"), rapidly fall to the charge of the novice on the much-quoted principle "See one, do one, teach one," which, as Klitzman ruefully points out, "ignores a beginner's anxiety, doubt, or clumsiness" (94). In his internship Klitzman goes through that most frightening passage from student to freshly qualified physician left solely responsible for the care of desperately sick patients. Though formally empowered by his M.D., he feels bereft of power because of his inexperience. He is especially nervous about making tough decisions on little sleep at night when the senior attending faculty member would hardly welcome a call (112). His anxiety blooms whenever he thinks he hears his name on the pager (9), and he notices the same "nervous insecurity" (112) in his fellow interns. Even on the last day, he admits that "the level of anxiety I felt at the beginning of the year when on call never fully dissipated" (218), although he has come to take for granted certain things and expressions that are alienating to his "timorous" (221) successor. Konner alone writes also of the increasing empowerment that is the reward for the fear overcome. Like the others, he has his "most anxious moment" (23) at his first encounter with patients; he is plain "frightened" (41) as he starts surgery and "more than a little apprehensive" (190) in the emergency room. He is even more categorically aware than the others of the doctor's "ready acceptance of responsibility, with all its practical, legal, and social consequences" (37), a responsibility that weighs heavily on him "although surrounded by people who could take over if I failed" (76). But the apprehension slowly yields to a sense of his growing competence and confidence, so that fear is tempered by exhilaration. Finally, he understands the power that medical knowledge confers, "the surge of almost spiritual energy that accompanies the successful clinical encounter" (367), and that is compensation for all the terrors and hardships.

Together with fear, all three suffer initially from the disturbing sense that they are merely enacting the role of doctor. The motif of role playing recurs frequently: "as an 'apprentice'" on clinical rotations, Klass explains, "you get to play, more or less, the role of doctor" (155). Klitzman is even more specific: "I played the doctor role and sought cues in following my part as much as they [patients] did. Sometimes more. I uttered lines that I thought a doctor would utter, acting with the model of the discreet, empathic professional in my mind" (111). His model is derived in part from the hospital dramas that patients love to watch on television, although he ruefully notes that the TV doctors seem "less harried than I, unscarred by years of medical training, . . . more leisurely, casual and friendly" (109) with their patients. Klitzman also realizes how he changes his role according to the needs of each patient: "I acted gentler, firmer, or more paternal depending on the patient. The characters influenced each other. The lines that I delivered to a patient affected how he understood his disease and his body, how he felt and replied" (110). Various words here—"acted," "characters," "lines"—are pointers to the presence of an unwritten script innate to the culture and interpreted by both doctors and patients in fulfillment of the expected etiquette. Konner regards the role as "a kind of game-playing, even a kind of lying" (20) as he begins his clinical work. He spells out in precise cognitive terms the cardinal components of the role and its accompanying gestures: "the physician must be firm and authoritative" (108); "in encountering any patient one must do whatever is necessary to give the patient the feeling that one is 'The Doctor'; if for a particular patient, for example, the doctor is the one who takes the blood pressure, then we must take the blood pressure, even if there is no rational reason for doing it" (19). This is an acknowledgment of the etiquette that determines the behavior of doctor and patient alike. The physician must assert power, if necessary by a superfluous act such as taking blood pressure, in order to establish in the patient's mind the image of the doctor in control.

Gradually, with the accumulation of skill and experience and the concomitant increase in self-confidence, the role turns from a consciously assumed posture into second nature. Konner repeatedly writes of occasions that make him "feel like a doctor" (194),[16] of his pride and gratification when he begins to "feel like an integral part of the team" (209), is consulted by relatives, friends, and neighbors, and does a good job of removing a large splinter from his landlady's thumb (296). The same self-assurance comes to Klass as she stitches up lacerations in the emergency room, an act that makes her "feel like a real doctor" (100). Konner concedes as well the comical underside of his new perspective when he zooms in on the good veins on the arms of a young woman sitting opposite him on the bus long before he notices how beautiful she is. Similarly, at a film version of *La Traviata*, one of his favorite operas, he catches himself "unable to banish medical thoughts" about Violetta's consumption (297). When he is consulted by his aunts at Thanksgiving, Klitzman also derives satisfaction from "beginning to think of myself as a physician, growing more confident, knowing what questions to ask of patients, what answers to give and what maneuvers to perform" (121). The absorption of the etiquette is an important concomitant of the acquisition of skills and knowledge in transforming the novice into the adept.

The apprentice physicians also learn from their occasional assumption of the patient's role. Klass does this imaginatively when she projects herself into the position of a patient at the mercy of a gauche medical student trying to do a spinal tap (118–19). At one point she is so exhausted that she indulges in a fantasy about trading places with the patient by getting into bed and being looked after. Interestingly, she equates the surrender of power with the bestowal of care as if power and care were counter poles, power being the doctor's right and care the patient's. When her pregnancy turns her into an actual patient, she is so informed as to be highly dissatisfied, particularly at the dearth of advice about such ordinary matters as nutrition and exercise. Konner's special interest in "the human dimensions of patient needs and patient care" (x), in addition to his age, inclines him throughout his training to identify "more with patients than with doctors" (xvi). He is himself thrust into the patient's part several times: when he takes his mother to consult a cardiologist, who proves a model of sagacity and courtesy; when his wife has to go to an emergency room because she has developed a high fever during a vacation; and when he himself is struck by agonizing pain on a Saturday evening following root canal treatment. His wife's long wait and his own difficulty in getting pain relief not only reinforce his understanding of the exasperated patient's angle but also make him query the prevalent etiquette of power. Only Klitzman cannot "imagine himself ever being a patient" (53), which is surely an unconscious defense mechanism. For as Dr. McKee in the film *The Doctor* reminds his imperious physician, who insists on scheduling solely at her convenience, sooner or later all medical personnel will in turn become patients. And then the tables of power will be turned.

The reminder is certainly timely, for nowhere is the balance of power portrayed in as adversarial a light as in the modern hospital. To grapple with the dominant indifference or hostility to patients is one of the major difficulties facing the initiates into the profession. Klitzman, for instance, is encouraged to regard each new patient as "a potential opportunity to learn" (96), which implies that the patients are there for his benefit, not vice versa. Konner notes quite early "that ignoring patients was normative" (56), for "the patient is on the lowest rung of the hospital ladder of authority" (83). Klass likewise emphasizes the power element inherent in the doctors' view of the patient's position: "Patients can be seen as territory, decisions as power, medical disagreements as personal challenges" (158–59). Consequently, "all too often the patient comes to personify the disease, and somehow the patient becomes the enemy" (81). This association of the patient with the disease underlies the patient's dehumanization and also spawns resentment in the physician if the patient fails to respond to treatment. "When the disease has essentially won and the patient continues to present the challenge, the macho doctor is left with no appropriate response. He cannot sidestep the challenge by offering comfort rather than combat, because comfort is not in his repertoire. And unable to do battle against the disease to any real effect, he may feel almost ready to battle the patient" (82). Although Klass imputes this behavior primarily to the "macho" male doctor, she finds it prevalent throughout the hospital and among women physicians too.

Konner also uses the word "enemy" (373), which evokes a battle between doctor and patient instead of the cooperation and friendship that were taken as the norm in the nineteenth century. If the tension stems in part from the reduction of patients to their diseases, it is also, as Konner grasps, the crux of a vicious circle, for "the sense of the patient as the cause of one's distress contributes to the doctor's detachment" (56). He cites time pressures on residents as a reason for their medical style: "They focused more narrowly on the present illness, showed less concern for the patient's or, certainly, the family's general health; paid less attention to behavioral and social factors in the patient's illness, were more abrupt and brusque and less responsive to the patient as a human being" (33). Repeatedly he castigates residents whose bedside manner betrays "listlessness, condescension, or patent fakery" (52). A similar exclusion of the human aspect, "tears shed, the slow acceptance of disability or death" as "secondary to the case" (110) is noted by Klitzman in senior physicians too. A woman with a rare progressive disease is demonstrated to students "as a sample of impaired neurological hardware, a malfunctioning computer" (165). Although Klitzman obviously condemns such a stance, he envisages the patient as having been forced to surrender autonomy, for "to be sick means to have used up one's resources" (85). To come to the hospital thus implies a readiness to submit to medical power because one's own psychological and physical reserves are exhausted. This seems like a late-twentieth-century psychologized reiteration of the nineteenth-century perception of hospital patients as self-selected victims of adversity, whose helplessness almost legitimates the churlishness meted out to them. That is certainly not Klitzman's personal view but a rationalization of the power structure he observes in the hospital, with its latent contempt for patients.

The indifference to the patient as a person that is a persistent leitmotif in these three autobiographies is confirmed by testimony from other sources. Twentieth-century doctors are said to have become "so laboratory-minded, so scientific, and so impersonal, that they forgot, or felt entitled to ignore, the patient as a person."[17] From a historicist perspective Starr points to the change from the nineteenth-century doctor's obligation to travel on visits to his twentieth-century successor's static location in office or hospital.[18] This change has both therapeutic and economic advantages for the doctor in that it gives him or her access to clinical equipment and ancillary personnel, as well as increased income because of the time saved. The physician's time becomes a precious commodity to which patients must defer. One of those interviewed in Mark L. Rosenberg's sensitive study complains: "My intern comes in at weird times, like ten or eleven o'clock at night. She seems more concerned about what other people are going to think of her than she is concerned about what is good for me." Medical students breeze in during breakfast and "expect you to do something when and because they want you to do it."[19] The hospital's organized routines have to take precedence over the patient's rhythms. But teamwork and delegation jeopardize the continuity of the doctor-patient relationship. In teaching hospitals, where patients are seen by a throng of "doctors," they often do not know who is in charge, who in effect is their doctor. The interaction of patients with hospital doctors is characterized by the absence of long-term relations. Physicians in training or those engaged in research, Starr points out, "do not require their patients' good will for future business."[20] This factor is mentioned by Konner in connection with Marty, an abrasive surgical resident: at least in private practice "a man like Marty would be as much at the mercy of his patients as they would be at his" (120). Outside the hospital, patients still retain some power as the payees, although with managed care they are increasingly being stripped of that element of choice.

An adversarial attitude toward patients is connected to the necessity for defense mechanisms to protect physicians from the pain they must confront every day. How to develop a proper degree of detachment is one of the main challenges in medical training with which all three writers constantly struggle. Konner is quite shocked that "making fun of patients" in the minor surgery room "was a regular part of the morning ritual" (60) for the residents. In another instance a chief resident makes fun of a patient by asking a series of completely unnecessary questions (135). In the emergency room a game is played, "The Wheel of Pain," on the analogy of television shows, to decide which pain medication to prescribe (70). All these bizarre episodes represent assertions of medical supremacy through unconscious but firm separation from the suffering of patients. Already in the preclinical lecture courses Konner had learned that "vulgar jokes about patients are a ubiquitous feature of medical social life, excused (and perhaps excusable) as a 'necessary defense mechanism' in the face of illness and death" (18). Konner's inner growth in the course of the year is indicated by his deeper understanding of the residents' alienating behavior. "As the days went by, I also began to understand more fully the bitterness and cynicism some of the residents in the field exhibited. It was brutally difficult to face these patients day by day, to see the extremity of their need, to know that they needed you to do whatever you could, and yet to be able to do so pathetically little for most of them" (136–37). Here it is the inadequacy of medical power and the unavowed sense of their own helplessness that underlies doctors' forbidding behavior. To avoid acknowledging the limitations of the physician's power is an even deeper mode of self-preservation than detachment from patients' pain.

Klitzman learns the same distancing "from a visceral reaction" (128) when he comes up against the failure of medicine in the autopsy of a patient of his:

> The pathologist, Dr. Spain, rolled out a cart stacked with what looked like cookie sheets. He pulled them out one by one and displayed them on the table. Each held a different organ. One tray exhibited the kidneys, another held slices of the liver neatly cut and laid out. "Here come the appetizers," Walt joked.
>
> The conference is nicknamed "The Man in the Pan."
>
> A cold air chilled my shoulders. My mind distanced these piles of flesh from the man who had been my patient, his brown eyes, and the smile I had once seen. (74)

This is his most testing experience, and it teaches him to resort in surgery to the intellectualization recommended by the psychiatrist who had addressed the interns during orientation: "I resumed my position, observing fat, flesh, and blood. This conglomeration wasn't soup, I told myself, but was anatomy. I tried to concentrate on how a surgeon must look at it. I began to see it as only 'tissue' and not as something human" (127). Yet he also chooses the word "numbed," in a negative connotation, to describe the process of desensitization (130) and does not conceal his own descent "to a scavenging beast, an automaton" when he gulps down, "emotionless and guiltless" (101), and incidentally unheated, the supper left uneaten by a patient who has just died. The process of taking possession of power exacts its toll.

The counterpart to Klitzman's toughening through pathology and surgery occurs for Klass in the pediatric intensive care ward, where she notices the staff's "self-protective mechanisms" (35). Detachment and the exercise of power are of particular concern to Klass as a woman entering what in the early 1980s was still a predominantly male profession. "Some of the women in my class . . . worry that they aren't tough enough, that they cannot afford to pass up any opportunity to prove, to themselves and to everyone else, that they have what it takes" (32). She herself, like many of the other women medical students, is "haunted by the prospect of crying in the hospital. . . . It seems to hover on the edge of our minds as something we are likely to do, something we must not do because it will confirm all the most clichéd objections to women as doctors. Crying will compromise our professionalism as well as our strength" (63–64). Nevertheless, she confesses that she did cry because she forgot to do things, or did not know how to do them, or found them to have been unnecessary, as well as out of sheer fatigue or sympathy admixed with self-pity, "but I took great care not to be seen at it" (64). When she asks her male fellow students whether they ever cried, they deny it; she wonders whether men are indeed slower to cry or maybe just too ashamed and therefore lying. To give in to tears is to subvert the image of power quintessential to the healer.

In the process of creating detachment from the patient language plays an important role. With her practiced writer's awareness of words, Klass has special insight into the function of medical jargon "to help doctors maintain some distance from their patients. By reformulating patients' pain and problems into a language that the patient doesn't speak, I suppose we are in some sense taking those pains and problems under our jurisdiction and also reducing their emotional impact" (76). Klass sees the translation of illness into professional terms of disease as an assumption of responsibility by physicians and at the same time a manifestation of power as knowledge and vice versa. For this reason all three writers insist upon the urgency of picking up colloquial usages as an essential facet of their initiation. Klass has a section entitled "Learning the Language" (73–77), Konner appends "A Glossary of House Officer Slang" (379–90), and Klitzman elaborates on pathology's preference for food names in describing diseased organs: "nutmeg tumors," "blueberry muffin lesions," "Swiss cheese endometrium" (76).

Hospital slang, which consists largely of acronyms and neologisms often derived from abbreviations, has a signification beyond its primary purpose as a kind of shorthand communication. It replaces the Latin formerly used in the medical world and now present only residually, for instance in "stat" (for *statim,* "immediately"). Like Latin, the current idiom satisfies the need for a private language that can be freely used in the presence of patients to discuss their problems openly but secretly. Besides this exclusionary purpose, it also has an inclusionary dimension in bonding those privy to the esoteric signals. Precisely because it is a mark of membership, it is pervasive among junior physicians, for whom the acquisition and adoption of this casual lingo is a step toward attaining professional empowerment. Mastery of this language denotes a particular sort of understanding that unites the medical community and endows it with the authority of knowledge.

A few of the acronyms have been absorbed into everyday parlance: "IV," "OD," and "D and C," for example, have become common terms, although laypeople may be unsure what the abbreviations stand for. Many belong simply to the conventions of record keeping: "sx" for "symptoms," "Nl" for "normal," "NAD" for "no apparent distress," and so forth. Others are more technical, pertaining to diagnoses or to procedures: "MI" for myocardial infarction, "COLD" for chronic obstructive lung disease, "BUN" for "blood urea nitrogen," a measure of heart failure, ""CHF" for congestive heart failure, "PCP" for "pneumocystic carinii pneumonia," and "FTT" for "failure to thrive." Procedural acronyms include "NG" for "nasogastric tube," "LP" for "lumbar puncture," "PFT" for "pulmonary function tests," "ECT" for "electroconvulsive therapy," "EKG" for "electrocardiogram," "CABG" (pronounced "cabbage") for "coronary artery bypass graft." More complicated are those acronyms with a didactic function, designed to help students to learn what ought to be done in case of certain symptoms. Konner calls these "alphabet soups," (344), citing "SOB = EKG + CXR + ABG," for "shortness of breath equals (requires) electrocardiogram plus chest x-ray plus arterial blood gases," or "AVUP" for "a cursory neurologic exam: A is Alert. V—not alert but responds to vocal stimuli. P—doesn't respond except to painful stimuli. U—unresponsive" (55). The same letters can also stand for "Awake, Vomiting, Pupils, Urination," important indicators of the level of brain or spinal cord damage.

More revealing than these technical abbreviations are those that drift from the denotative to the judgmental: "FLK" for "funny looking kid," "LOL" for "little old lady," "007s" for "licensed to kill," that is, bad doctors, "GOK" for "God only knows," an admission of inability to establish a diagnosis, and "gomer," originally an acronym for "get out of my emergency room," applied to any old, decrepit, hopeless patient whose care will be a thankless task. Like "gomer," many of the slang terms are indicative of the doctors' perception of patients, often crossing quite inventively into the realm of metaphor. Drawing on sporting terminology, every patient is a "player," and one who has a problem difficult to remediate is deemed "hard-wired." A "hit" is a newly admitted patient whose workup may well take a good hour; a "wall" is a house officer on duty in the emergency room who knows how to prevent unnecessary admissions; a "sieve" is the opposite, one who easily permits admission, and a "pump" pushes for the hospitalization of patients who do not really need it. To "buff" and to "turf" mean respectively to make patients look so much better that they can be transferred to another service. If the "turf" is unsuccessful, the patient is said to "bounce," like a bad check. Black humor creeps in when a patient given to hematomas is described as a "hematomato" or when an extremely rare disease, read about in textbooks and much in the minds of medical students, is called a "zebra." Much of this medical slang, like the judgmental acronyms, expresses feelings, generally of a negative nature, about those so designated. Apart from "gomer," various other terms of contempt are used to characterize patients: a "dirtball" may be a chronic alcoholic, drug abuser, bag lady, or street person who rarely washes, has frequent infectious contacts, and is likely to be host to a multitude of threatening microorganisms; a "worm" is a hateful, treacherous, dishonest patient; a "boarder" is one who has been "turfed" from another unit; a "crock" is a hypochondriac or a somatizer; and a "dud" is one with no medically interesting findings. The only grudgingly benign term for a patient is "rose," for one who is completely "buffed," not necessarily well but ready to be moved on. The striking feature of this vernacular is the barely repressed aggression against patients who are seen as challenges or even threats to the physician's rule. The subtext is one of discord between doctor and patient in which the doctor has to fight to maintain sovereignty.

The power structure within the profession is also formulated in slang: a "twit in the pit" is a house officer in the emergency room; "fleas" is the term applied by surgeons to medical doctors because they are thought to be the last to leave a dying body; a parallel pejorative used by surgeons of nonsurgeons, "mope," is, like "gomer," a neologism developed from the acronym MOP, for medical outpatient physicians, who take care of trivial conditions by slow and uncertain methods under no pressure; "money changers" are private physicians, often in prosperous group practices, whose work cannot be trusted because of the profit motive. A slightly self-aggrandizing image is projected by the terms "metabolic rounds" for food breaks and "liver rounds" for a social gathering. Though humorous, both terms suggest that medical personnel, while in the hospital, are always engaged in patient care, so that eating and socializing are turned into another kind of "rounds."

Much of this "deleterious terminology" centers on bad occurrences in treatment that disempower the doctor.[21] There are multiple euphemisms for dying: she "boxed"; he is "crumpling on me"; she "coded," that is, required full emergency measures for resuscitation. A patient close to death may be said to be "circling the drain" or, in another phrase derived from the arena of sport, "dribbling off the court." Less catastrophic happenings are conveyed in the same style: he "dropped his pressure"; she "bumped her enzymes"; he "failed chemotherapy"; she "blew her IV." The crucial factor in all these locutions is the active tense of the verb, with the patient as the subject. In other words, the patient is cast as the actant, as the responsible and culpable agent for any turn for the worse. By this means the physician is, by syntax and so by implication, absolved of any blame as the grammatical construction imposes it on the patient. The resort to the active voice of the verb at one and the same time exculpates the physician and expresses an unmistakable hostility toward the patient for failing to respond positively to medical interventions. Hospital language is, therefore, not only a convenient means of rapid communication and an oblique defense mechanism but also a robust affirmation of medical power.

The detachment and the struggle for domination discernible in hospital slang do not, however, exclude genuine caring allied to the primary purpose of curing. How to achieve the necessary equipoise between distance and humaneness is another recurrent problem for novices to the profession. Despite their explicitly or implicitly critical stance, all three of the accounts contain heartening examples of humane solicitude for patients through the tactful use of medical power. Konner expresses admiration for a number of the senior teaching faculty, notably the "simple human decency" of one excellent internist: "He was simply *with* patients. . . . He had a penetrating gaze that was medically critical yet full of convincing practical warmth. . . . He cared, professionally, about the nonmedical aspects of his patients' problems—their characters, their families, their situations, their incomes" (38). He has similar praise for both a pharmacological psychiatrist whose bedside manner "*was* wonderful" (162), putting some of the most seriously ill patients at their ease, and the pediatric endocrinologist who is "the most sensitive clinician" (203). He also notes the considerate neurosurgical resident who carries a flashlight pointed at the ceiling on 6:00 A.M. rounds "instead of flipping the lights on and parading in with the troops to a dazed, half-asleep, psychologically stunned patient" (128). He contrasts the "curt officialese peppered with medical jargon" (300) used by one woman doctor in speaking to the daughter of a recently deceased patient with the conduct of another physician who, in a parallel situation, "went to the waiting room to talk with [the family]. He sat down close to them, facing the wife directly. He spoke slowly and softly. He looked straight into her eyes. And . . . he took her hand" (315). This genuineness is the opposite of the mechanistic behavior of those who "smile at their patients, when they can, in something like the way flight attendants smile at their passengers" (375). Konner very much emphasizes the value of listening, and his belief that medical students, because they have more time, can give significant support to patients by a willingness to lend an attentive ear: "I sat down and listened to him" (145); or with a patient who is facing the prospect of imminent death: "You just sit there and stay there and listen and say a few words. Mainly you listen" (153), sitting back in the chair and not looking at one's watch.

Klitzman too appreciates the importance of listening.[22] He shows a compassionate understanding of difficult, noncompliant patients and far exceeds the call of duty in tracking down the background of an aphasic old woman whom he later even visits in a nursing home. Like Konner, he encounters a wide spectrum in physicians' attitudes, ranging from the chief resident who is "looking for good patient material" (31) to present as teaching specimens to the neurologist who urges: "Don't treat lab tests or CAT scans. . . . Treat the patient first" (158). Klitzman evolves his own compromise: "I divided my work up by individual patients and thought in terms of a disease acting itself out in somebody's body" (30), but there are occasions when his desire to deal with patients as persons is frustrated by sheer time pressures. Klass, who seems far more competitively minded than Konner or Klitzman, has least to say about humaneness, writing it off with a certain flippancy as an insoluble problem: ". . . what about the students who are simply incompetent at dealing with people? That, after all, is a much harder skill to teach. In medical school my classmates used to joke about taking up a collection for a scholarship fund to pay all the future training expenses of a certain student, as long as he went into research and promised never to talk to or touch a patient" (121). It seems as though Klass, because she is a woman, needs throughout her training to demonstrate the toughness that makes her fear crying.

In these three works talking to patients emerges as a crucial and largely neglected aspect of care. Konner, probably because of his consciousness as an anthropologist of verbal exchange, dwells most insistently and most critically on the problem of communication. He sees the primacy of technological procedures as leading to an atrophy of human contact through speech. The maxim taught as "a categorical imperative"—Touch the patient—even if it is not strictly necessary, is drained of its communicative meaning in the hurly-burly haste of hospital routine: "The laying on of hands was reduced to the carrying out of procedures, and words exchanged with the patient were basically viewed as tools to make those procedures go more smoothly" (26). One of the most shocking incidents Konner records is the visit of the medical group to a woman who had attempted suicide and now

> lay completely constrained, weak and helpless, in a lower body cast and in one arm and shoulder cast, with tubes in her nose and in her free arm. Her face was nonetheless distressingly alert.
>
> Mark presented her to the group, and Marty asked a few perfunctory questions. No one spoke to the patient, touched her, even met her eyes during the five minutes we spent in her room. Marty was making a move to gesture the group out when she began speaking. She was looking around at the white coats in abject fear and confusion. She said wanly, in a thick regional working-class accent, "Can I have something for the pain?"
>
> Marty stopped and looked at her from where he stood about four feet from the bed. "You bet!" he barked. This was the single exchange that occurred between this patient and a physician during the daily period at bedside. (115)

The psychological interaction is complicated here by the fact that the patient's abject condition is self-inflicted, probably both provoking guilt on her part and further goading this physician's notorious insolence. In another case, an old woman hospitalized with heart disease is discharged with appropriate medications but without adequate instructions about dangerous symptoms, so that she delays returning to the emergency room until it is too late. Konner spells out the lesson that *an act of communication can sometimes be a lifesaving intervention* (277); full treatment requires words to accompany drugs and procedures. In the laments of a demented ninety-five-year-old man, "Why you do this to me? What I did to you? I never did nothing to you," Konner reads "a superb ironic commentary on the doctor-patient relationship and . . . an exaggerated symbol of failure of communication" (292).

Hospital etiquette, in Konner's eyes, comprises brusqueness, embarrassment at "acts and gestures that are other than completely instrumental" (26), attention to the immediate disease without heed to the patient's or the family's general health or to behavioral or social factors, and unresponsiveness to the patient as a human being. All these, though attributable in part to immediate time pressures, add up to a distinctive style of medicine: "humane acts not directly affecting 'care'—a word meaning neither more nor less than medical and surgical intervention for the purpose of favorably altering the course of an illness—are in short supply in the hospital world; . . . the patient's mental status is only marginally relevant to the effort at helpful verbal or nonverbal communication" (26). The quotation marks surrounding the word "care" here and the carefully interpolated explanation of its limited meaning reveal how perverted and drained the concept has become. Konner admits to being himself tongue-tied with a young paraplegic waiting in the hallway to be demonstrated to a class; although he recognizes that "patients almost always want to be spoken to by doctors (including medical students)" (24), he is at a loss what to say and relieved when an athletic-looking fellow student exclaims: "Pretty tough break." The patient's face brightens perceptibly as the emotional tension is broken. The soothing impact of a few words is vividly brought out when Konner recalls an acute, alarming illness some years back that finally led his wife to call the emergency room. "Yes, that's the flu that's going round this season. It causes nausea and vomiting. It lasts a few days" (202). "A transfer of the simplest information had healing power," Konner comments (202). The value of the "'therapeutic alliance'—a doctor-patient relationship tending to promote understanding of the illness and compliance with the treatment" (130) is a grossly underestimated factor in the balance of power within and beyond the hospital.

This atrophy of communication between doctor and patient can be traced back to the development of a specific medical discourse. As the patient's subjective story is rewritten into the ritualistic, standardized format of medical records the discrepancy between the patient's experience of illness and the doctor's perception of disease becomes an obstacle to colloquy. What Fissell describes as "the disappearance of the patient's narrative" is abetted by current conventions of medical writing as much as by the primacy of the objective evidence of tests. In the eighteenth and early nineteenth centuries "the patient's and the doctor's words are one. It is easy to hear the patient's voice in the doctor's case report."[23] By the twentieth century, however, the patient's individuality has been effectively squelched by the formal conventions of medical charting. Physicians themselves have in several recent instances commented trenchantly on the pejorative effect of the prevailing mode of case presentation. The formulaic format "turns the sick person as *subject* into *object*," Arthur Kleinman laments in his penetrating study of a series of personal narratives by the chronically ill, which he compares to the stark medical account of them.[24] Like Konner, Kleinman is an anthropologist as well as a psychiatrist. Another physician with anthropological leanings, Oliver Sacks, is even more emphatic: "There is no 'subject' in a narrow case history; modern case histories allude to the subject in a cursory phrase ('a trisomic albino female of 21') which could as well apply to a rat as a human being."[25] In translating illness into disease the physician is indeed taking the patient under medical jurisdiction as a step toward cure or alleviation. Klass conceives of this practice as a benign acceptance of responsibility on the doctor's part. But it has an equivocal concomitant since patients' transposition into medical power results in the discounting of their personality.

The change in the way the patient is described has been examined in two recent studies that analyze contemporary models of medical discourse. In a comparison of the writing of case history and literary biography, Anne Hunsaker Hawkins observes that the "depersonalizing focus on the disease rather than the diseased person" immediately becomes evident.[26] She characterizes the case history as "nomothetic" (6), that is, directed to the apprehension of general laws, and biography as "idiographic" in its interest in uniqueness. So the physician's medicalized report is episodic, pragmatic, and rational, in contrast to the patient's personal story, which is holistic, historical, and imaginative. The hospital, where most likely an acute crisis is handled, is conducive to case history. On the other hand, the family practitioner or, even more, the psychiatrist, while still remaining within a stylized format, is at greater liberty to adopt a longer-term, more comprehensive view that partakes of both case history and biography.

More extensive research in this field is presented in *Doctors' Stories*, by Kathryn Montgomery Hunter, a medical humanist who accompanied hospital teams on their rounds, attended conferences, and scrutinized the ways in which patients' illnesses were discussed and charted in order to ascertain how the actual narrative structuring of medical knowledge affects the etiquette between doctor and patient. Even more than Klass, Klitzman, and Konner, she is "an outsider, far more observer than participant" (xii) in the processes she analyzes, a listener par excellence. Her ulterior purpose, namely, to investigate "the interaction between patient and physician" (xiv) in a teaching hospital, makes her book a singularly illuminating cognitive commentary on the incidents related in the three autobiographies. Hunter gives a clear definition of the aim of medical discourse as always "to eliminate or control the purely personal and subjective, whether its source be patient or physician, so that the physical anomalies that characterize illness can receive the attention their successful treatment requires. Illness is a subjective experience, and the examining physician faces the task of translating it, locating the malady in the medical universe and conveying its characteristics and their meaning to others who know the medical language well but this particular patient not at all" (52). Hunter here relates medicine's scientific character directly to the necessity for a deliberate disregard of patients as idiosyncratic individuals in favor of their existence as one of a series of similar cases. Thus the identification with science has adverse consequences for both the education of physicians and their interaction with patients, two facets that are interdependent. Physicians and patients alike are encouraged "to focus narrowly on the diagnosis of disease rather than attend to what is even more necessary, the care of the person who is ill" (xix). This conflict between cure and care is a continuation of the tendency already apparent in the nineteenth-century hospital of treating diseases rather than diseased people. The mistaken underlying assumption is that the two are mutually exclusive.

Hunter draws on terms derived from the nature of vision to render the shortcomings in physicians' view of patients: she writes of "professional shortsightedness that sees maladies rather than people as the objects of medical attention" (61) and of "the sort of epistemological scotoma in medicine" that has created the "hope of achieving a minimal, streamlined scientific account in every instance of disease" (104). The minimalism stems from the ideal of the chart as a "regular, patterned, self-effacing plot" (63), whose essence resides precisely in the eradication of personal detail as intrusive and distracting from the medical picture. So "the chart refuses awareness of the pain of human existence" (91); it strives to be a variant on the scientific report in its "plain and flat and dry" style, which seeks to banish personal involvement and to keep the medical face calm by controlling—or, in fact, repressing—"the subjectivity of the observer" (90). Consequently, the patient's and the doctor's versions of the malady are "fundamentally, irreducibly different narratives" (123). Once it has yielded its diagnostic information, the patient's version is often ignored, for much subjective experience of suffering, uncertainty, helplessness, fear of death, and anxiety over loss of autonomy is dismissed as medically irrelevant. The frequently noted proclivity in hospitals to think and speak of patients as if they had become their diagnoses, "an object with only a medical existence and only a diagnostic meaning" (137), is a direct outcome of the scientific approach predominant in twentieth-century practice.

Hunter paints a discouraging, indeed frightening picture of the patient's reification. She steers a careful if somewhat tricky course between reification and impersonality, which she characterizes as "a virtue of medicine" (82). "Impersonality is not inattention" (133); similarly, "the objective gaze," whereby the patient is "flattened" and the narrative made "relentlessly passive," far from being "cruelty," is exactly what the patient has come for in order to have established "with relative certainty what the matter is" (162). The argument is convincing to a point, yet the cumulative weight of Hunter's evidence contravenes it. The imperative of the objective gaze is beyond question, but it has a "tendency to hypertrophy," which, she avows, "is potentially harmful" (136). The complement to objectivity is not its opposite, subjectivity, but the kind of compassion that Konner in particular finds in the most outstanding of his teachers.

The precarious contradictoriness of hospital medicine in its dual allegiance to science and the patient emerges from the conflicting statements made by Klass. At one moment she insists that "there's a thread-fine line that good doctors must walk, a desperately sensitive balance to preserve, which consists of understanding for each individual patient" (214), especially in imparting deadly diagnoses. This endorsement of humaneness stands uneasily next to her jubilation at a scientific rarity: "A great case is a great case, even when it's dying" (71). Klass concedes that such an attitude "can be disturbing to a medical student who has come to see the patient as something more than a teaching exercise" (71). In her own resolution of such dissonances, she comes to realize that in the first two years already, along with the basic science and pathophysiology, "values were being taught, though not explicitly" (27). Significantly, she applies the same adjective that she uses to describe a medical student's response to a great case, "disturbing," to her own reactions to being socialized into medicine. Although she feels anger at being "at the very bottom of a fairly rigid hierarchy, . . . being treated like someone who doesn't matter, . . . being made to wait constantly" (57), she soon accepts these humiliations, along with such hardships as sleep deprivation and isolation, as integral to the toughening process "intended . . . to divide me from ordinary normal people" (32). She shows a streak of pride in likening it to an initiation "into a priesthood" (36). "Like any other subculture, medicine develops its own internal systems of values, its own hierarchies of prestige and power. And these don't necessarily have anything to do with helping patients" (69). Klass's evolution confirms Lipkin's observation: "Most students enter training intending to learn how to take care of patients. By the time they graduate, many have become more interested in the mechanisms and diagnoses of disease than in all the other activities involved in the care of the ill."[27] Put even more cynically by the dean of the medical school in *A Year-Long Night:* "Students enter medical school wanting to do good. They leave hoping to do well" (6).

Klitzman, as an intern already on a slightly higher rung of the ladder, is less concerned than Klass about hierarchy. He mentions "the politics of medicine" (5) and is aware of the tensions in the power structure, but he does not seem to be personally involved in issues. His major anxiety is how to survive the "year-long night," and his primary orientation is toward his patients. He comes across as more of a loner than the two medical students, Konner and Klass, who write of their work as members of a team. Klitzman sees the hospital as an exclusive and exclusionary microcosm with "the laws and language of a foreign country" (6). The priority of scientific pursuits over patient welfare is a reiterated theme: one instance is the physician who refuses the dying patient's wish to go home with the announcement: "I'm not giving her up now—not yet" (47), as if she were his possession. Even more crass is the doctor who persists in continuing his chemotherapy research, "indifferent" to both the patient's suffering and the fact that the treatment is ineffective (59). Usually so reticent, Klitzman interjects this laconic, unvarnished statement: "He didn't want to lose his research subject. He wanted to find out whether his concoction worked. Research studies require research subjects" (57). Strictly speaking, such practices are not misuses of medical power, but they are abuses of patients, whose personal well-being is subordinated to a stubborn pursuit of treatment literally to the bitter end. These physicians put their own interests—and pride—above those of the patient, and they are technically, if not ethically, authorized to do so by the etiquette of power, which puts them in control. For a patient to defy such control takes more energy and courage than most very sick people can muster. And it entails a challenge to the conventional wisdom that "the doctor knows best" that is tantamount to a resistance to scientific medicine and its prestige.

Of the three, Konner is by far the most troubled by the system and the most trenchant in his criticisms. "American medicine," he concludes, "is a spiritual wasteland and its practitioners impotent to confront matters of life and death other than with a test or a scalpel" (361). His previous training in social science and his maturity enable him to place experience in a wider context and to probe the values motivating the actions. His assessment of the hospital comes closest to Jewson's conceptualization of it as a collective order where authority is inherent in occupational status rather than in individually proven worth, so that moral and personal qualities recede before "strictly prescribed patterns of deference" in a hierarchical etiquette.[28] The defining thrust toward certainty and order is immediately evident to Konner in the contrast between a good graduate seminar, "arguing generously with itself, teaching itself, learning," and the single-mindedness of hospital instruction, "rigid, authoritarian, intolerant of ambiguities and constantly searching for certainties, reliable rules, unchallengeable procedures, incontrovertible facts" (56). Such stringency can result in "bad teaching" and "bad medicine" (97), a lack of flexibility detrimental to patients. Konner follows for some time a patient he names Charlotte (299 ff.), who has an organic disease for which she refuses a treatment antagonistic to the severe, active bulimia she also has. The gastroenterologist in charge resolutely denies her a psychiatric consultation—which does finally take place while he is away attending a conference. Even then he rejects any suggestion of a connection between her eating disorder and her colitis. The entire staff, from the nurses upward, are contemptuous of the treatment he orders yet obliged to carry it out. This is the grossest example in these three autobiographies of a power structure pushed to its extreme as patient and medical personnel are all coerced by the will of a single imperious physician obdurate in imposing the supremacy to which he is in fact entitled.

Konner is glad to leave internal medicine, with its "interminable hairsplitting conferences, without humane sensibility and without ethics beyond legally defensive medicine" (310–11). Yet however sharp his criticisms and however negative his ultimate verdict, he never loses a sense of proportion. His hospital comprises simply "the usual mix of marvelous, terrible, and ordinary people" (208): the terrorizing resident is neutralized by another who is "full of kindnesses" (279), and within "the emptiness of hospital medicine" he finds reassuring examples of physicians who are "real" (295) in their warmth. As if in response to the common reproach that doctors like to play God, he characterizes them as "healing artisans": "Doctors are craftspeople of the highest order. Sometimes, like engineers, they lean very heavily on science. Sometimes, like diamond cutters, they seem to be coasting along on pure skill. And occasionally, like glassblowers or goldsmiths, what they do verges on art" (xvii). The striking images in this passage affirm the possibility that, when practiced in an ideal manner, medicine can transcend its own internal contradictions in a confluence of science and art.

8.
BALANCING THE POWER

— · — · — · — · — · — · — · — · — · — · — · — · — · — · — · — · — · —

In default of health, we manage by *care,* and control, and cunning,
and skill and luck.—OLIVER SACKS

— · — · — · — · — · — · — · — · — · — · — · — · — · — · — · — · — · —

Patient empowerment. Need help understanding your disease and treatment options? Yale University trained physician reviews case and provides synopsis of world literature search with simple, clear, unbiased explanation of your choices. Reasonable rates. Call (619) 535-1313." This announcement appeared on 25 June 1992 in the *New York Review of Books* under the heading "Services." The advertisement is quite startling for a number of reasons: it reflects an acknowledgment of patients' bewilderment in the face of a proliferation of possible treatments; it propounds the need for a wholly new type of professional advice to mediate between patients and their personal physicians, thereby insinuating that those physicians are in default in their counseling obligations; and it unabashedly envisages the doctor-patient interaction today as pivoting on power.

The power element is much less prominent a constituent in traditional definitions of the etiquette between doctor and patient. The Hippocratic oath, indeed, binds physicians to a series of limitations on their power: to desist from giving deadly medicine on request, to desist from providing an abortive remedy, to desist from cutting persons laboring under the stone,[1] and to desist from taking advantage of access to homes by instigating mischief or indulging in seduction. Taken as a whole, the Hippocratic oath devotes a surprisingly large proportion of its imperatives to prohibitions.[2]

A more positive line was taken by the British physician Thomas Percival in *Medical Ethics,* which he was asked to compile in 1791 by the trustees of the Manchester Infirmary to settle a dispute among its staff. Printed for private circulation in 1794, it appeared in 1803 under the title *Medical Ethics; or, a*

Code of Institutes and Precepts, Adapted to the Professional Conduct of Physicians and Surgeons. As the subtitle suggests, Percival is not concerned with ethics in the contemporary sense of specific dilemmas of conscience that arise in connection with such decisions as the possibility of terminating life under certain circumstances. He concentrates instead on the rules of etiquette in the conduct of physicians toward one another, including the tenets of professional courtesy, no doubt because of the origins of his work in response to episodes of friction within the medical community. But the notion of medical ethics also denotes for Percival the conduct of physicians toward their individual patients and toward society as a whole. His is, therefore, a substantial work of more than a hundred pages that addresses in its four chapters professional conduct relative to hospitals or other medical charities, in private practice, toward apothecaries, and duties that require a knowledge of law. The second and longest chapter, devoted to private practice, sets out a combination of moral and practical guidelines: it advocates strict observance of "secrecy and delicacy" (90), temperance, punctuality, avoidance of "officious interference" (92), respect for seniority, judicious regulation of visits, promotion of consultations in difficult cases, continued attendance on the incurable, the necessity for solidarity, discouragement of quack medicines, the prohibition of secret nostrums, and the collection of what Percival euphemistically calls "the *pecuniary acknowledgments* of their patients" (99) in accordance with local custom. The impression that emanates from Percival's prescriptions is of a still rather unruly and certainly not powerful profession.

Nor is power openly projected as a central issue in the "Code of Ethics" formulated in 1847 by the newly founded American Medical Association.[3] As in Percival's work, *ethics* here denotes desirable conduct in general. Many of the topics discussed by Percival recur here, at times almost verbatim. For example, mid-nineteenth-century American physicians are enjoined strictly to observe "discretion" as well as "secrecy and delicacy" (219) and also to continue to alleviate the pain and to soothe the mental anguish of those beyond cure. But important new elements are introduced too, notably the ideal of the physician as engaged on a "mission." That is the salient word in the first article of the opening section, "The Duties of Physicians to their Patients": the physician's mind ought "to be imbued with the greatness of his mission" (219). This is in keeping with the conceptualization of the doctor at that time as a "missionary to the bedside," or, as the AMA code puts it, in similarly religious terms, "the minister of hope and comfort to the sick" (220). When "authority" and "firmness" are mentioned, they are in immediate alliance with "tenderness" and "humanity" so as "to inspire the minds of patients with gratitude, respect and confidence" (219). Significantly, it was "respect" that medical men sought at a period when the profession's status and prestige were far lower than today.

The prevailing insecurity is implicit as a subtext in the second part of the 1847 code, "Obligations of Patients to their Physicians." This is a novel departure, unique to the 1847 code and never replicated. The tenor of this second part, which is one and a half times as long as "The Duties of Physicians to their Patients," is quite defensive. The doctors straightaway proclaim themselves as performing "so many important and arduous duties towards the community, and as required to make so many sacrifices of comfort, ease, and health for the welfare of those who avail themselves of their services" that, they argue, they "have a right to expect and require, that their patients should entertain a just sense of the duties they owe to their medical attendants" (221–22). This declaration, tactful and cautiously phrased though it is, introduces into the etiquette between doctor and patient the principle of reciprocity absent in the Hippocratic oath and in Percival's *Medical Ethics*. Some of the following nine clauses deal with practical arrangements such as sending for the doctor in the morning, if possible, not delaying consultation until the condition has advanced to a violent stage, and giving reasons for dismissal. Others devolve from conditions in that period, notably the injunction to select as medical adviser "one who has received a regular professional education" (222). Similarly, the argument for confiding the care of the family to one physician over the long term is grounded in the mid-nineteenth-century belief in the patient specificity of treatment, "for a medical man who has become acquainted with the peculiarities of constitution, habits, and predispositions, of those he attends, is more likely to be successful in his treatment, than one who does not possess that knowledge" (222). The mind-body connection, strongly upheld at that time, is cited as the reason for the faithful and unreserved communication of the supposed cause of the disease to the physician so that he may spot a possible "mental origin" (222). Yet the patient is at certain points addressed with categoric directives and firmly placed in a subordinate position, for instance, when "prompt and implicit obedience" to the physician's prescriptions are ordered without allowing the patient's "crude opinions as to their fitness to influence his attention to them" (223). Here the doctrine that "the doctor knows best" makes an early appearance, conjoined to a demand for the suspension of judgment on the patient's part. In the same vein, the patient is urged to give "clear answers to interrogatories" rather than an "acount of his own framing" (222). In other words, even then physicians preferred closed questions, that is, those aimed at and limited to a target area, to open-ended ones. The combination of defensiveness and self-justification characteristic of the entire document is very apparent in the closing clause: "A patient should, after his recovery, entertain a just and enduring sense of the value of the services rendered him by his physician; for these are of such a character, that no mere pecuniary acknowledgement can repay or cancel them" (225).

The very length of this 1847 code, which runs to fifty-six hundred words, points to the number and complexity of the uncertainties in the etiquette between doctor and patient that it endeavors to clarify. By contrast, the Hippocratic oath consists of a mere three hundred fifty-eight words, and the American Medical Association's 1980 "Principles of Medical Ethics"[4] contains just two hundred fifty. The latter document, instead of comprising laws, lays down the standards of conduct for the honorable behavior of physicians. The eight articles deal directly and cogently with the major facets: "compassion and respect for human dignity" comes first, and honesty second; safeguarding patients' confidences is also a high priority. These are, by and large, modern restatements of the ethos underlying the Hippocratic oath. The oath's obligation to teach is reformulated into the imperative "to continue to study, apply and advance scientific knowledge, make relevant information available to patients, colleagues, and the public" (238). The new provisions deal with the freedom to choose whom to serve, responsibility to participate in activities contributing to an improved community, and, while respecting the law, to seek changes in requirements that are contrary to the best interests of patients. In its very brevity and assertiveness the "Principles" is a much more self-confident declaration than the 1847 code. Power is not invoked by name, but it is clearly assumed in the wider ameliorative responsibilities that stem from a base of strength in the social system.

Doctors' special position in the twentieth-century social structure, together with their relationship to patients, was examined by the social philosopher Talcott Parsons in chapter 10 of *The Social System,* entitled "Social Structure and Dynamic Process: The Case of Modern Medical Practice." Although in some respects, of course, Parsons's analysis has become dated as a result of both sociological and epidemiological changes such as the now widespread prevalence of third-party insurance payments, the recent rise of managed care, the AIDS epidemic, and the recognition of the noxiousness of smoking, nonetheless it remains a fundamentally sound description and assessment. Parsons begins by designating the factors at stake: first, the quality of illness as "partly biologically and partly socially defined" (431); second, the physician's characteristic "affective neutrality," "collectivity orientation," and the "ideology" that puts the "welfare of the patient" above personal interests and regards "commercialism" as the "most serious and insidious evil with which it has to contend" (436); and third, the institutionalized expectations of the "sick role" (436), such as exemption from normal social responsibilities, the acceptance of "help" (437), and cooperation with such help in a desire to get well. However, no sooner has Parsons set out the "pattern elements" (439) in the relationship between doctor and patient than he has to concede "the intricacy of the social forces operating on this superficially simple sub-system" (439). The most problematic of these intricacies is what Parsons calls a "communication gap" (441), that is, the grave disparity between the sick person's qualifications to judge what needs to be done and the expert's capacity to do just that by virtue of knowledge and experience. This is the primary source of the imbalance in power between patient and doctor. As Parsons points out, "The combination of helplessness, lack of technical competence, and emotional disturbance make [the sick person] a peculiarly vulnerable object of exploitation" (445). "Exploitation" is not a felicitous term here, as Parsons seems to realize: in his apologia in the next two sentences he argues that it is not an "exploitation" that befalls a sick person but rather a subjection to medical power. The way in which that necessary power is exercised has been, and is, the major difficulty in the etiquette between doctor and patient. Parsons argues that, taken together, the interactions of patients, their intimates, and the physician "present a very considerable set of complications of the functioning of medical practice on the level of human adjustment" (453). These complications, in transcending "the simple common-sense view," create "another order of functional problems to the social system" (453). They also present functional problems in the doctor-patient interaction that turn on degrees of empowerment or disempowerment.

While Parsons eschews the word *power* even as he delineates the concept, Starr, a sociologist, posits it as the central element in the social evolution of medicine.[5] Medicine is not only "a sovereign profession," the title he gives to his opening chapter, but also "a world of power" (4). Starr concurs with Parsons in seeing the origins of this power as dependent upon knowledge and competence. The authority of medicine has been greatly enhanced, in comparison to that of the law and the church, by its close bonds with modern science, which "has held a privileged status in the hierarchy of belief" (4). For this reason the dominance of the medical profession extends beyond its rational foundation, spilling "over its clinical boundaries into arenas of moral and political action for which medical judgment is only partially relevant and often incompletely equipped" (5). This comment, which seems to imply a certain arrogance on the part of the medical profession, recalls its self-appointed task of responsibility for improvement in the community. Presumably that improvement would focus on health-related matters, but Starr sees it as spreading outward into areas not specifically under medical jurisdiction. His stance is at least partly explained by his fundamental purpose of discerning how medicine rose "from a relatively traditional profession of minor economic significance" to its current predominance. "This transformation has not been propelled solely by the advance of science and the satisfaction of human needs. The history of medicine has been written as an epic of progress, but it is also a tale of social and economic conflict over the emergence of new hierarchies of power and authority, new markets, and new conditions of belief and experience" (4). Starr therefore concentrates mostly on public and socioeconomic factors. However, his insistence on the increasingly high prestige and wide-ranging power of the medical profession has implications for the etiquette between individual doctor and patient in that it underscores the growing inequality between the two sides.

The question of power is approached from an entirely different angle by the medically qualified Howard Brody, who seeks to analyze the workings of the healer's power in terms of the personal transaction between physician and patient. Of the three sources of power that he discerns, the third, social power, is akin to what preoccupies Starr insofar as it arises from social status and becomes manifest in "cultural power" in the implied contract between the medical profession and society.[6] But the other two sources of power are more important to Brody. The first he designates as "Aesculapian power" (16),

which devolves from possession of specialized knowledge and skills and experience in their practical application. On this there is universal agreement:
expertise of a particular kind, concerned with life and death, is the ultimate
foundation of the doctor's power. And it also occasions the imbalance between doctor and patient because "the physician is likely to hold a near monopoly on Aesculapian power, having the necessary knowledge and skills
(which the patient usually lacks) to diagnose and treat diseases" (62). But
alongside this impersonal type of power, transferable to other physicians,
Brody identifies another sort of power, which he calls "charismatic" (16) since
it is based on the physician's personal qualities of courage, decisiveness, firmness, kindness, and so forth. It is often this power, not transferable to others,
that carries persuasive weight in the doctor-patient encounter.

Brody's three strands of power are closely interconnected, and they are
reinforced by the unconscious processes of transference and countertrans-
ference that tend to exalt the physician in the patient's wish image into an
omnipotent healer and, as a corollary, may lead to "an underevaluation of
the patient as a competent adult" in the doctor's eyes.[7] This overestimation
of medicine contains the potential for "the dark side of the force, the misuse
and abuse of power" (31) in the form of domination through a mystification
that controls and intimidates patients, especially those perceived as recalci-
trant. However, in Brody's view the opposite trend is in the ascendant: the
shift from control to cooperation following the realization that patients more
actively involved in their treatment are likely to prosper better.[8] According to
Brody, "The new ethics has focused on how to promote patient autonomy
and contain or eliminate physician paternalism" (44). So Brody argues for the
cultivation of a group of three further powers in the doctor-patient interaction: "aimed power" to set realistic goals for therapy and appropriate means
to achieve them; "shared power" in anticipatory decision making; and "owned
power" through a high degree of awareness and self-awareness (155–56). This
schematic categorization, obviously intended as a complement to the physician's three powers, appears rather artificial. The difference in persuasiveness
between the two sets of powers signals the fact that the physician's powers
are in force, whereas those in which doctor and patient are to participate
jointly can hardly attain Brody's ideal because of the virtually insuperable discrepancy in knowledge, which becomes harder to overcome as medicine continues to grow more complex and technological. Yet the desirability of a

switch from an authoritative to a consultative mode is frequently asserted by theoreticians of medical practice in pleas for less passive, better educated, questioning patients capable of more equal participation.[9] Instead of being "self-regulating" and "authoritarian," "albeit benign,"[10] the physician should educate patients, involve them in decision making, and adjust recommendations according to patients' values and wishes.

A parallel argument in favor of a more person-centered perspective is made by Allen Barbour in *Caring for Patients*. Basing his recommendations on his long experience in the Department of Internal Medicine at Stanford Medical Center, he cites the damage done by unnecessary surgeries that failed to remove the pain of which patients had complained. He asserts that in many such cases the problem is psychogenic, stemming from the patient's personal situation, which is totally ignored in the course of a thorough—and costly—physical workup. He envisages a set of dualisms that doctors must heed: patients/persons, disease/illness, understanding the biological situation/understanding the personal situation, diagnosis/clinical judgment, curing/healing, treatment/collaboration, eradicating sickness/ achieving health (32).

Nevertheless, patients continue to have a troubling sense of disempowerment. To some degree, of course, disempowerment is intrinsic to sickness, which undermines self-confidence, diminishes control and autonomy, and may distort judgment and so induce a frightening helplessness. It is because patients are in the grip of the power of disease that they submit to medical power. Some do indeed prefer the exercise of authority by physicians over the burden of choice. Patients' resentment is often directed less at medical power per se than at the style in which it is exercised as if the patient were merely a biomedical being without a distinctive personality. Disregard for the person surfaces in various ways. Anecdotally, it has been reported that a junior medical student, when asked what a patient was, replied: "some values on a chart."[11] On the chart the subject/object dichotomy is institutionalized in current methods of recording where the patient's "subjective" account of pain or disturbance is to be immediately superseded by the "objective" findings of the physical examination and laboratory tests. Thus the patient's voice is considered "an 'unreliable narrator' of bodily events, a voice which must be bypassed as quickly as possible so that they [the doctors] can get round and behind it to the physical events themselves."[12] Pain, however tormenting and disruptive to the patient, is of significance only as an indicator of pathology; once diagnosed, it loses interest for medical thinking and is to be remediated in separate "pain clinics" by such means as biofeedback and self-hypnosis, which work well for some sufferers and not at all for others. The consequent discongruity between the patient's and the doctor's perception of the same situation has been vividly illustrated in the research of a group who interviewed a sixty-nine-year-old black woman in a rehabilitation facility after a stroke.[13] Her personal story of struggle, frustration, and discouragement is interleaved with her medical chart of treatment and progress: "The optimistic voices of the physician and other caregivers combined with the unfolding details of the patient's story produce an almost eerie dissonance" (18). In this instance the stories exchanged between patient and physician, instead of relieving suffering, actually exacerbate it.

The aggravation of the patient's distress by established medical etiquette is the subject of a hard-hitting article by the philosopher Alisdair MacIntyre, "Medicine Aimed at the Care of Persons Rather Than What?" Rational though his contentions are, they barely conceal the anger that inspires his observations. In asking what it means "to treat the patient as a *person*" (18) MacIntyre sets up a series of contrasts, beginning with that between persons and the roles they happen to be playing. Coexistent with the patient, who consults a doctor about a syndrome, there is a person—a husband, a father, a professor of philosophy—with a justified claim to recognition that is all too often denied. For this habit of not seeing the person behind the patient MacIntyre faults medicine as bureaucracy and as applied science, both of which distance and depersonalize the patient. "As a result," he says, "the patient experiences not only impersonality, but also a continuously recurring divorce between expectation and reality. This is perhaps why the appropriate word to express the attitude of many patients is *disappointment,* a disappointment grounded less in bad diagnosis or failures of treatment than in the absence of an anticipated but necessarily unavailable form of human relationship" (86). MacIntyre is more successful in pinpointing how the individual comes to be "emptied of human substance" (93) by the prevailing system than at putting forward a solution. He himself applies the word "utopian" (95) to the amendment he suggests, namely, to make the home, the family, the workplace the locus of medical practice. Impressive in its exposé of the system's shortcomings, the article peters out into unrealistic nostalgia.

It is interesting to juxtapose this patient's view with that of the physician David Hilfiker in his *Healing the Wounds*. As a family doctor in a small northern Minnesota town Hilfiker certainly ran a personal practice insofar as he knew his patients as individuals with families, jobs, histories, and worries. He takes as his starting point the climate of hostility to the profession manifest in "the rising tide of criticism against physicians as a group, criticism of our attitude toward patients and of our general behavior. . . . We are too preoccupied with disease and not concerned about the whole person. We don't listen to our patients, won't communicate with them. We are authoritarian, dictatorial. We are told that we place too much reliance on science and technology, and that we don't put enough energy into personal, caring contact with our patients" (12). Without directly refuting these criticisms, Hilfiker shows, by writing of his own experiences, how physicians themselves are constrained and consumed by the pressures under which they work. He comes across as a thoroughly caring doctor, aware not only of his patients' feelings ("scared and angry" [4]) but also of those of "an anxious spouse" (5), of his office staff's "emotional fatigue" (9) as well as his own: "I'm tired, irritable" (5). He is conscious too of his "insecurities" (5), of "constantly confronting our own ignorance" (37), and of having to steer a compromise course between the idealistic precepts of his training ("if we even *thought* of the possibility of meningitis, we should do a lumbar puncture" [20]) and the practicalities of routine care. Even more disturbing to him are "the degree of perfection expected of physicians" (77) and his realization that he requires psychological skills he was never taught. Often the chief limitation is simply time, as on the occasion when he cannot spend more than fifteen minutes with the mother of a child just drowned because of "my feelings of responsibility to those who have appointments. Which is more important?" (24). But despite his goodwill, misunderstandings abound: for instance, when a patient's main concern is to get better by the weekend whereas the doctor needs to rule out a serious illness, or when a patient has acquired a simplified knowledge of diseases through newspapers, magazines, and television and cannot understand the necessity of working with probabilities and uncertainties. Hilfiker candidly admits that it is easier for a doctor to "retreat behind a mask of stony indifference" (69) and issue reassurances that the doctor knows best than really to engage with patients. Yet the very fact that he wrote *Healing the Wounds*—the wounds that he has sustained during his professional work—

reveals the seriousness with which he confronts the issues he is accused of avoiding. Still, he avows bluntly that "it is, in fact, one of the basic dilemmas of the physician—to be caught between a desire to be of service and a need for respite. This conflict surfaced in many different ways throughout any given day, producing a long-term sense of alienation from my patients and encouraging me to deal with them as problems to be handled rather than as persons in need of care" (32).

Hilfiker touches tangentially on another area that has been changing the balance between doctor and patient: that in the last thirty years medicine has been "monetarized." It has come to speak "much more the language of business, with cost/benefit analyses, time management, and financial profiles being an important part of any practice" (170). In the name of "modernizing" and "streamlining," there is a "trade-off between efficiency and deeper personal relationship, between productivity and medicine as art" (144). The doctor has been turned into "society's gatekeeper" (144) by such charges as the physical examination for insurance purposes to authorize absence from work or to certify fitness to drive, which tend to engender "mutual feelings of suspicion" (94). The commercialization, of which Hilfiker was already complaining in the early 1980s, not only has grown far more pronounced as a result of the escalating costs associated with the latest technologies but has entered an entirely new phase with the emergence of managed care, which transfers decision-making power from the physician to the insurance company. There can be no doubt, Hunter maintains, that "the welter of contemporary economic arrangements estranges patient and physician and encourages distrust on both sides."[14] Although a financial dimension to medicine through the payment of fees has always been a factor (and, incidentally, one that used to empower patients), its configuration has undergone radical change through the intervention of a third party between physician and patient. This matter is beyond the scope of this book, and besides, the situation is at present in a constant state of flux. But the terminology itself tells much of the story: "As a physician, I am somewhat distressed at being called a *health care provider*," writes David A. Worth, M.D., P.A., of Union, New Jersey, "rather than a doctor, a physician or a professional."[15] When a health care provider delivers services to a consumer, the relationship between doctor and patient is converted into that between a purveyor and a customer.[16] Irrespective of the specifics of the pecuniary reckoning, such a shift is reductive as the "management" of patients replaces care. The climate of hostility toward current medical practice is attributable in considerable measure to the bureaucratization to which the profession has had to submit in an attempt to curb the astronomical increases in cost faced by insurance companies through the wider use of new, expensive technologies. Physicians themselves are being "managed," to their own resentment as well as to the detriment of their relationship to their patients.

The anger at moves to substitute management for care has created a backlash: "I don't want to manage clients, I want to care for patients," protests a psychiatrist employed by a health maintenance organization (HMO).[17] The persistence of the exclusive focus on the disease model and the utter neglect of the human is amply illustrated in several of the cases recorded by Kleinman, who works at the interface of psychiatry and anthropology. Most striking is that of Mrs. Flowers, a black, single, thirty-nine-year-old mother who is seen by her doctor for worsening hypertension.[18] Throughout the interview Dr. Richards asks clipped, closed questions about physical symptoms such as shortness of breath, chest pain, swelling of the feet, nausea, and so forth. When he comes to headaches, Mrs. Flowers responds with: "Sometimes I think my life is one big headache" (133) and begins to speak of the recent death of her friend Eddie Johnson. At other points she brings up her anxieties about her two pregnant teenage daughters, her sons' getting into trouble, her mother's drifting into senility, and her money problems. All these pressing worries, which might well affect her blood pressure, are totally ignored by the doctor, who proceeds with his programmatic interrogation. He goes over Mrs. Flowers like a steamroller, uncomprehending of the metaphoric force of "headache." At best, he refers her to a social worker to discuss her finances. On her chart he enters hypertension and evidence of mild congestive heart failure, along with the ironic notation "No other problems" (134). The misprision here reflects the doctor's perception of her disease as a copy of textbook examples despite her attempts to expound the particularity of her situation.

Counterbalancing the insensitive Dr. Richards in Kleinman's *Illness Narratives* is Dr. Paul Samuels, a fifty-two-year-old internist in a large Midwestern city, whose patients cannot find sufficient praise for his "humanness" (212). "Medicine," he declares, "doesn't interest me nearly as much as people"; to be technically first-rate is a prerequisite, but "what really counts is the human aspect" (214). If medical school made him a doctor, life experience has made him "a *healer*" (212) to whom the practice of medicine "is a way of life, a moral discipline" (214). Like this exemplary physician, Kleinman himself strongly believes in "a moral core to healing" and in "the art of medicine" (253), although he acknowledges this to be "a term of ambivalence and even disparagement in a profession for which the preferred self-image is decidedly that of science" (272). Perhaps the best compromise is Brody's conception of medicine "as a practical craft that applies scientific knowledge to individual cases toward the end of a right and good healing action."[19] This is an attempt to bring into consonance the diverse elements of practicality, science, the individual, and healing.

A crucial factor in the achievement of "a right and good healing action" is precisely the quality of the doctor-patient interaction. Brody designates such an "ongoing personal relationship with each patient" as the "tool of the trade for the primary-care physician" (58), corresponding to the surgeon's scalpel or the gastroenterologist's endoscope. The annual checkup can be useful not only in establishing baselines for future comparison when illness strikes but also in reinforcing the patient-physician relationship.[20] "Sensitivity to patients," hailed by Brody as the new medical style, in contrast to the old way, which emphasized "technical skill and scientific knowledge,"[21] connects back, somewhat ironically, to the oldest, pretechnological mode of patient-centered therapeutics. The challenge now is to reconcile disease-specific treatment with the maintenance of a sense of the patient as a person. Such a stance creates a whole new set of problems for physicians, most of whom would naturally prefer to deny the patient's demoralization and pain because it represents a threat or a reproach to their healing power. Particularly in the case of chronic illness with a relentless downhill movement, practitioners often feel as frustrated and impotent as patients, so that "a duet of escalating antagonism ensues, much to the detriment of the protagonists."[22] Kleinman uses the same term as Hilfiker, "the mask of medicine" (216), to denote the deliberate distancing of the professional persona who meets human suffering with silence, as does Dr. Richards with Mrs. Flowers. He also cites a research-oriented gastroenterologist who admits: "I feel the need to protect myself, my involvement with patients. If I could only do, just do the cognitive side, and leave the emotions, the family, the whole mess to someone else" (214). The retreat from suffering behind "the cognitive side" is the donning of the mask as a self-defensive gesture. "Listening to him makes me feel so bad," confesses the medical student who wonders whether he is too sensitive and who adds: "Maybe that's why doctors don't listen" (220).

But the absolute necessity of listening more has been forcefully asserted by such humanistic physicians as William Carlos Williams: "Doctors should keep their mouths shut more than they do—including me! We should look more; we should listen more. Patients are our teachers."[23] This kind of listening means more than merely applying the stethoscope to detect the physical signs of disease; much rather it requires lending an ear and time to the patient's narrative of distress in the way that Konner does for the moribund. As Eric Cassell puts it, listening involves "hearing not only what the symptoms are, but what they mean to the patient."[24] But precisely such listening is actually negated by medical education which begins with the dissection of a cadaver, a rite of passage that "teaches primacy of the eye over the ear" and makes students "learn that the patient is passive."[25] Yet such attentive listening is an important prelude and means to empowering patients: "the empathetic auditing of their stories of illness must be one of the clinician's chief therapeutic tasks."[26] For "the doctor-patient relationship is always and inevitably a compromise between the patient's 'offers' and demands and the doctor's responses to them."[27] That compromise can only be the product of what Kleinman calls "negotiation": "Of all the tradecraft of the physician, nothing more effectively empowers patients. The very act of negotiation, if it is genuine and not a grudging pseudomutuality, necessitates that at the very least the health professional show respect for the patient's point of view. The real challenge is for the physician to engage in negotiation with the patient as colleagues involved in care as collaboration" (242). Kleinman's proposition adumbrates an ideal that is necessarily contingent on—and restricted by— each patient's intelligence and willingness to accept the responsibility for meaningful cooperation. Successful negotiation in turn creates the conjunctive foundations of care by bridging the communication gap identified by Parsons as a major obstacle to a better doctor-patient rapport.

The recognition that "all medical care flows through the relationship between physician and patient" and that "the spoken language is the most important tool in medicine" has prompted a considerable volume of writing in the past fifteen to twenty years on doctor-patient communication.[28] This work falls into two main categories: prescriptive advocacy and descriptive recording and discussion of actual doctor-patient interviews. In the advocacy of the benefits of better communication there is unanimity. Some of the arguments, notably on the function of listening, have already been cited. But equally important is the physician's role in talking with patients in order to explain diagnosis and proposed treatment. This is a fairly new trend in the twentieth century, although again it represents a continuity with early-nineteenth-century prescientific days, when therapeutics were a matter of discussion between patients and their attendants. In that period, however, the disparity in knowledge and hence power between the two parties to the medical encounter was relatively small. Through the later nineteenth century and most of the twentieth "we have spared no effort to make better tools but we have paid little attention to learning how to communicate better with one another."[29] "With" is the crucial word here, for "talking *to* the patient about medical facts may be much more common than it used to be, but talking *with* patients about medical facts remains rare."[30] The problem stems partly from doctors' difficulty, or at times inability, to translate professional into lay terms. Technical phrases, so familiar to doctors as to seem self-explanatory, may be incomprehensible to patients. Examples of such misunderstanding abound; often comic on the surface, they are nonetheless a source of distress, as in the case of a patient put on a low-sodium diet who is upset at having to cut down on salt too,[31] or the man who takes "lumbar puncture" to denote surgery to remove fluid from the lungs.[32] Even in the absence of technical jargon, Balint notes instance after instance of "a dangerous confusion of tongues, each party talking in a language not understood and apparently not understandable by the other."[33]

Balint's findings are especially striking because they are derived from a self-selected group of physicians strongly committed to better practice through good communication. Ironically, however, again and again they turn out to have misinterpreted their patients' appeals, slipping into a tacit collusion by accepting the frustrations and irritations caused by each other's limitations. So these doctors voice reassurances, for example, about cancer when their patients' anxieties lie elsewhere or give vague, "nothing wrong" answers that leave patients stranded in disappointment. This is the context for Balint's experiment in the early 1950s, when he convened a number of general practitioners for weekly meetings at the Tavistock Clinic in London throughout a year for a frank discussion of their cases. His "chief aim" was a "reasonably thorough examination of the ever-changing doctor-patient relationship, that is, the study of the pharmacology of the drug 'doctor'" (1). Its main effect, he argues, stems from the nature of the doctor's response to the patient's "offer" (18). "Reassurance" and "advice" are found to be "the most frequent forms in which the drug 'doctor' is administered" (116). So Balint advocates, with considerable idealism, especially given the extreme time pressures under the National Health Service in Great Britain, that practitioners institute what he calls a "long interview," which he defines as "a kind of give-and-take affair" (136) with obvious similarities to a psychotherapeutic meeting. While Balint concedes that "it is exceedingly difficult to state exactly what it is that restores the balance," the outcome of even a single long interview is that "the patient feels understood, relieved, or even enriched, instead of being despoiled or cheated" (136). However, the doctor "has to learn to *listen*" (121) in a new and more subtle way in order to pick up what is indirectly hinted rather than openly expressed by patients, who may themselves be hardly aware of the underlying issue. If this method is applied successfully, as Balint's group discovers, the whole atmosphere of the clinical encounter changes when the doctor comes to be perceived as "a real friend, who makes things right by his understanding of the hidden problems" (126).

More than thirty years later a somewhat parallel plea, this time for "a rhetoric of explaining to patients," has been put forward by Kleinman as a remedy for the miscommunication between well-meaning but ineffectual doctors and their patients.[34] Because they "are poised at the interface between scientific and lay cultures" (241), physicians have a special obligation, though little training or even incentive, to develop such communicative skills. The downgrading of "talking with patients" is closely linked to the overwhelming dominance in modern medicine of a technical bioscience orientation. The behavioral scientist Elliot Mishler offers, if not a solution, at least a theoretical framework for dealing with the "communication gap" by envisaging the doctor-patient encounter as an interplay—or a clash—between two entirely different kinds of discourse.[35] The one is "the voice of medicine" (90), articulated by the doctor from the normative perspective of the biomedical model. Interacting with this voice is that "of the lifeworld" (90), spoken by patients as they "sometimes talked about problems in their lives that were related to or resulted from their symptoms or illnesses. The meanings expressed in this voice differed from those framed within the biomedical perspective and physi-

cians tended to treat this material as nonmedically relevant. In a typical interview, this other voice was quickly suppressed and the physician restored
the voice of medicine to its position of dominance in the discourse" (91).
(This passage is an exact description in theoretical terms of the exchange
between Dr. Richards and Mrs. Flowers.) The dominance and interruption
by the voice of medicine "leads to an 'objectification' of the patient, to
stripping away of the lifeworld contexts of patient problems" (128). In hopes
of evolving a "non-coercive discourse based on norms of reciprocity rather
than dominance-subordination" (6), Mishler proposes a greater use of open-
ended questions that leave space for the patient's input in the voice of the lifeworld in place of the closed questions in the voice of medicine that enable
the doctor to maintain tight control. The obvious and very real stumbling
block to the implementation of such an approach lies in the time constraints
that govern clinical practice.

Between these idealistic, forward-looking blueprints for the improvement
of doctor-patient communication and the records of what has actually been
taking place there is a painful contrast. Systematic efforts have been made
in the last two decades to document the dynamics of the doctor-patient interaction by means of tape and video recordings. In the transcription of the
tapes coding is used to convey phonetically and visually on the printed page
the pace and progression of talk between doctors and patients, which differs
markedly from the fluency of the literary text in its repetitions, silences, non-
lexical utterances, false starts, and incomplete phrases. This method undoubtedly comes closer than any other to revealing the realities of medical
encounters because the mediating vehicle is a machine, which eliminates the
participants' inevitable subjectivity. All these studies, in Great Britain as in the
United States, uncover generally unsatisfactory and at times downright bad
situations.

The most thorough and extensive of these inquiries is that by Candace
West, a sociolinguist who scrutinized doctor-patient interactions in an outpatient family medical center in Charleston, South Carolina, and published
the results in *Routine Complications: Troubles with Talk between Doctors and Patients* (1984). This title, which seems at first just witty, is actually a telling brief
summary of the outcome of West's research. Her design involves scrupulous
analyses of a number of crucial variables, such as interruptions in encounters
between patients and male physicians (table 1, 57), similar interruptions be-

tween patients and female physicians (table 2, 58), the proportion of questions initiated respectively by patients and by physicians (table 3, 81), and the terms of address used (table 7, 130). Patients' age, gender, social status, and color are related to the ways in which they are handled; by and large, in this experiment as in others older patients, women, those of lower social status, and the colored are found to be liable to greater condescension. Like Parsons, West locates the fundamental problem in the essential asymmetry in knowledge and standing that underlies the practitioner's situational authority and the patient's situational dependency. The relationship is *"predicated* on institutionalized inequality" (18), which entitles doctors to command and receive deference as "dominants" while relegating patients as "subordinates" (92) in need of help. So West argues that the "script" (16) is already written for both physicians and patients. Not only are patient-initiated questions "dispreferred" (78), they are less frequently answered than those posed by doctors, tend to be formulated with hesitations that betray anxiety, and in fact seem to be regarded by the patients themselves as troublesome because they may appear to be querying doctors' godlike status (83–99). West's investigation is remarkable for the attention she devotes to the manner as well as the matter of the interchange: the problems of opening up a state of talk, sustaining an ongoing conversation, and terminating an exchange, the tone in which things are said (a whisper, a shout, with a stutter or a drawl), and such channels of nonverbal communication as eye contact, facial expression, and body orientation. West ascertains that there is "very little explaining time" (99) and that fear is aroused in patients as a means to achieve compliance.[36] Little seems to have changed since Parsons's opinion some thirty years earlier that the practitioner must exercise rigid control over the interaction so as to ensure that the patient will follow the desired regimen. Whether these tactics have the desired effect or, instead, explanation and understanding result in better cooperation is a major area of contention.

Parallel tapings and interpretation of the doctor-patient interview were undertaken in Great Britain in a survey of office visits to 1,850 physicians under the National Health Service. Despite the difference in context, the findings are quite similar to West's. The style of consulting is described as "highly mechanistic," with a predominance of closed questions that elicit a yes or no reply.[37] Consultations are seen as structured into six phases: relating to the patient; discovering the reason for the patient's attendance; conducting verbal and physical examination; considering the patient's condition; detailing treatment or further investigation; and terminating. The total average time span was a mere five and one-half to seven minutes, with the diagnosis made after three minutes and the final two and one-half minutes given to advice, prescription, and closure. This echoes West's observation that "talk, in short, is not cheap"[38] as practitioners' practical concerns (with time and, in the United States, money) have a negative impact on communication with patients.

Doctors' therapeutic behavior includes advice, explanation, discussion, and listening, but listening as such is not an integral part of medical training. The "apparent unwillingness to enter into any relationship with patients," very evident in "the way in which these doctors prevent and stifle an expression of feeling in the consultation,"[39] recalls once more the paradigm of Dr. Richards and Mrs. Flowers. Insensitivity surfaces in the doctors' lack of insight into the possible consequences of recommending that patients change jobs, retire, or rest. The patients' inhibitions deter them from disputing advice of this kind and also cause them to introduce very late, and often obliquely, the real reason for the visit. This curious tendency is mentioned by Balint and West too. "Talking down" to patients is another recurrent feature, although "jargon" is more common in the United States,[40] whereas baby talk is more prevalent in Great Britain.[41] Whatever the local circumstances, failure to communicate adequately thwarts the very purpose of the visit.

The impact on patients of the communication gap is explored with great finesse by Mark L. Rosenberg in *Patients: The Experience of Illness,* a vivid attempt by a physician to enter into "what it feels like to be a patient and receive medical care" (11). Rosenberg conducted in-depth interviews with six hospitalized patients at different life stages and suffering from different diseases in order to solicit their responses not so much to their illnesses as to the way they had been treated by their doctors. The interviews are supplemented in some cases by input from the patients' families and are enriched by photographs revealing body language. When the book appeared in 1980, doctors traditionally conveyed little information to patients about their diseases; at most, one or two minutes out of twenty were given to providing information. Time pressure was the usual excuse; however, Rosenberg contends that the reticence to speak may also reflect doctors' uncertainty and consequent reluctance to risk any conjecture about outcome, especially as these patients all suffered from life-threatening conditions. Nor were the three prerequisites for communication, namely, the desire on both sides to do so, the ability to transmit information, and receptiveness by the listener, always fulfilled. The listener here is the patient and, in some instances, the family; one of the points brought out by Rosenberg's interviews is the wide variation in patients' capacity as listeners and the resultant difficulties faced even by those doctors who strive to communicate. For instance, Sandy, a black woman with kidney failure, says that at first she did not want to talk to doctors and nurses because she did not know what they were talking about. When she finally asks, "And how come I wasn't going to the bathroom," her physician replies, "Didn't anybody tell you that when your kidneys are out you don't urinate?" (56). This is a patient not at all savvy medically and a doctor lacking the imagination to empathize with her. The same shortcoming in appreciating the patient's individuality can produce the equally unsatisfactory result of imparting more information than the patient is able to tolerate. This happened to Jeanne's husband, whose physician "insisted on telling him that he had cancer. I didn't want them to tell him but they did. He is not the type that can handle it, and this is one of the reasons he's so despondent. . . . The doctor insisted on telling him" (152). Jeanne approaches her own breast cancer in the opposite manner in the belief that the way to "answer" it is to "bring it out," to "talk about it and face it" (153). In command of her options, she chooses a simpler procedure than her doctor recommends because she wants to get back to work quickly on account of her sick husband. Although the doctor has told her that the decision is strictly up to her, when she goes against his preference, "I had a feeling he was angry with me. He didn't really say anything—he just turned and walked away" (148). Clearly, in the doctor's view medical considerations outweigh social ones, and he does not tolerate kindly the rebuff to his power represented by Jeanne's choice.

Despite these cross-communications, most of the doctors in Rosenberg's sample seem thoughtful and caring. A possible exception is the oncologist in charge of Kay, an elderly woman with massive tumors in both breasts that have metastasized extensively. The bluntness reported alike by the patient and her sister is perhaps less the brutality it may appear than a manifestation of frustration at having to admit defeat. Bluntness is used to good purpose by Edwin's cardiologist to force him to overcome his denial and to convince him to agree to bypass surgery. As Edwin blithely plans a summer trip and reiterates a glib "no problem," Dr. Collins tells him point-blank that he thinks he will not be around "to go on any trip this summer" (106). That Dr. Collins is deliberate in his shock tactic is suggested by his comment that "the physician has to a be a little careful in his technique of telling the truth" (117). While this may sound ironic in light of his forthrightness, it supports the hypothesis that his bluntness was calculated. Often, as with Edwin, dealing with the patient's family is an added complication. Kay's oncologist meets with family opposition to his wanting to keep her out of a chronic care facility. The most complex case, Joel, a twenty-six-year-old man who has had a stroke and a heart attack, develops differing relationships to his two physicians. Joel's cardiologist is evasive, wanting to spare the patient the stress that discussion might generate. Joel, in turn, responds by not confiding in him; for instance, he does not tell him that his wife has left him because he wants to avoid "the hassle of having to explain" (192). This reciprocal silence contrasts with the same patient's warm, open, and trusting rapport with his neurologist, who takes the time to sit down, talk, and explain. Nowhere does the delicate mutuality of the doctor-patient interaction become as manifest as in the contradictory pattern of this one patient's dealings with his two doctors.

Joel's antithetical experiences with his two doctors at the same time, during the same hospitalization, raises the tricky issue of a good or bad match between a particular patient and a particular doctor. Because of physicians' superior knowledge and authority compared with that of their patients, it is invariably they who are held responsible for the communication gap. But Joel's cardiologist is reticent for legitimate reasons: the problem he wants to avoid discussing is his emotionally charged counsel that Joel not have children. On the other hand, the patient's role as listener is generally underestimated, partly because it is harder to assess than the physician's performance as speaker. Some patients may not know how to become listeners. For example, Michael Crichton, who completed medical training before becoming a writer, describes a man who "never asked what was in his lung that required surgery. He never asked anything at all. And nobody volunteered to tell him."[42] Convinced that he has cancer, he jumps out of the window—a spectacular instance of the communication gap, with shared blame for the silence.

Although the doctor-patient relationship is in many ways a special one, both especially privileged and especially tense, it is nevertheless still affected

by the same partly irrational likes and dislikes that govern other social interactions. Just as nineteenth-century patients were influenced by appearance—
the shape of a mustache, for example—and manners in their choice of
medical attendants, so also nowadays congruence of personal style between
doctor and patient probably plays a greater part than is usually acknowledged.
Indeed, one pitfall may be patients' inability to distinguish between doctors'
competence and their "bedside manner"; mere affability does not make for
effectiveness and may even serve to cover ineffectiveness. Contrariwise,
brusqueness is by no means inimical to expert treatment. It is true, as Balint
maintains, that "self-selection of patients" occurs "according to the doctor's
apostolic beliefs."[43] However, apart from the rational evaluation of expertise
and "apostolic beliefs," a subconscious preference on the patient's part for a
certain style of behavior or a dislike of another is a significant element in the
establishment of a sound, trusting rapport. "The intimate, paternalistic
doctor-patient relationship is little more than a historical curiosity," according
to many feminists.[44] Paternalism may well be anathema to some patients but
balm to others. Along similar lines, it has been claimed that "the trust relationship that doctors prefer in interactions with patients mirrors the one that
prevailed at the first stage of parent-child interaction."[45] That type of relationship, a welcome regression from adult responsibility for some sick people,
may be violently resented by others. A fundamental, often unavowed consonance between physician and patient is of primary importance in enabling a
doctor, on the basis of understanding and reciprocal good faith, to function
as the "comforter."[46]

Such intuitive harmony is more operative than any intellectual input in the
"placebo effect," which Kleinman defines as "the non-specific therapeutic effect of the doctor-patient relationship."[47] He cites patients with chronic pain
who know that "medicine doesn't do much for us" yet realize that going back
to the doctor is "one way of asking for help, for protection, for someone big-
ger and stronger to take care of us" (83). Balint actually elevates this trait to
the potency of a drug: *"One of the most important side effects—if not the main
effect—of the drug 'doctor' is his response to the patient's offer."*[48] It is no more than
a small step from this perception of the doctor-patient interaction to one that
singles out its magical aspects in the "rescue fantasy" of an omnipotent figure
able to dispel suffering, as a parent conjures away a child's hurt.[49] This desire
to invest doctors with quasi-magical powers is an archetypal, self-preserving

tendency in all patients and an overarching continuity in the balance of power between doctor and patient through the ages. For the physician too "the rescue fantasy is a power trip" that supports the drive to certainty, contributes to the necessary reassuring demeanor, and fosters the patient's dependent gratitude.[50]

What if this idealized scenario breaks down? Since trust and confidence are essential to the medical enterprise, and we want the magic to work, "we tell ourselves the comforting story. But the fear, distrust, and resentment remain because we are unable to believe it totally."[51] The idea of acknowledging to patients the limitations of medical knowledge and of doctors' capacity to cure or even to relieve effectively is opposed by both ancient tradition and the observation that faith in the drug "doctor" enhances the prospect of healing. With the advances in therapeutics and surgery over the past two hundred years, expectations of the power of medicine have risen incrementally. We are loath to remember that physicians can provide not immortality, only "endless deferrals"[52]—and "endless" is patently the wrong adjective here.

When the excessively positive credence in medicine's ability to provide such "endless deferrals" turns out to be in vain in the face of a poor outcome or death, it can capsize into an equally negative attitude. So what West calls, with some exaggeration, "the flood of 'hate' books" can be interpreted as the obverse of the rescue fantasy.[53] Gone askew, the rescue fantasy provokes virulent criticisms and indictments of physicians—the psychological precipitate of disappointed hopes. This is most readily evident in the spate of pathographies written in the last twenty years or so by patients or family members to recount medical adventures or, more frequently, misadventures. A few, in the wake of Cousins's *Anatomy of Illness,* strive to be constructive by tracing their own battle for restoration to a modicum of functionality together with acceptance of their condition. An outstanding example of this type is *At the Will of the Body,* by Arthur Frank, a Canadian academic, an account of his struggle to recover from the heart attack and cancer that hit him in rapid succession in the very prime of life. Similarly, in *A Whole New Life* the novelist Reynolds Price chronicles with great frankness his devastation by a malignant tumor wound around his spinal cord. Although he remains confined to a wheelchair as a paraplegic, his story is subtitled "An Illness and a Healing." Both Frank and Price have harsh, in fact horrifying things to report about certain of their doctors, but they also find humaneness and generosity allied to high expertise. The heroic, inspirational strain in these works makes them transcend mere "hate" books. In these pathographies the sufferers themselves are more able to come to terms with their own illness and even impending death than are their relatives and survivors, whose sense of loss is aggravated by their anger at a system whose failure is in some instances directly implicated in the debacle. The bitterness in Sandra Gilbert's *Wrongful Death* at her husband's bleeding to death following successful surgery for prostate cancer is surely justified.

More troubling than the pathographies that grow out of individual experience are the systematic attacks on diverse aspects of the medical profession that appear under the guise of investigative journalism or advice manuals for patients. The former have their model in Illich's *Medical Nemesis,* which caused quite a sensation when it appeared in 1976 because of its vehement accusation that current medicine actually represents a "threat" (7) to the health of populations through iatrogenesis as a result of over- and mistreatment. In sections with such provocative titles as "Doctors' Effectiveness—an Illusion," "Useless Medical Treatment," "Doctor-Inflicted Injuries," and "Diagnostic Imperialism" Illich argues that "the medicalization of life" has created "defenseless patients" (32) at the mercy of doctors who "conspire in an attempt to produce, as if it were a commodity, something called 'better health'" (34). This state of affairs, "medical nemesis" consequent to "the expropriation of health" by professional experts, places patients "in the grip of pernicious techniques" (33). Illich's lurid phraseology is hardly neutralized by the mass of scholarly footnotes to back his contentions. His perception of the medical world stands in the tradition of the evil doctor and prefigures the negative images in contemporary films and novels.

In a similar vein, the investigative journalist Walt Bogdanich in *The Great White Lie* takes on, as its cover announces in red capital letters, "dishonesty, waste, and incompetence in the medical community." Through his investigation of a series of well-documented scandals, many of which were hushed up or left unresolved, Bogdanich acts as a whistle-blower on negligence and, above all, fraudulent misuse of public funds for private gain. His accounts of unqualified personnel passed off as registered nurses by greedy agencies, Pap smears hardly glanced at and pronounced normal, doctors disbarred for malfeasance in one state obtaining positions of authority and doing further damage elsewhere, and substandard hospitals managing to stay in business and reaping huge profits from grossly inflated Medicare reimbursements while bandying patients around like goods are shocking horror stories. But they emanate from the criminal margins of the medical industry and attempt to pass off muckraking in the name of patient empowerment.

Another category of "hate" books originates within the medical community in the form of advice manuals for patients. There are noticeably fewer of these than there are textbooks advising doctors how to handle their patients. This clearly reflects the asymmetry of power, the assumption that physicians will take the lead and that patients are destined for the passive part. It is precisely as a tool to redress this imbalance that books such as Stuart Berger's *What Your Doctor Didn't Learn in Medical School* and Richard Podell's *When Your Doctor Doesn't Know Best* are presented to the general public. Both Berger and Podell, doctors who purport detachment from the medical establishment, seek to teach patients how to protect themselves from the "medical mistakes that even the best doctors make," "how to be more effective as patients, better communicators with your doctors and appropriately assertive on your own behalf in all your dealings with your health care providers."[54] The word "providers," like Berger's dedication to making medicine "become more consumer-oriented,"[55] bespeaks the implicit vision of medicine as a marketplace where the rule is Caveat emptor. Berger, whose folksy manner put his book on the *New York Times* bestseller list, attacks the entire medical system as putting us all at risk: *"All of us, patient and practitioner alike, are caught in a vast, expensive, elaborate medical machine, one that very often works against our health and well-being"* (17). This is a reiteration of Illich's thesis, except that doctors too are seen as caught in the meshes of the system rather than as bad guys themselves—a clever, tactical amendment that avoids offending patients' well-known loyalty to *their* own physician.

Nevertheless, Berger's catalog of dangers—iatrogenesis, drug reactions, nosocomial infections, excess surgery, greed, commercialism, and dirt—is more than enough to strike terror in any prospective patient. Likewise, Podell's suggestion that physicians are ignorant in their approach to many common conditions and therefore guilty of harmful oversights is likely to make patients wary to the point of suspiciousness. Both manuals in fact trade on the arousal of anxiety and claim to help patients not to become "victims" by the salutary advice they give. However, the counsel Berger offers is undermined not only by overdramatization and exaggeration but also by his magic-bullet solution of appropriate diet as the answer to sundry medical syndromes.[56] Podell's pointers to specific "mistakes" that the patient can catch presuppose incompetent physicians. The sole certain outcome of his precepts would be to wreck the doctor-patient relationship as patients openly display their mistrust. Both Berger and Podell pass themselves off as twentieth-century versions of the patient's best friend. But far from inducing security, their books will only alarm patients by furnishing them with half-baked information. These self-appointed watchdogs with their formulaic directives are parodistic successors to the nineteenth-century patient's personal "confidential friend." Yet it is significant that many of the most searing criticisms of current medical practice come from within the profession, from outstanding practitioners with high ideals such as Kleinman, Robert Coles, and the neurologist Oliver Sacks.

The only hope of attaining patient empowerment is not by any kind of adversarial trickery such as Berger and Podell outline but by a sincere cooperation between doctor and patient based on mutual respect for each other's integrity. No panaceas will generate this ideal rapport. "Humanistic medical care" has become, in Lipkin's words, "a kind of rescue theme for halting the continuing decline of mutual trust between the sick and those who would heal them."[57] Like so many slogans and fashions in medical beliefs that are greeted with enthusiasm, Lipkin adds, this will escalate into overexpectations and disappointment without ultimately "increasing clarity about the proper blending of science and art" (4). One key factor in that blending must be an ongoing awareness of the patient as a person with a life beyond the disease, however severely the disease may have impinged on and distorted that life. In an attempt to induce such awareness Rita Charon, who is both a physician and a literary scholar, has set her medical students to writing stories about their patients after interviewing them as medical cases. Some of these "stories" are couched in the first person as if from the patient's point of view; others adopt a third-person format.[58] The aim of the exercise is to implant "the empathic stance" by coaxing "medical students away from the detached and objectifying stance inevitably produced in them through the reductionism of most of the medical curriculum, without disarming them or rendering them ineffective through over-identification with the patient" (139). In other words, narratology, by activating the imagination, is harnessed to counteract objectification of the patient. Charon reports that although the students find the task difficult, "they emerge from writing their stories with a sense of sadness, dread, even victory" (140).[59]

A similar endeavor to bring the imagination into greater play is described by the child psychiatrist Robert Coles in *The Call of Stories,* in which he argues that the reading and discussion of fiction by budding professionals in law and business as well as in medicine can open up greater sensitivity in relating to others. The advantages—and disadvantages—of empathy, "the feeling that 'I might be you,'" as "a balance to equanimity"[60] are extensively discussed in the recent collection of essays *Empathy and the Practice of Medicine.* The concept is enthusiastically endorsed by all the contributors (most of whom are physicians). The one exception is Richard Landau, who holds both an M.D. and a Ph.D. and who argues with considerable fervor that physicians should be sensitive and even "sympathetic" but that those who deliberately cultivate empathy will forfeit the authority expected by the patient and will not be able reliably to give "the decisions of a scholarly, experienced expert."[61] Yet this does not happen to Konner, Klass, and Klitzman, who go through the same process of reflectiveness innate to writing as Charon's students in eyeing their institutions and the wider institution of the etiquette of medicine with a questioning gaze.

The cardinal role of narratology in humanizing medicine is nowhere more brilliantly illustrated than in Oliver Sacks's series of books about his patients. Although they tell of bizarre medical syndromes, they have attracted so large a readership as to become bestsellers. This success must be attributed to Sacks's recognition of his neurologically impaired patients as persons and his ability to present them in graphic language. What is distinctive about Sacks is his ability to respond simultaneously as a scientist and a humanist. He returns repeatedly to this twofold impulse in his personality: "When I was young, I was torn between two passionate, conflicting interests and ambitions—the pursuit of science and the pursuit of art. I found no reconciliation until I became a physician. I think all physicians enjoy a singular good fortune, in that we can give full expression to both sides of our nature, and never have to suppress one in favour of the other."[62] Likewise, in the preface to *The Man Who Mistook His Wife for a Hat* he writes of "a certain doubleness in me: that I feel myself a naturalist and a physician both; and that I am equally interested in diseases and people; perhaps, too, that I am equally, if inadequately, a theorist and dramatist, am equally drawn to the scientific and the romantic" (vii).

The term "romantic" is open to misunderstanding if it is taken in a narrow literary sense; Sacks invests it with a more ample denotation as referring to the mysterious, that is, the nonscientific facets of personality. Thus in considering the world of mental defectives he comments on his perception: "This is science, this is romance too."[63] Romance therefore comprises precisely what scientific medicine ignores as irrelevant to disease: "an inner perspective, an existentialist perspective,"[64] the endeavor on the physician's part empathetically to sound the patient's interior psychological realm. Sacks envisages himself as a "neuroanthropologist" (xx) who employs "an intersubjective approach" to supplement "the objective approach of the scientist" (xxi).

This dualism has a profound effect on Sacks's whole conceptualization of disease and the diseased, notably in his unremitting consciousness of the human dimension of any pathology: "Animals get diseases, but only man falls radically into sickness."[65] He objects with vehemence to the "mechanistic concepts of neurology," which envision the nervous system "as a sort of machine or computer" (57), for such "mechanicalness" forecloses exploration of the "life of the mind" (89). Indeed, he claims that "traditional neurology" actually "conceals from us the very life of the mind" (89) and propagates instead "the ugliest exemplars of assembly-line medicine: everything human, everything living, pounded, pulverized, atomized, quantized, and otherwise 'processed' out of existence."[66] Little wonder that *Awakenings* encountered opposition and rejection by the medical establishment: it calls into question not only "the militant ideology of cure that has dominated medicine in the latter part of the twentieth century"[67] but also the very foundations of scientific medicine in its assertion that objectivity alone is wholly unequal to the challenge of understanding the sick. Sacks goes so far as to attack with outspokenness "the Newtonian-Lockean-Cartesian view . . . which reduces men to machines, automata, puppets, dolls, blank tablets, formulae, ciphers, systems, and reflexes."[68] "The therapeutic correlate of such notions is the idea that one must *attack* the disease with all the weapons one has, and that one can launch the attack with impunity, without a thought for the *person* who is ill." Instead of this divorce of "disease as purely *alien* and bad, without organic relation to the person who is ill," Sacks sees his patients not just as "cases" caught in a "uniform process" but as "physiology as it is embedded in people, and people as they are embedded in living in history" (267). This rehumanization can only be achieved, however, if mechanicalness is "supplemented by concepts more dynamic, more alive," that enable the physician to register "a 'who' as well as a 'what,' a real person, a patient in relation to disease."[69] From this perspective, accounts of pathologies are "a form of natural history—but they tell us nothing about the individual and *his* history, they convey nothing of the person, and the experience of the person, as he faces, and struggles to survive, his disease" (viii).

To redress this imbalance, which amounts, in Sacks's eyes, to a travesty, "to restore the human subject at the center—the suffering, afflicted, fighting, human subject—we must deepen a case history to a narrative or a tale" (viii). "Tales," "fables," "stories," and "studies" (ix) are the unconventional words Sacks uses to describe his style of writing about his cases. He seeks to recuperate the person within the disease by heeding the voice of life to return to the "tradition by which patients have always told their stories to doctors" (viii). This is not, of course, to exclude the voice of modern medicine, as is apparent from Sacks's advanced drug use on his postencephalitic patients in *Awakenings,* but rather to rehumanize it by reinstating the importance of the patient's narrative. For like Mishler, Sacks conceives two types of discourse in answer to even such apparently simple questions as "How are you?" and "How are things?"[70] The first, essentially logical and mathematical, consists of measurements, data, vital signs, urinalysis, and so forth, while the second, dependent on "the delicacy of one's senses and intuitions," creates "a direct human confrontation, an 'I-Thou' relation between the discoursing worlds of physicians and patients" (204). Each type of discourse is complete in itself, yet they are complementary, and both are essential to understanding the patient's world. Equally essential, according to Kleinman, is physicians' posture toward the patient: "The way they nod their head, fidget, or look at the patient influences how the patient tells the illness story," for "how they listen to these accounts constrains the telling and the hearing."[71] Such reciprocity is generally disregarded when misunderstandings are attributed to either the doctor or the patient, whereas their source is most likely in the absence of consonance between the two parties.

Sacks's attitude of positive and respectful attentiveness is fundamental to his success in eliciting such a degree of responsiveness and in establishing a relationship not only to retarded but even to autistic patients. In *An Anthropologist on Mars* he sees the subjects, whatever their handicaps, as human beings who have, besides their "defects," a "personal center," a "self," an "I"

(227) struggling to express itself and in so doing to accommodate to what is missing, be it visual intelligence, as with Virgil (108–52), or a sense of color, as with the painter, Mr. I (3–41), vision and awareness of time, as with Greg F (42–76), or "social junction" (257) as with the autistic Temple Grandin (244–96) and Stephen Wiltshire (188–243). In all these instances Sacks is intent on neurological disturbances of function, but the way he phrases his interest is highly revealing: "It is, then, less deficits, in the traditional sense, which have engaged my interest, than neurological disorders affecting the self."[72] So he always strives to seek out that underlying, often hidden self and its coping strategies. From his own experiences with his injured leg, recorded in *A Leg to Stand On,* and with his right shoulder after surgery he knows that "adaptation follows a different path in each person."[73] He reaches beyond the mere outward processes of accommodation for an imaginative sense of patients' feelings in these particular, frequently peculiar situations. Thus in *Awakenings* he deplores the absence in the medical literature of any "picture of what it *feels* like to have Parkinsonism, to receive L-DOPA, and to be totally transformed" (207). Even more persistently, in *An Anthropologist on Mars* he tries to penetrate the world of the autistic, to intuit why Grandin "often feels excluded, an alien" (272) despite her really amazing success as an assistant professor of animal sciences. Similarly, with Stephen Wiltshire, the autistic drawing prodigy, Sacks wonders repeatedly "what he was feeling" (219), whether he feels sad about "his deep lack of human and social knowledge" (236), how he sees things (229), "following his gaze" so as "to see [the Grand Canyon] through his eyes, relinquishing my own intellectual knowledge of the rock strata below, and seeing them in purely visual terms" (231). He contrasts these endeavors to see him "as a human being, as a whole, . . . as a mind and person" (213–14) with the disquiet aroused in himself by days spent "in reducing Stephen to defects and gifts" (213).

The desire to see his patients as persons and to find out how they manage "in real life" leads Sacks to doff his white coat, to leave the hospital and the office in order to visit his subjects in their home environments.[74] While previously he had occasionally called on patients at home, for instance, on Rebecca as soon as he heard of her grandmother's death,[75] he makes it a consistent practice with his subjects in *An Anthropologist on Mars.* He learned the value of observing patients in their natural habitat from his father, who decided, when reluctantly considering retirement at the age of ninety, to "keep the house calls—I'll drop everything else instead."[76] He emphasizes what "a remarkable human and clinical experience" (104n) it is to go canoeing with Shane F; to fly in a small plane with Dr. Carl Bennett, who, like Shane, has Tourette's syndrome; to travel through Holland, Russia, and the United States with Stephen Wiltshire; or to take Greg F to a concert of his favorite band. Clearly, such excursions are a privilege Sacks the neurologist enjoys as a writer; they would be incompatible with routine practice. Nevertheless, the principle animating these trips is of paramount importance insofar as it represents a reprise of the doctor's old role of missionary to the bedside that fosters his capacity, in this personal context, to relate to patients as human beings.

Sacks's acknowledgment of his neurologically handicapped patients as persons is underscored by his freely reiterated expressions of affection for them. "One cannot," he explains in *Awakenings*, "make a minute study for many years of any group of patients without coming to love the patients one studies" (254). In arguing for the need to include "the emotional part of our nature" he affirms feeling as not standing "in the way of scientific precision"; instead, each acts as "the generator of the other" (254). His approach in *An Anthropologist on Mars* to Virgil, who has recently regained some sight after more than forty years of virtual blindness, is a good example of his method. Sacks goes to Virgil's home in the Midwest together with a specialized ophthalmologist, armed with a welter of test objects—color charts, letter charts, pictures, and illusions—as well as a video camera. His purpose is to "look not merely at his eyes and perceptual powers but at the whole tenor and pattern of his life" (116), especially at any "psychological difficulties that Virgil might encounter" (115). He goes through the same sequence of scientific testing and clinical observation with all the cases about whom he writes in *The Man Who Mistook His Wife for a Hat* and *An Anthropologist on Mars*. Yet he comes to realize that the testing alone captures merely one aspect of these idiosyncratic patients, namely, their departure from the norm. Only a wholly different apperception of them will restore their human side. The dichotomy is most evident in the case of Rebecca, who "had a partial cleft palate, which caused a whistling in her speech; short, stumpy fingers, with blunt, deformed nails; and a high, degenerative myopia requiring very thick spectacles—all stigmata of the same congenital condition which had caused her cerebral and mental defects. She was painfully shy and withdrawn, feeling that she was, and had always been, a 'figure of fun.'"[77] Sacks sets his negative, medicalized first impression against his second, humanistic view of her:

> When I first saw her—clumsy, uncouth, all-of-a-fumble—I saw her
> merely, or wholly, as a casualty, a broken creature, whose neuro-
> logical impairments I could pick out and dissect with precision: a
> multitude of apraxias and agnosias, a mass of sensorimotor im-
> pairments and breakdowns, limitations of intellectual schemata
> and concepts similar (by Piaget's criteria) to those of a child of
> eight. A poor thing, I said to myself, with perhaps a "splinter skill,"
> a freak gift, of speech; a mere mosaic of higher cortical functions,
> Piagetian schemata—most impaired.
>
> The next time I saw her, it was all very different. I didn't have
> her in a test situation, "evaluating" her in a clinic. I wandered
> outside—it was a lovely spring day—with a few minutes in hand
> before the clinic started, and there I saw Rebecca sitting on a bench,
> gazing at the April foliage quietly, with obvious delight. Her pos-
> ture had none of the clumsiness which had so impressed me before.
> Sitting there, in a light dress, her face calm and slightly smiling, she
> suddenly brought to mind one of Chekov's young women—Irene,
> Anya, Sonya, Nina—seen against the backdrop of a Chekovian
> cherry orchard. She could have been any young woman enjoying
> a beautiful spring day. This was my human, as opposed to my neu-
> rological, vision. (180)

Within the clinic, the tests "had given no inkling of anything *but* the defects, of anything, so to speak, *beyond* the deficits" (181). Rebecca's absorbed pleasure in the spring garden leads Sacks to explore her "strangely moving, poetic power" (179) and her capacity for "warm, deep, even passionate attachments" (178). Pressed into various workshops and classes under the aegis of the clinic's "Developmental and Cognitive Drive" (183), Rebecca does as appallingly badly as on the tests. On the other hand, she finds her own niche in a special theater group, where "she became a complete person, poised, fluent, with style, in each role" (185) because she has a scenic and narrative structure to guide her. Sacks remembers her "warmly" (177), citing her as an example of the validity of "narratology" over "defectology" (183).

A parallel instance is Martin, a sixty-one-year-old man with brain damage and intellectual limitations but such extraordinary musical retentiveness that Sacks calls him "A Walking Grove" after Grove's immense, nine-volume *Dictionary of Music and Musicians,* which he knows by heart. Like Rebecca, Martin is at one level a disaster: "He was often childish, sometimes spiteful, and prone to sudden tantrums—and the language he then used was that of a child. 'I'll throw a mudpie in your face!' I once heard him scream, and, occasionally, he spat or struck out. He sniffed, he was dirty, he blew snot on his sleeve—he had the look (and doubtless the feelings) at such times of a small, snotty child."[78] But he becomes "a different man" once "he returned to song and church—recovered himself, recollected himself, became real again" (191). It is a measure of Sacks's wisdom and genuine empathy that he can refrain from imposing a medical will on these retardates and instead lets them follow their own path to "poignant innocence, transparency, completeness, and dignity" (174). Of these patients he cherishes an especially "warm sense" (173).

In the way in which he writes about these uncommon people Sacks's humaneness and his dualism become very apparent. He uses technical terms such as *apraxias* and *agnosias, cerebral achromatopsia,* and *cystoid macular edema* to give as precise as possible a diagnostic designation of the physical manifestations of impairment. *Awakenings* contains a glossary of "unfamiliar words" referring to the book's special subject matter, "designed as a reader's companion, to help him visualize the peculiar disorders of movement, posture, will, appetite, sleep, etc." (324) characteristic of the conditions described. These are the terms that would appear on the patients' charts. But instead of just leaving the highly depersonalized notations of the chart, Sacks also gives a very individualized image of each of his patients, so that they emerge vividly as persons in their own right, notwithstanding their pathologies. The examples just cited of Rebecca and Martin are typical of Sacks's evocative insight. This trait is most striking in *Awakenings,* where all the patients are afflicted with the same syndrome yet each is granted a personality, a history, a self. Like Rebecca, Sacks himself is endowed with a "strangely moving, poetic power," an artist's imaginative and linguistic faculty that is perhaps itself a compensation for the "incorrigible clumsiness" that prevented him from becoming a surgeon, as he had originally wished.[79] This necessity of having to accommodate to his own limitations and develop his narratological talent may well have predisposed him to a fuller understanding of his patients' situation. Certainly his writing, notably in *Awakenings,* is alive with—and touching for—a metaphoricity that enters into both his patients' exigencies and the expression of his own reactions. Theirs is postulated as "a very mixed landscape, partly familiar, partly uncanny, with sunlit uplands, bottomless chasms, volcanoes, geysers, meadows, marshes, something like Yellowstone—archaic, prehuman, almost prehistoric, with a sense of vast forces simmering all round one" (208). Their disease is "an ontological ghoul" (212) that causes a "singularly complex . . . brain weather . . . full of inordinate sensitivities and sudden changes, no longer susceptible to an item-by-item analysis, but requiring to be seen as a whole, as a *map*" (228). Lacking a "feeling *at home* in the world" (239), the patients—and their physicians—have to take "arms by learning how to negotiate or navigate a sea of troubles, by becoming a mariner in the seas of one's self" (234–35). For Sacks too, in the process of his patients' awakening and relapse, goes through an experience of dislocation and wonder: "I felt like a slum child suddenly transplanted to Africa or Peru" (207). "These seven years," he summarizes, "have seemed like a single long day: a long night of illness, a morning awakening, a high noon of trouble, and now a long evening of repose" (240). Such poetic phraseology is the linguistic incarnation of his humanistic recognition of his patients not as freaks but as people grappling with their lot as best they can. And in this struggle he is as much their partner as their doctor.

Not least because of his writerly gifts, Sacks is an exceptional doctor whose interactions with his patients can serve as an ideal, though hardly as a practical model. Nevertheless, implicit in his stance are the fundamental issues about power, respect, compassion, and reciprocity central to every doctor-patient encounter. While continuing to draw on modern technological tools, Sacks manages to bridge the distance they have interjected between doctor and patient, literally and figuratively. In a symbiotic mixture of resistance and desire, patients simultaneously resent that distance and want the diagnostic and therapeutic benefits of contemporary scientific modalities. The outcome, the archetypal wish dream of entrusting one's welfare to an omniscient, omnipotent physician, is counterbalanced nowadays by a distrustful fear that produces a deeply conflicted transference. "Paradoxically doctors have not become more popular through their improved means of helping."[80] The simplistic "myth of uninterrupted medical heroism and inevitable progress," the perception of modern medicine as "a victory of reason over superstition, knowledge over ignorance, life over death,"[81] is increasingly being queried along with the idealization of the old-style doctor, who concentrated on the patient's personal profile. That he did so largely because little effective therapeutic intervention was available to him is overlooked in the favorable scenario of the "missionary at the bedside." Yet the ideals of the medical humanists, represented by the likes of Sacks, Kleinman, and Coles, rest on the desire to recuperate into contemporary practice the therapeutically valuable aspects of the older style, notably the personal doctor-patient alliance. The advances of medicine, beneficial though they were in totality, have, however, also undoubtedly complicated the balance of power between doctor and patient through the intervention of new quandaries such as the quality of life in terms of well-being as against its quantity in longevity.

This may perhaps be one of those dichotomies that doctors are said to prefer: "right or left, up or down, physician or patient, you or I."[82] Such antipodal thinking conforms to the scientific model; human relations, however, are rarely if ever so clearcut. The patient's pain will be right or left, up or down, but the discussion of it must be physician *and* patient, you *and* I. For as Sacks reminds us, medicine is not only "the oldest of the sciences" but also "the oldest of the arts."[83] And because "it is human relations which carry the possibilities of proper being-in-the-world" (238), medicine must be "collaborative," joining "the physician and his patient together in learning, teaching, communicating, and understanding" (247). The balance of power cannot be even, but it must at least strive to be fair.

NOTES

PREFACE

1. Warner, *Therapeutic Perspective,* 2.

1. "THE DOCTOR KNOWS BEST"

1. Parsons, *Social System,* 436.

2. Starr, *Social Transformation,* 92.

3. Ibid., 8.

4. Reynolds, "Enhancing Doctor-Patient Interactions," 72.

5. Beier, *Sufferers and Healers,* 3.

6. King, *Transformations in American Medicine,* 17.

7. See, e.g., Anderson and Helm, "Physician-Patient Encounter"; Byrne and Long, *Doctors Talking to Patients;* Freeling and Harris, *Doctor-Patient Relationship;* and Stewart and Roter, *Communicating with Medical Patients.*

8. There are, of course, other types of study, including the essentially humanistic work of Kleinman and the consideration of what genuine care of patients means by Brody, Cassell, Lipkin, and Mishler. These will be discussed in chapter 8.

9. See Katz, *Silent World of Doctor and Patient.*

10. Klass, *A Not Entirely Benign Procedure,* 73–74.

11. Barbour, *Caring for Patients,* 260, 152.

12. Williams, *Autobiography of William Carlos Williams,* 356.

13. See Hawkins, *Reconstructing Illness.*

14. Shryock, *Development of Modern Medicine,* 332.

15. Foucault, *Birth of the Clinic,* xii.

16. Rosenberg, *Explaining Epidemics,* 10.

17. Warner, *Therapeutic Perspective,* 7.

18. Crichton, *Five Patients,* 45.

19. Zola, *Thérèse Raquin,* 23.

20. See Furst, *All Is True,* 1–27.

21. See Rothfield, *Vital Signs.*

22. See Kramer, "Literature, Criticism, and Historical Imagination," 98.

23. For instance, Morantz-Sanchez on Sinclair Lewis's *Arrowsmith* in *Science and*

Sympathy, 309–10; Walsh on late-nineteenth-century American novels about the "doctress" in *"Doctors Wanted,"* 180–81; Peterson on Conan Doyle's *Stark Munro Letters* in *The Medical Profession in Mid-Victorian London,* 93–98; Newman on Mrs. Gaskell's *Wives and Daughters* in *The Evolution of Medical Education in the Nineteenth Century,* 25; Porter on Virginia Woolf's *Mrs. Dalloway* in "The Body and the Mind," 247.

24. See Furst, "Realism and Hypertrophy."

25. See Furst, "Struggling for Medical Reform in Middlemarch."

26. See Akerknecht's *Medicine at the Paris Hospital,* vii, and idem, *Short History of Medicine,* 146.

27. de Kruif, *Microbe Hunters,* 153–58.

2. "MISSIONARY TO THE BEDSIDE"

1. Cited in Warner, *Therapeutic Perspective,* 17.

2. See Peterson, *Medical Profession in Mid-Victorian London,* chapter 3, "Careers in General Practice," 90–138.

3. Waddington, *Medical Profession in the Industrial Revolution,* 7.

4. Peterson, *Medical Profession in Mid-Victorian London,* 102–6.

5. See Murphy, *Enter the Physician,* 32–69.

6. Rosenberg, *Explaining Epidemics,* 32.

7. For an exemplary study of the impact of one of these see ibid., 57–73.

8. Ibid., 132.

9. Ibid., 67.

10. See Furst, "Realism and Hypertrophy"; Galérant, *Médecine de campagne;* Léonard, *La France médicale;* idem, *La Médecine;* and idem, *La Vie quotidienne.*

11. Starr, *Social Transformation,* 70.

12. Ibid., 69.

13. Rosenberg, *Explaining Epidemics,* 132.

14. Early in the century overdependence on the opinions of the family's medical attendant was exposed to gentle satire in Jane Austen's *Emma* (1816). The elderly, ailing Mr. Woodhouse solicits the views of Mr. Perry on every domestic as well as health matter and constantly urges his married daughter, Mrs. Isobel Knightley, to consult her London surgeon, Mr. Wingfield, on the most favorable air in the city and the choice of a vacation spot (71–74).

15. Reiser, *Medicine and the Reign of Technology,* 5.

16. Rosenberg, *Explaining Epidemics,* 74–89.

17. Parsons, *Social System,* 478.

18. Starr, *Social Transformation,* 31.

19. Pellegrino, "Philosophy, Medical Ethics, and the Physician's Image," 83–84.

20. Murphy, *Enter the Physician,* xiii.

21. Rosenberg, *Explaining Epidemics*, 63.

22. Katz, *Silent World of Doctor and Patient*, 35.

23. Murphy, *Enter the Physician*, 70 ff.

24. Warner, *Therapeutic Perspective*, 85.

25. Cathell, *Book On the Physician Himself*, 1.

26. Hooker, *Physician and Patient*, 393.

27. Belkin, "New Wave in Health Care"; Karinch, *Telemedicine*.

3. SEEING—AND HEARING—IS BELIEVING

1. The prevalence of this custom is confirmed by the paragraph in Thomas Percival's *Medical Ethics* (1803) that lays down the financial etiquette on such occasions: "As the first *consultation* by *letter* imposes much more trouble and attention than a personal visit, it is reasonable on such an occasion, to expect a gratuity of double the usual amount. And this has long been the practice of many established physicians. But a subsequent epistolary correspondence, on the further treatment of the same disorder, may justly be regarded in the light of ordinary attendance, and may be compensated, as such, according to the circumstances of the case, or of the patient" (Leake, *Percival's Medical Ethics*, 102).

2. See Nuland, *Doctors*, 206–37, for an excellent biography of Laënnec and an assessment of his work.

3. Akerknecht, *Medicine at the Paris Hospital*, 90.

4. Ibid., 90.

5. Jarcho, "Early Review of Laënnec's Treatise."

6. Rosenberg, *Explaining Epidemics*, 144.

7. Newman, *Evolution of Medical Education*, 91–92.

8. The *Lancet*, founded in 1823 by the radical Thomas Wakley, was initially an organ for political campaigning for the Doctors' Registration Movement.

9. See Akerknecht, *Medicine at the Paris Hospital*, 191–93; Huard and Grmek, "Les Élèves étrangers de Laënnec"; and Maulitz, "Channel Crossing."

10. Warner, "Idea of Science in English Medicine," 198.

11. See ibid., 138–40.

12. Jacyna, "Robert Carswell and William Thomson," 111.

13. See Maulitz, "Channel Crossing," 492.

14. For an overview of the development of the microscope see Guthrie, *Janus in the Doorway*, 208–21.

15. See Reiser, *Medicine and the Reign of Technology*, 76–77.

16. Lydgate actually explains to him that this "was first divined and explored by Laënnec, the man who gave us the stethoscope, not so many years ago" (461).

17. Hunter, *Doctors' Stories*, 129.

18. Reiser, *Medicine and the Reign of Technology*, 4.

19. Foucault, *Birth of the Clinic*, xii.

20. Nuland, *Doctors*, 221.

21. For a speculative analysis of these five practioners see Cline, "Qualifications of the Medical Practitioners in *Middlemarch*."

22. Peterson, *Medical Profession in Mid-Victorian London*, 134.

23. Cartwright, *Social History of Medicine*, 53.

24. Eliot makes ironic reference to "the expensive and highly rarified medical instruction obtained by graduates of Oxford and Cambridge [, which] did not hinder quackery from having an excellent time of it" (175).

25. Parry and Parry, *Rise of the Medical Profession*, 104. For the history of the Edinburgh Medical School and its emphasis on clinical experience see Cartwright, *Social History of Medicine*, 47–48.

26. According to Jeanne Peterson, "The term 'general practitioner' emerged in the first thirty years of the century to refer to men who practised medicine and surgery, whether dually licensed or not" (*Medical Profession in Mid-Victorian London*, 17).

27. Waddington, *Medical Profession in the Industrial Revolution*, 54–68.

28. Porter and Porter, *Patient's Progress*, 69.

29. Anatomical pathology had advanced far more rapidly in France than in England because postmortem examinations were legal. For an illuminating exploration of the ramifications and implications of the Anatomical Act see Richardson, "'Trading Assassins' and the Licensing of Anatomy," 74–91.

30. Abel-Smith, *Hospitals*, 5.

31. Peterson, *Medical Profession in Mid-Victorian London*, 116–18, 139–41.

32. Ibid., 123.

33. ibid., 143.

34. Akerknecht, *Medicine at the Paris Hospital*, 102.

35. Cartwright, *Social History of Medicine*, 97–101. There were virtually no public hospitals for infectious diseases before mid-century (cf. Abel-Smith, *Hospitals*, 153).

36. Rosenberg, *Cholera Years*, 37–75.

37. W. J. Harvey, in Eliot, *Middlemarch*, notes to the Penguin edition, 902.

38. Peterson, in *Medical Profession in Mid-Victorian London*, 107, writes of the qualities of the "good 'medical wife,'" who preferably would come from a medical background, so that she would know the rigors of practice and the inroads they might make on family routine.

39. References in the text to popular religious works of the period suggest that the internal time of the action is in the 1830s. Thomas Noble writes in *George Eliot's "Scenes from Clerical Life"* that the "story is laid in the market town of Milby, around the years 1830–32" (9).

4. "A WOMAN'S HAND"

1. Nathanael West, quoted in the *Cincinnati Lancet and Observer* 38 (1877): 317, cited in Warner, *Therapeutic Perspective,* 11.

2. See Starr, *Social Transformation,* 90–92.

3. See Kett, *Formation of the American Medical Profession,* 181–84.

4. Ibid., 185–86.

5. Starr, *Social Transformation,* 99.

6. Akerknecht, *Short History of Medicine,* 223.

7. Rosenberg, *Cholera Years,* 154.

8. Ibid., 155.

9. Warner, "Fall and Rise of Professional Mystery," 112.

10. Shryock, *Development of Modern Medicine,* 240.

11. T. C. Minor, *Cincinnati Lancet and Observer* 37 (1876): 842, quoted in Warner, "Fall and Rise of Professional Mystery," 182.

12. Cathell, *Book On the Physician Himself,* 175.

13. Rothstein, *American Physicians in the Nineteenth Century,* 152–74, 230–46; Kett, *Formation of the American Medical Profession,* 132–64.

14. Kett, significantly, counts "female physicians" among the "irregulars" on the grounds that at the time of his census in 1858 they were "mainly botanic" (*Formation of the American Medical Profession,* 185).

15. An earlier example of this theme is found in *The Gilded Age* (1873), by Mark Twain with Charles Dudley Warner, which portrays a female medical student, Ruth Bolton, from a Quaker family in Philadelphia. As a rebel against the useless and dependent life that was the norm for women, Ruth is a foil to the novel's heroine, Laura Hawkins, a socialite femme fatale in Washington. Ruth takes up medicine, against her mother's wishes, as "the only method of escape" from "the clutches of the old monotony" (179) of her dour, stiff home. Although medical study is draining for her, she shows "the utmost coolness," "skillful hands," and "a gentle firmness" (247) in tending a patient's wound. However, after nearly dying of a fever contracted in the hospital, Ruth ends up by admitting her love for Philip Sterling. Her future is left open, but presumably it is marriage. *The Gilded Age* also makes mention of a successful female practitioner, Mrs. Dr. Longstreet, who "has a great income" (344). The novel is not included in my study because its primary focus is satire of social mores; Ruth is no more than a subsidiary figure. A female physician also occurs in Louisa May Alcott's *Jo's Boys* (1886); she shares many features with the others, but since this novel was directed at a juvenile audience, the issues are rather simplified.

16. Kamm, *Hope Deferred,* 176.

17. See, e.g., Peterson, "Victorian Governess"; Charlotte Brontë, *Jane Eyre* (1847) and *Villette* (1853); and Anne Brontë, *Agnes Grey* (1847).

18. Starr, *Social Transformation,* 40.

19. Ibid., 43.

20. Ibid., 80.

21. Lerner, "The Lady and the Millgirl," 6.

22. James Compton Burnett, M.D., in 1895, reprinted in Hellerstein et al., *Victorian Women,* 94.

23. Clarke's treatise is reprinted in Bell and Offen, *Women, the Family, and Freedom,* 1:429.

24. Elizabeth Garrett Anderson, reprinted in ibid., 1:435.

25. For the history of women in U.S. medicine see Morantz-Sanchez, *Science and Sympathy;* and Walsh, *"Doctors Wanted."*

26. Starr, *Social Transformation,* 81.

27. Jex-Blake, *Medical Women,* 44.

28. For a recent feminist interpretation of this tendency see Kent, *Sex and Suffrage in Britain:* "The reluctance of women to seek help from male doctors—stemming not from prudery or false modesty but from their experience of violation—had serious ramifications" (124).

29. Jex-Blake, *Medical Women,* 41.

30. Blackwell, "The Influence of Women," in *Essays in Medical Sociology,* 1:5.

31. Morantz, "Feminism, Professionalism, and Germs," 463. Some of this article is incorporated into chapter 7 of Morantz-Sanchez, *Science and Sympathy,* 184–202.

32. Blackwell, *Essays in Medical Sociology,* 2:98, 42.

33. For a late twentieth-century version of this postulate see Sheridan, *Pain in America:* "Male domination of health care institutions establishes a value system that prefers science to humanism and tends to be concerned about issues of power and competition" (101).

34. Anne Preston, quoted in Allsop, *History of the Women's Medical College,* 81.

35. Jacobi, "Description of the Early Symptoms of Meningeal Tumor," reprinted in *Mary Putnam Jacobi,* 501–4.

36. Jacobi, "Shall Women Practice Medicine?" reprinted in ibid., 367–90.

37. William Osler, quoted in ibid., xiv.

38. See ibid., xxviii.

39. Jacobi, "Inaugural Address," reprinted in ibid., 337–38.

40. Jacobi, "Shall Women Practice Medicine?" 373.

41. Jacobi, "Addressed Delivered at the Commencement of the Woman's Medical College," reprinted in *Mary Putnam Jacobi,* 392.

42. Jex-Blake, *Medical Women,* 44.

43. See Price, *A Whole New Life,* for a patient's account of both scientific and redemptive treatment in the same major medical center recently.

44. Cathell, *Book on the Physician Himself,* 143.

45. Mitchell, *Characteristics,* 264.

46. Kenton, "The Pap We Have Been Fed On," 287.

47. Walsh, *"Doctors Wanted,"* 186.

48. In 1900 women constituted 5 percent of the students in regular medical schools, 9 percent in eclectic schools, and 17 percent in homeopathic schools (Rothstein, *American Physicians in the Nineteenth Century,* 300n).

49. Jex-Blake, *Medical Women,* 41.

50. Jacobi, *Mary Putnam Jacobi,* 353.

51. The tension between marriage and a profession is played out in *The Bostonians* in Verena Tarrant, who opts to marry Basil Ransom in preference to continuing as the star speaker of the feminist movement.

52. *Helen Brent, M.D.* is just one vehicle—the least felicitous—of Meyer's ardent campaigning for women's rights, above all to higher education, which culminated in a signal victory when she not only raised the funds for a women's college but also persuaded the Columbia University trustees to approve the plans for Barnard College, which opened in October 1889.

53. See Blake, *Charge of the Parasols,* 207–10, for a chronological overview.

54. Conan Doyle, *Round the Red Lamp,* 294.

55. One concrete instance of the tendency to idealization and romance can be documented by comparison of the course of the fictive Dr. Edith Romney's life with that of the woman who served as a model for her, Dr. Edith Pechey, one of the first seven women who fought for admission to Edinburgh. Attractive, pretty, calm, with a quiet manner and a sense of humor, she was also highly gifted. She scored top in the chemistry exam in 1870 and so was entitled to the Hope Scholarship, but she was deprived of it when only males were deemed eligible. Already holding an M.D. from Bern, she was chosen to be among the first to take the exams in Dublin in 1877 because she was charming, modest, and not a bluestocking. But rather than finding a perfect partner, as Dr. Edith Romney does, Dr. Edith Pechey went out to India in 1883 and became senior medical officer at the Cama Hospital in Bombay.

56. Kenton, "The Pap We Have Been Fed On," 287.

5. DISEASES AND DISEASED PEOPLE

1. Zola, *L'Assommoir,* 126.

2. Rosenberg, *Care of Strangers,* 26.

3. Vogel, *Invention of the Modern Hospital,* 2.

4. Akerknecht, *Short History of Medicine,* 186.

5. Akerknecht, *Medicine at the Paris Hospital,* 77.

6. Karl Wunderlich, *Wien und Paris* (1841), 16, quoted in Akerknecht, *Medicine at the Paris Hospital,* 15.

7. Abel-Smith, *Hospitals*, 2.

8. Ibid., 1.

9. Vogel, *Invention of the Modern Hospital*, 1.

10. Cathell, *Book On the Physician Himself*, 172–73.

11. Rosenberg, *Care of Strangers*, 4.

12. Abel-Smith, *Hospitals*, 1.

13. Vogel, *Invention of the Modern Hospital*, 1.

14. Williams, *Age of Agony*, 89.

15. Abel-Smith, *Hospitals*, 46–65, 83–100.

16. Williams, *Age of Agony*, 89.

17. Bynum, "Hospital, Disease, and Community," 41.

18. Abel-Smith, *Hospitals*, 99.

19. Warner, *Therapeutic Perspective*, 102–14.

20. Vogel, *Invention of the Modern Hospital*, 13.

21. Rosenberg, *Explaining Epidemics*, 226.

22. *British Medical Journal*, 28 January 1853, 76, quoted in Abel-Smith, *Hospitals*, 104.

23. Peterson, *Medical Profession in Mid-Victorian London*, table 15.

24. Foucault, *Birth of the Clinic*, 125.

25. Bynum, "Hospital, Disease, and Community," 110.

26. Shryock, *Development of Modern Medicine*, 186.

27. Rosenberg, *Care of Strangers*, 82–83.

28. An English translation under the title *The Mysteries of Paris* was published in six volumes in Boston; neither the date of publication nor the translator's name is mentioned. It is so free a translation, with such significant omissions and elisions, as to be very unreliable. I therefore give references to the French text.

29. Bory, *Eugène Sue*, 243.

30. Akerknecht, *Medicine at the Paris Hospital*, 3.

31. Warner, *Therapeutic Perspective*, 195.

32. See Nuland, *Doctors*, 232.

33. "A Letter from Vienna," *Boston Medical and Surgical Journal* 86 (1872): 214–15, quoted in Warner, *Therapeutic Perspective*, 199.

34. *Boston Evening Transcript*, 24 February 1888, quoted in Vogel, *Invention of the Modern Hospital*, 13–14.

35. Cunningham and Willis, *Laboratory Revolution in Medicine*, 2.

36. Foucault, *Birth of the Clinic*, 42.

37. Rosenberg, *Care of Strangers*, 83.

38. Sir Dyce Duckworth, "Prognosis of Disease," *British Medical Journal* 2 (1896): 251, quoted in Reiser, *Medicine and the Reign of Technology*, 90.

39. Starr, *Social Transformation*, 112, 169.

40. Peterson, *Medical Profession in Mid-Victorian London,* app. D.

41. Ibid., 174.

42. Jewson, "Disappearance of the Sick-Man," 235.

43. Cathell, *Book On the Physician Himself,* 51.

44. Rosenberg, *Care of Strangers,* 118.

45. Foucault, *Birth of the Clinic,* 136.

46. See Peterson, *Medical Profession in Mid-Victorian London,* 136 ff.; and Akerknecht, *Medicine at the Paris Hospital.*

47. Jewson, "Disappearance of the Sick-Man," 237, 236.

48. Jacobi, "Inaugural Address," reprinted in *Mary Putnam Jacobi,* 335.

49. Reiser, *Medicine and the Reign of Technology,* ix.

50. Akerknecht, *Medicine at the Paris Hospital,* 22.

51. In "The Origins of Anaesthesia," chapter 10 of Nuland, *Doctors,* the bizarre rivalries surrounding the early uses of ether and the final attribution of this discovery to Morton are traced.

52. Guthrie, *Janus in the Doorway,* 235–42; Rosenberg, *Care of Strangers,* 147–49.

53. Shryock, *Development of Modern Medicine,* 173.

54. Nuland, *Doctors,* 346.

55. Joseph Lister, in *Lancet,* 8 January 1870, cited in ibid., 366.

56. Akerknecht, *Short History of Medicine,* 191.

57. Rosenberg, *Care of Strangers,* 97–98. See also Alcott, *Hospital Sketches,* for an account of Alcott's work as a volunteer nurse in a field hospital from December 1862 to January 1863.

58. Peterson, *Medical Profession in Mid-Victorian London,* 152 ff. For patterns of hospital growth in the United States see Rosenberg, *Care of Strangers,* 109 ff.

59. See Abel-Smith, *Hospitals,* 133–51, for a detailed account of the debate in Britain.

60. Ibid., 190.

61. Ibid.

62. Foucault, *Birth of the Clinic,* 137.

6. THE QUESTIONABLE SANCTUARY

1. Bernard, *Introduction to the Study of Experimental Medicine,* 146.

2. Cunningham and Williams, *Laboratory Revolution in Medicine,* 3.

3. de Kruif, *Microbe Hinters,* 75–101.

4. Ibid., 101–40.

5. Akerknecht, *Short History of Medicine,* 179.

6. See ibid., 180, for a complete list.

7. King, *Transformations in American Medicine,* 226.

8. Institutes for physiological research had existed since the middle third of the century, notably in Germany (see Kremer, "Building Institutes for Physiology in Prussia).

9. See Weindling, "Scientific Elites and Laboratory Organisation."

10. King, *Transformations in American Medicine*, 221.

11. See Chen, "Laboratory as Business."

12. Shryock, *Development of Modern Medicine*, 211.

13. Pellegrino, "Sociocultural Impact of Twentieth-Century Therapeutics."

14. *Le Docteur Pascal*, in *Les Rougon-Macquart*, 5:923.

15. Baguley, "Du naturalisme au mythe."

16. Léonard, *La France médicale*, 31 ff.

17. Rosenberg, "Martin Arrowsmith," 449.

18. It has been argued that *Arrowsmith* is a *roman à clef*, with Gottlieb corresponding to Jacques Loeb as well as Alexis Carrel, Terry Wickett in part to J. H. Northrop, and A. DeWitt Tubbs to Dr. Simon Flexner (see Schorer, Afterword to *Arrowsmith*, 432).

19. Markowitz and Rosner, "Silicosis and the Politics of Disability," esp. 188–202.

20. Morantz-Sanchez, *Science and Sympathy*, 310.

21. Schorer, Afterword to *Arrowsmith*, 437.

22. Rosenberg, "Martin Arrowsmith," 51.

23. Ibid.

24. Cunningham, "Transforming the Plague," 218.

25. Ibid., 224–36.

26. Ibid., 236.

27. Chen, "Laboratory as Business," 178–79.

28. Griffin, Introduction to *Twentieth Century Interpretations of "Arrowsmith,"* 12.

29. Maulitz, "Physician versus Bacteriologist," 98.

30. Jewson, "Disappearance of the Sick-Man," 239.

31. Rosenberg, *Explaining Epidemics*, 30.

32. King, *Transformations in American Medicine*, 231.

33. Warner, *Therapeutic Perspective*, 249.

34. Jewson, "Disappearance of the Sick-Man," 238.

35. Conan Doyle, *Round the Red Lamp*, 50.

36. Schorer, Afterword to *Arrowsmith*, 435.

37. Ober, "*Arrowsmith* and *The Last Adam*," 58.

7. EYEING THE INSTITUTION

1. Peabody, "Care of Patients," 878.

2. Konner, *Medicine at the Crossroads,* 29.

3. Rosenberg, *Care of Strangers,* 325.

4. Ibid., 290.

5. Peabody, "Care of Patients," 878.

6. Vogel, *Invention of the Modern Hospital,* 133.

7. For a history see Katz, *Silent World of Doctor and Patient.*

8. Reiser, *Medicine and the Reign of Technology,* ix.

9. Lipkin, *Care of Patients,* ix.

10. Ibid., xiii.

11. Charon, "To Render the Lives of Patients," 64; see also idem, "Doctor-Patient/Reader-Writer."

12. Angier, "From Dr. Welby to Dr. Giggles," 14.

13. Rosenberg, *Care of Strangers,* 3.

14. Joanne Trautman argues in "The Image of the Physician in Twentieth-Century Literature" that the negative image was more common before the nineteenth century. Obviously, it was easier for quacks to flourish before the the profession was regulated by law.

15. Angier, "From Dr. Welby to Dr. Giggles."

16. See also Konner, *Becoming a Doctor,* 185, 201, 302.

17. Akerknecht, *Short History of Medicine,* 235.

18. Starr, *Social Transformation,* 76.

19. Rosenberg, *Patients,* 89, 189.

20. Starr, *Social Transformation,* 362.

21. Monroe, Holleman, and Holleman, "Is There a Person in This Case?" 46.

22. He went on to become a psychiatrist, a professional listener, so to speak, in New York City.

23. Fissell, "Disappearance of the Patient's Narrative," 99.

24. Kleinman, *Illness Narratives,* 131.

25. Sacks, *Man Who Mistook His Wife for a Hat,* xiv. See also idem, *Anthropologist on Mars;* and Nuland, *Doctors,* 163.

26. Hawkins, "A. R. Luria and the Art of Clinical Biography," 2.

27. Lipkin, *Care of Patients,* xiv.

28. Jewson,"Disappearance of the Sick-Man," 232.

8. BALANCING THE POWER

1. For an explanatory comment on the prohibition from cutting persons laboring under the stone see Nuland, *Doctors,* 28.

2. The Hippocratic oath was replaced at Tufts University Medical School in 1986

by a new oath with a more positive charge that included such clauses as: "I will prevent disease whenever I can, for prevention is preferable to cure," and "I will remember that there is art to medicine as well as science, and that warmth, sympathy,
and understanding may outweigh the surgeon's knife or the chemist's drug" (Berger,
What Your Doctor Didn't Learn, 60).

3. The "Code of Ethics" is reprinted in Leake, *Percival's Medical Ethics,* 219–38.

4. The "Principles of Medical Ethics" are reprinted in Katz, *Silent World of Doctor
and Patient,* 238–39.

5. Starr, *Social Transformation.*

6. Brody, *Healer's Power,* 17.

7. Katz, *Silent World of Doctor and Patient,* 142.

8. "Among the recent discoveries in the practice of medicine is the fact that human
beings come equipped with resources for healing that are best mobilized not by detached scientific efficacy but by communication and supportive human outreach"
(Cousins, *Physician in Literature,* xxi; see also idem, *Anatomy of an Illness*).

9. Reynolds, "Enhancing Doctor-Patient Interactions," 78.

10. Pellegrino, "Philosophy, Medical Ethics, and the Physician's Image," 87.

11. Monroe, Holleman, and Holleman, "Is There a Person in This Case?" 45.

12. Scarry, *Body in Pain,* 6–7.

13. Poirier et al., "Charting the Chart."

14. Hunter, *Doctors' Stories,* xix.

15. David A. Worth, quoted in Safire, "Health Care Provider, Heal Thyself."

16. Reeder, "Patient-Client as a Consumer."

17. Kleinman, *Illness Narratives,* 219.

18. Ibid., 132–34.

19. Brody, *Healer's Power,* 174.

20. Lipkin, *Care of Patients,* 187.

21. Brody, *Healer's Power,* 2.

22. Kleinman, *Illness Narratives,* 57.

23. Williams, *Autobiography,* 128.

24. Cassell, *Healer's Art,* 94.

25. Spiro, "What Is Empathy and Can It Be Taught?" 9.

26. Kleinman, *Illness Narratives,* 130.

27. Balint, *The Doctor, The Patient, and His Illness,* 217.

28. Cassell, *Talking with Patients,* 1:1.

29. Katz, *Silent World of Doctor and Patient,* xiv.

30. Brody, *Healer's Power,* 89.

31. Silver, "Medical Terms," 4.

32. Cicourel, "Language and Medicine," 409.

33. Balint, *The Doctor, the Patient, and His Illness,* 26.

34. Kleinman, *Illness Narratives,* 240.

35. Mishler, *Discourse of Medicine,* 10.

36. See also Paget, "On the Work of Talk."

37. Byrne and Long, *Doctors Talking to Patients,* 14.

38. West, *Routine Complications,* 1.

39. Byrne and Long, *Doctors Talking to Patients,* 117.

40. West cites jargon in 50 percent of eight hundred visits, adding that "it seems that patients do not like medical jargon, but physicians do not know what constitutes it" (*Routine Complications,* 24).

41. Baby talk may be motivated in part by the need to communicate with immigrant patients who have little English and different cultural assumptions (see Freeling and Harris, *Doctor-Patient Relationship*).

42. Crichton, *Travels,* 61.

43. Balint, *The Doctor, the Patient, and His Illness,* 265.

44. Ehrenreich and English, *Complaints and Disorders,* 78.

45. Katz, *Silent World of Doctor and Patient,* 100.

46. Balint, *The Doctor, the Patient, and His Illness,* 225

47. Kleinman, *Illness Narratives,* 245.

48. Balint, *The Doctor, the Patient, and His Illness,* 18.

49. Brody, *Healer's Power,* 141.

50. Ibid., 139.

51. Ibid., 22.

52. Cousins, *Physician in Literature,* xv.

53. West, *Routine Complications,* 36.

54. Podell, *When Your Doctor,* jacket and foreword.

55. Berger, *What Your Doctor Didn't Learn,* dedication.

56. Berger is also the author of *How To Be Your Own Nutritionist* and *Forever Young.*

57. Lipkin, *Care of Patients,* 4.

58. Charon, "Doctor-Patient/Reader-Writer," 141–42.

59. Charon has restated her arguments for improving narrative competence in "The Narrative Road to Empathy."

60. Spiro, "Empathy: An Introduction," 2.

61. Landau, " . . . And the Least of These Is Empathy," 108.

62. Sacks, *Awakenings,* 253–54.

63. Sacks, *Man Who Mistook His Wife for a Hat,* 177.

64. Sacks, *Anthropologist on Mars,* 79.

65. Sacks, *Man Who Mistook His Wife for a Hat,* vii.

66. Sacks, *Awakenings,* 207.

67. Hawkins, "Myth of Cure," 11.

68. Sacks, *Awakenings*, 205.

69. Sacks, *Man Who Mistook His Wife for a Hat*, 87, viii.

70. Sacks, *Awakenings*, 203.

71. Kleinman, *Illness Narratives*, 52.

72. Sacks, *Man Who Mistook His Wife for a Hat*, 6.

73. Sacks, *Anthropologist on Mars*, xvi.

74. Ibid. 116.

75. Sacks, *Man Who Mistook His Wife for a Hat*, 182.

76. Sacks, *Anthropologist on Mars*, xx.

77. Sacks, *Man Who Mistook His Wife for a Hat*, 178.

78. Ibid, 190

79. Sacks, *Anthropologist on Mars*, 93.

80. Akerknecht, *Short History of Medicine*, 240.

81. Beier, *Sufferers and Healers*, 2.

82. Spiro, "What Is Empathy and Can It Be Taught?" 14.

83. Sacks, *Awakenings*, 26.

BIBLIOGRAPHY

PRIMARY SOURCES

Alcott, Louisa May. *Hospital Sketches.* 1863. Reprint, edited by Bessie Z. Jones, Cambridge: Belknap Press of Harvard Univ. Press, 1960.

———. *Jo's Boys.* 1886. Reprint, New York: New American Library, 1987.

Alexander, G. G. *Dr. Victoria: A Picture from the Period.* London: Tinsley, 1881.

Austen, Jane. *Emma.* 1816. Reprint, New York: Bantam, 1958.

Balzac, Honoré de. *La Comédie humaine.* Ca. 1830–50. Critical edition by Marcel Bouteron. 8 vols. 1948. Reprint, Paris: Gallimard, 1976.

———. *Eugénie Grandet.* 1833. In *La Comédie humaine,* ed. Bouteron, 3:480–649. Translated by Ellen Marriage (New York: Dutton, 1968).

———. *Le Médecin de campagne.* 1833. In *La Comédie humaine,* ed. Bouteron, 8:317–535. Translated by Ellen Marriage under the title *The Country Doctor* (New York: Dutton, 1911).

———. *Le Père Goriot.* 1835. In *La Comédie humaine,* ed. Bouteron, 2:847–1085. Translated by Marion A. Crawford under the title *Old Goriot* (Harmondsworth: Penguin, 1975).

Beeton, Isabella. *Book of Household Management.* 1861. Reprint, New York: Exeter, 1986.

Berger, John. *A Fortunate Man.* New York: Holt, Rinehart & Winston, 1967.

Berger, Stuart M. *Forever Young: Twenty Years Younger in Twenty Weeks.* New York: Avon, 1988.

———. *How To Be Your Own Nutritionist.* New York: Avon, 1988.

———. *What Your Doctor Didn't Learn in Medical School.* New York: Avon, 1988.

Bernard, Claude. *Introduction à l'étude de la médecine expérimentale.* 1865. Edited by Paul F. Cranefield. New York: Science History Publications/USA, 1976. Translated by Henry Copley Greene under the title *Introduction to the Study of Experimental Medicine* (1927; reprint, New York: Macmillan, 1957).

Blackwell, Elizabeth. *Essays in Medical Sociology.* 1902. Reprint, 2 vols. in 1, New York: Arno Press & The New York Times, 1972.

———. *Pioneer Work in Opening the Medical Profession to Women.* 1895. Reprint, New York: Schocken, 1977.

Bogdanich, Walt. *The Great White Lie*. New York: Touchstone, 1991.

Cabanis, Georges. *Du degré de certitude dans la médecine*. Paris, 1797.

Cathell, Daniel Webster. *Book On the Physician Himself*. Philadelphia: Davis, 1881.

Conan Doyle, Arthur. *Round the Red Lamp; Being Facts and Fancies of Medical Life*. 1894. Reprint, London: Appleton, 1921.

Cook, Robin. *Coma*. New York: Putnam, 1977.

———. *Godplayer*. New York: Penguin, 1984.

———. *Harmful Intent*. New York: Putnam, 1990.

———. *Vital Signs*. New York: Putnam, 1991.

Cronin, A. J. *The Citadel*. 1937. Reprint, Boston: Little, Brown & Co., 1965.

Davies, Robertson. *The Cunning Man*. 1994. Reprint, New York: Penguin, 1996.

Dr. Edith Romney. London: Richard Bentley & Son, 1883.

Eliot, George. "Janet's Repentance." In *Scenes from Clerical Life*, 167–301. 1858. Reprint, New York: Oxford Univ. Press, 1988.

———. *Middlemarch*. Edited by W. J. Harvey. 1872. Reprint, Harmondsworth: Penguin, 1965.

———. *Quarry for "Middlemarch."* Edited by Anna T. Kitchel. Berkeley: Univ. of California Press, 1957.

Flaubert, Gustave. *Madame Bovary*. 1857. Reprint, Paris: Gallimard, 1947. Translated by Merloyd Lawrence (Boston: Houghton Mifflin, 1969).

Fontane, Theodor. *Effi Briest*. 1895. Reprint, Munich: Droemer, 1956. Translated by Douglas Parmée (Harmondsworth: Penguin, 1956).

Frank, Arthur. *At the Will of the Body*. Boston: Houghton Mifflin, 1992.

Gaskell, Elizabeth. *Mary Barton*. 1848. Reprint, New York: Norton, 1958.

———. *Wives and Daughters*. 1866. Reprint, New York: Penguin, 1969.

Gilbert, Sandra. *Wrongful Death: A Medical Tragedy*. New York: Norton, 1995.

Hilfiker, David. *Healing the Wounds: A Physician Looks at His Work*. New York: Pantheon, 1985.

Holmes, Oliver Wendell. *Elsie Venner*. 1861. 31st ed. Boston: Houghton Mifflin, 1886.

Hooker, Worthington. *Physician and Patient; or, A Partial View of the Mutual Duties, Relations and Interests of the Medical Profession and the Community*. 1849. Reprint, New York: Arno Press & The New York Times, 1972.

Howells, William Dean. *Dr. Breen's Practice*. Boston: Osgood, 1881.

Huxley, Aldous. *Brave New World*. 1932. Reprint, Harmondsworth: Penguin, 1955.

Jacobi, Mary Putnam. *Mary Putnam Jacobi, M.D.: Pathfinder in Medicine*. 1882. Reprint, New York: Putnam, 1925.

James, Henry. *The Bostonians*. 1886. Reprint, New York: New American Library, 1974.

———. *Washington Square*. 1881. Reprint, New York: Bantam, 1959.

Jewett, Sarah Orne. *A Country Doctor.* 1884. Reprint, New York: New American Library, 1986.

Jex-Blake, Sophia. *Medical Women.* 1886. Reprint, New York: Source Books, 1970.

Johnson, Diane. *Health and Happiness.* New York: Fawcett, 1990.

Klass, Perri. *A Not Entirely Benign Procedure.* New York: Signet, 1987.

Klitzman, Robert. *A Year-Long Night.* New York: Penguin, 1989.

Konner, Melvin. *Becoming a Doctor.* New York: Penguin, 1987.

Leake, Chauncy D., ed. *Percival's Medical Ethics.* Baltimore: Williams & Wilkins, 1927.

Lessing, Doris. *A Proper Marriage.* 1952. Reprint, New York: Plume, 1970.

Lewis, Sinclair. *Arrowsmith.* 1925. Reprint, New York: Signet, 1961.

Mann, Thomas. *Buddenbrooks.* 1901. Reprint, Frankfurt: Fischer, 1961. Translated by H. T. Lowe-Porter (New York: Vintage, 1952).

Mason, Mary. *The Young Housewife's Counsellor.* Philadelphia: Lippincott, 1871.

Maugham, Somerset. *Of Human Bondage.* 1915. Reprint, New York: Penguin, 1963.

Meyer, Annie Nathan. *Helen Brent, M.D.* 1891. Reprint, New York: Cassell, 1894.

Millet-Robinet, Cora-Elisabeth. *La Maison rustique des dames.* 10th ed. Paris: Librairie agricole de la maison rustique, n.d.

Mitchell, Silas Weir. *Characteristics.* New York: Century, 1915.

Moore, George. *Esther Waters.* 1894. Reprint, New York: Dutton, 1962.

Mosher, Eliza M. "The Human in Medicine, Surgery, and Nursing." *Medical Woman's Journal* 32, no. 5 (1925): 117–19.

Peabody, Frances W. "The Care of Patients." *Journal of the American Medical Association* 88, no. 2 (1927): 877–81.

Phelps, Elizabeth Stuart. *Dr. Zay.* Boston: Houghton Mifflin, 1882.

Podell, Richard N. *When Your Doctor Doesn't Know Best.* New York: Simon & Schuster, 1995.

Price, Reynolds. *A Whole New Life.* New York: Atheneum, 1994.

Reade, Charles. *A Woman-Hater.* 1877. Reprint, Boston: Colonial, n.d.

Rosenberg, Mark L. *Patients: The Experience of Illness.* Philadelphia: Saunders, 1980.

Sacks, Oliver. *An Anthropologist on Mars: Seven Paradoxical Tales.* New York: Knopf, 1995.

———. *Awakenings.* 1973. Reprint, New York: Dutton, 1983.

———. *A Leg to Stand On.* New York: Summit, 1984.

———. *The Man Who Mistook His Wife for a Hat and Other Stories.* 1970. New York: Basic, 1986.

Shem, Samuel. *The House of God.* 1978. Reprint, New York: Dell, 1988.

Stevenson, Robert Louis. *Dr. Jekyll and Mr. Hyde.* 1886. Reprint, New York: Dutton, 1962.

Sue, Eugène. *Les Mystères de Paris*. 4 vols. Brussels: Meline, Cans, 1844. Translated under the title *The Mysteries of Paris*, 6 vols. (Boston: Nicolls, n.d).

Svevo, Italo. *La coscienza di Zeno*. 1923. Reprint, Pordenone: Studio Tesi, 1985. Translated by Beryl de Zoete under the title *The Confessions of Zeno* (Harmondsworth: Penguin, 1964).

Travers, Graham. *Mona Maclean, Medical Student*. Edinburgh: Blackwood & Sons, 1893.

Trollope, Anthony. *Dr. Thorne*. 1858. Reprint, New York: Penguin, 1991.

Turgenev, Ivan. *Fathers and Sons*. 1862. Translated by Ralph Matlaw. New York: Norton, 1989.

Twain, Mark, and Dudley, Charles Warner. *The Gilded Age*. 1873. Reprint, New York: Trident, 1964.

Williams, William Carlos. *The Autobiography of William Carlos Williams*. 1948. Reprint, New York: New Directions, 1951.

Zola, Emile. *L'Assommoir*. 1877. In *Les Rougon-Macquart,* ed. Mittérand, 2:371–796. Translated by L. W. Tancock (Harmondsworth: Penguin, 1970).

———. *Les Rougon-Macquart*. 1871–93. Edited by Henri Mittérand. 20 vols. in 5. Paris: Gallimard, 1956–67.

———. *Le Docteur Pascal*. 1893. In *Les Rougon-Macquart,* ed. Mittérand, 5:913–1220. Translated by Ernest A. Vizetelly under the title *Doctor Pascal* (London: Caxton, 1893).

———. *Le Roman expérimental*. 1880. Reprint, Paris: Garnier-Flammarion, 1971. Translated under the title *The Experimental Novel*, in *Documents of Modern Literary Realism,* edited by George J. Becker (Princeton: Princeton Univ. Press, 1963), 162–96.

———. *Thérèse Raquin*. 1866. 2d ed. 1867. Translated by L. W. Tancock (Harmondsworth: Penguin, 1962).

SECONDARY SOURCES

Abel-Smith, Brian. *The Hospitals, 1800-1940*. Cambridge: Cambridge Univ. Press, 1964.

Akerknecht, Erwin H. *A Short History of Medicine*. 1955. Rev. ed. Baltimore: Johns Hopkins Univ. Press, 1982.

———. *Medicine at the Paris Hospital*. Baltimore: Johns Hopkins Press, 1967.

Allsop, Giulielma Fell. *History of the Women's Medical College of Philadelphia, Pennsylvania, 1850-1950*. Philadelphia: Lippincott, 1950.

Anderson, W. Timothy, and David T. Helm. "The Physician-Patient Encounter: A

Process of Reality Negotiation." In *Patients, Physicians, and Illness,* edited by E. G. Jago, 259–71. 3d ed. New York: Free Press, 1979.

Angier, Natalie. "From Dr. Welby to Dr. Giggles, a Steep Slide." *New York Times,* 23 August 1993, sec. H, pp. 9 and 15.

Baguley, David. "Du naturalisme au mythe: L'alchimie du docteur Pascal." *Cahiers naturalistes* 48 (1974): 141–83.

Bailin, Miriam. *The Sickroom in Victorian Fiction: The Art of Being Ill.* New York: Cambridge Univ. Press, 1994.

Balint, Michael. *The Doctor, the Patient, and His Illness.* New York: International Press, 1957.

Barbour, Allen. *Caring for Patients: A Critique of the Medical Model.* Stanford: Stanford Univ. Press, 1995.

Beier, Lucinda McCray. *Sufferers and Healers: The Experience of Illness in Seventeenth-Century England.* New York: Routledge & Kegan Paul, 1987.

Belkin, Lisa. "New Wave in Health Care: Visits by Video." *New York Times,* 15 July 1993, sec. A, pp. 1 and 15.

Bell, Susan Groag, and Karen M. Offen. *Women, the Family, and Freedom.* 2 vols. Stanford: Stanford Univ. Press, 1983.

Biasin, Gian-Paolo. *Literary Diseases: Theme and Metaphor in the Italian Novel.* Austin: Univ. of Texas Press, 1975.

Blake, Catriona. *The Charge of the Parasols: Women's Entry into the Medical Profession.* London: Free Press, 1990.

Bory, Jean-Louis. *Eugène Sue.* Paris: Hachette, 1962.

Brody, Howard. *The Healer's Power.* New Haven: Yale Univ. Press, 1992.

Bynum, W. F. "Hospital, Disease, and Community: The London Fever Hospital, 1801–50." In *Healing and History,* edited by Charles E. Rosenberg, 97–115. New York: Dawson Science History Publications, 1979.

Byrne, Patrick S., and Barrie E. L. Long. *Doctors Talking to Patients: A Study of the Verbal Behaviour of General Practitioners in Their Surgeries.* London: Her Majesty's Stationery Office, 1976.

Carson, Ronald A., Richard C. Reynolds, and Harold Gene Moss, eds. *Patient Wishes and Physician Obligations.* Gainesville: Univ. of Florida Press, 1979.

Cartwright, Frederick A. *A Social History of Medicine.* New York: Longman, 1977.

Cassell, Eric J. *The Healer's Art: A New Approach to the Doctor-Patient Relationship.* New York: Penguin, 1976.

———. *Talking with Patients.* 2 vols. Cambridge: MIT Press, 1985.

Charon, Rita. "Doctor-Patient / Reader-Writer: Learning to Find the Text." *Soundings* 72 (1989): 137–52.

————. "The Narrative Road to Empathy." In Spiro et al., *Empathy and the Practice of Medicine,* 147–59.

————. "To Render the Lives of Patients." *Literature and Medicine* 5 (1986): 58–74.

Chen, Wai. "The Laboratory as Business." In Cunningham and Williams, *Laboratory Revolution in Medicine,* 245–92.

Cicourel, Aaron V. "Language and Medicine." In *Language in the USA,* edited bu Charles A. Ferguson and Shirley Brice Heath, 407–29. New York: Cambridge Univ. Press, 1981.

Cline, C. L. "Qualifications of the Medical Practitioners in *Middlemarch.*" In *Nineteenth-Century Perspectives: Essays in Honor of Lionel Stevenson,* edited by Clyde D. L. Ryals, 271–81. Durham NC: Duke Univ. Press, 1974.

Coles, Robert. *The Call of Stories: Teaching and the Moral Imagination.* Boston: Houghton Mifflin, 1989.

Cousins, Norman. *Anatomy of an Illness as Perceived by the Patient.* New York: Norton, 1979.

————, ed. *The Physician in Literature.* Philadelphia: Saunders, 1982.

Crichton, Michael. *Five Patients.* New York: Knopf, 1970.

————. *Travels.* New York: Knopf, 1988.

Cunningham, Andrew. "Transforming the Plague: The Laboratory and the Identity of Infectious Diseases." In Cunningham and Williams, *Laboratory Revolution in Medicine,* 209–44.

Cunningham, Andrew, and Perry Williams, eds. *The Laboratory Revolution in Medicine.* Cambridge: Cambridge Univ. Press, 1992.

de Kruif, Paul. *Microbe Hunters.* 1926. Reprint, New York: Harcourt Brace, 1945.

Drachman, Virginia. *Hospital with a Heart: Women Doctors and the Paradox of Separatism at the New England Hospital, 1862-1969.* Ithaca: Cornell Univ. Press, 1984.

Ehrenreich, Barbara, and Deirdre English. *Complaints and Disorders: The Sexual Politics of Sickness.* Old Westbury NY: Feminist Press, 1973.

Fissell, Mary E. "The Disappearance of the Patient's Narrative and the Invention of Hospital Medicine." In French and Wear, *British Medicine in an Age of Reform,* 92–109.

Foucault, Michel. *The Birth of the Clinic.* 1963. Translated by A. M. Sheridan Smith. New York: Vintage, 1975.

Freeling, Paul, and Conrad M. Harris. *The Doctor-Patient Relationship.* 3d ed. Edinburgh: Churchill Livingstone, 1984.

French, Roger, and Andrew Wear, eds. *British Medicine in an Age of Reform.* London: Routledge, 1991.

Furst, Lilian R. *All Is True: The Claims and Strategies of Realist Fiction.* Durham NC: Duke Univ. Press, 1995.

————. "Halfway up the Hill: The 'Doctress' in Late Nineteenth-Century American

Fiction." In *Women Healers and Physicians: Climbing a Long Hill,* edited by Lilian R. Furst, 221–38. Lexington: Univ. Press of Kentucky, 1997.

———. "Realism and Hypertrophy: A Study of Three Medico-Historical 'Cases.'" *Nineteenth-Century French Studies* 22, nos. 1 and 2 (1993–94): 29–47.

———. "Struggling for Medical Reform in Middlemarch." *Nineteenth-Century Literature* 48, no. 3 (1993): 341–61.

Galérant, Germain. *Médecine de campagne: De la Révolution à la Belle Epoque.* Paris: Plon, 1988.

Griffin, Robert J., ed. *Twentieth-Century Interpretations of "Arrowsmith."* Englewood Cliffs: Prentice-Hall, 1968.

Guthrie, Douglas. *Janus in the Doorway.* Springfield IL: Charles C. Thomas, 1963.

Hawkins, Anne Hunsaker. "A. R. Luria and the Art of Clinical Biography." *Literature and Medicine* 5 (1986): 1–15.

———. "The Myth of Cure and the Process of Accommodation: *Awakenings* Revisited." *Medical Humanities Review* 8, no. 1 (1994): 9–21.

———. *Reconstructing Illness: Studies in Pathography.* West Lafayette IN: Purdue Univ. Press, 1993.

Hellerstein, Erna Olafson, Leslie Parker Hume, and Karen M. Offen, eds. *Victorian Women.* Stanford: Stanford Univ. Press, 1981.

Howarth, William. "Oliver Sacks: The Ecology of Writing Science." *Modern Language Studies* 20, no. 4 (1990): 103–20.

Huard, Pierre, and Mirko D. Gremk. "Les Élèves étrangers de Laënnec." *Revue d'histoire des sciences et de leurs applications* 26 (1973): 315–37.

Hunt, Lynn, ed. *The New Cultural History.* Berkeley: Univ. of California Press, 1989.

Hunter, Kathryn Montgomery. *Doctors' Stories: The Narrative Structure of Medical Knowledge.* Princeton: Princeton Univ. Press, 1991.

Illich, Ivan. *Medical Nemesis: The Expropriation of Medical Care.* London: Boyar's, 1976.

Jacyna, Stephen. "Robert Carswell and William Thomson at the Hôtel-Dieu of Lyons: Scottish Views of French Medicine." In French and Wear, *British Medicine in an Age of Reform,* 110–35.

Jarcho, Saul. "An Early Review of Laënnec's Treatise." *American Journal of Cardiology* 9 (1962): 962–69.

———. "A Review of Auenbrugger's *Inventum Novum.*" *Bulletin of the History of Medicine* 33 (1959): 470–74.

Jewson, N. D. "The Disappearance of the Sick-Man from Medical Cosmology, 1770–1870." *Sociology* 10 (1976): 225–44.

Kamm, Josephine. *Hope Deferred: Girls' Education in English History.* London: Methuen, 1965.

Karinch, Maryann. *Telemedicine: What the Future Holds When You're Ill.* Far Hills NJ: New Horizon, 1994.

Katz, Jay. *The Silent World of Doctor and Patient.* New York: Free Press, 1984.

Kent, Susan Kingsley. *Sex and Suffrage in Britain, 1860-1914.* Princeton: Princeton Univ. Press, 1987.

Kenton, Edna. "The Pap We Have Been Fed On." *Bookman* 44, no. 3 (1916): 280–87.

Kett, Joseph. *The Formation of the American Medical Profession: The Role of Institutions, 1780-1860.* New Haven: Yale Univ. Press, 1968.

King, Lester S. *Transformations in American Medicine: From Benjamin Rush to William Osler.* Baltimore: Johns Hopkins Univ. Press, 1991.

Kleinman, Arthur. *The Illness Narratives: Suffering, Healing, and the Human Condition.* New York: Basic, 1988.

Konner, Melvin. *Medicine at the Crossroads: The Crisis in Health Care.* New York: Pantheon, 1993.

Kramer, Lloyd S. "Literature, Criticism, and Historical Imagination." In Hunt, *The New Cultural History,* 97–128. Berkeley: Univ. of California Press, 1989.

Kremer, Richard L. "Building Institutes for Physiology in Prussia, 1836–1846." In Cunningham and Williams, *Laboratory Revolution in Medicine,* 72–109.

Landau, Richard L. " . . . And the Least of These Is Empathy." In Spiro et al., *Empathy and the Practice of Medicine,* 103–9.

Léonard, Jacques. *La France médicale au XIXè siècle.* Paris: Juillard, 1978.

———. *La Médecine entre les savoirs et les pouvoirs.* Paris: Aubier-Montaigne, 1981.

———. *La Vie quotidienne du médecin de province au XIXè siècle.* Paris: Hachette, 1977.

Lerner, Gerda. "The Lady and the Millgirl: Changes in the Status of Women in the Age of Jackson." *Mid-Continent American Studies Journal* 10 (spring 1969): 5–15.

Lipkin, M. *The Care of Patients: Perspectives and Practices.* 2d ed. New York: Oxford Univ. Press, 1987.

MacIntyre, Alisdair. "Medicine Aimed at the Care of Persons Rather Than What?" In *Changing Values in Medicine,* edited by Eric J. Cassell and Mark Siegler, 83–96. Washington DC: University Publications of America, 1979.

Markowitz, Gerald, and David Rosner. "Silicosis and the Politics of Disability." In Rosenberg and Golden, *Framing Disease,* 185–205.

Maulitz, Russell. "Channel Crossing: The Lure of French Pathology for English Medical Students, 1816–36." *Bulletin of the History of Medicine* 55 (1981): 475–96.

———. "Physician versus Bacteriologist: The Ideology of Science in Clinical Medicine." In Rosenberg and Vogel, *The Therapeutic Revolution: Essays in the Social History of American Medicine,* 91–107.

Mishler, Elliot G. *The Discourse of Medicine: Dialectics of Medical Interviewing.* Norwood NJ: Ablex, 1984.

Monroe, William Frank, Warren Lee Holleman, and Marsha Cline Holleman. "Is There a Person in This Case?" *Literature and Medicine* 11, no. 1 (1992): 45–63.

Morantz, Regina Markell. "Feminism, Professionalism, and Germs: The Thought of Mary Putnam Jacobi and Elizabeth Blackwell." *American Quarterly* 34 (winter 1982): 461–78.

Morantz-Sanchez, Regina Markell. "Feminist Theory and Historical Practice: Rereading Elizabeth Blackwell." *History and Theory,* Beiheft 31 (December 1992): 51–69.

———. *Science and Sympathy: Women Physicians in American Medicine.* New York: Oxford Univ. Press, 1985.

Murphy, Lamar Riley. *Enter the Physician: The Transformation of Domestic Medicine, 1760-1860.* Tuscaloosa: Univ. of Alabama Press, 1991.

Newman, Charles. *The Evolution of Medical Education in the Nineteenth Century.* New York: Oxford Univ. Press, 1957.

Noble, Thomas A. *George Eliot's "Scenes from Clerical Life."* New Haven: Yale Univ. Press, 1965.

Nuland, Sherwin B. *Doctors: The Biography of Medicine.* 1988. New York: Vintage, 1995.

Ober, William. "*Arrowsmith* and *The Last Adam.*" In Griffin, *Twentieth-Century Interpretations of "Arrowsmith,"* 57–60.

Paget, Marianne A. "On the Work of Talk: Studies in Misunderstandings." In *The Social Organization of Doctor-Patient Communication,* edited by Sue Fisher and Alexandra Dundas Todd, 55–74. Washington: Center for Applied Linguistics, 1983.

Parry, Noel, and José Parry. *The Rise of the Medical Profession.* London: Croom Helm, 1976.

Parsons, Talcott. *The Social System.* New York: Free Press, 1961.

Payer, Lynn. *Medicine and Culture.* New York: Penguin, 1989.

Pellegrino, Edmund D. "Philosophy, Medical Ethics, and the Physician's Image." In Carson, Reynolds, and Moss, *Patient Wishes and Physician Obligations,* 80–107.

———. "The Sociocultural Impact of Twentieth-Century Therapeutics." In Rosenberg and Vogel, *The Therapeutic Revolution,* 245–66.

Peterson, Jeanne M. *The Medical Profession in Mid-Victorian London.* Berkeley: Univ. of California Press, 1978.

———. "The Victorian Governess: Status Incongruence in Family and Society." In *Suffer and Be Still,* edited by Martha Vicinus, Bloomington: Indiana Univ. Press, 1972.

Poirier, Suzanne, Lorie Rosenblum, Lioness Ayres, Daniel J. Brauner, Barbara F. Sharf, and Anne Folwell Stanford. "Charting the Chart—An Exercise in Interpretation(s)." *Literature and Medicine* 11, no. 1 (1992): 1–22.

Porter, Roy. "The Body and the Mind, the Doctor and the Patient." In *Hysteria Beyond Freud,* edited by Sander L. Gilman, Helen King, Roy Porter, G. G. Rousseau, and Elaine Showalter, 225–66. Berkeley: Univ. of California Press, 1993.

————, ed. *Patients and Practitioners: Lay Perceptions of Medicine in Pre-Industrial Society*. Cambridge: Cambridge Univ. Press, 1986.

Porter, Roy, and Dorothy Porter. *Patient's Progress: Doctors and Doctoring in Eighteenth-Century England*. Cambridge: Polity, 1989.

Reeder, Leo G. "The Patient-Client as a Consumer: Some Observations on the Changing Professional-Client Relationship." *Journal of Health and Social Behavior* 13, no. 4 (December 1972): 406–12.

Reiser, Stanley Joel. *Medicine and the Reign of Technology*. Cambridge: Cambridge Univ. Press, 1978.

Reynolds, Richard C. "Enhancing Doctor-Patient Interactions." In Carson, Reynolds, and Moss, *Patient Wishes and Physician Obligations*, 68–79.

Richardson, Ruth. "'Trading Assassins' and the Licensing of Anatomy." In French and Wear, *British Medicine in an Age of Reform*, 74–91.

Rosenberg, Charles E. *The Care of Strangers*. New York: Basic, 1987.

————. *The Cholera Years: The United States in 1832, 1849, and 1866*. 1962. Reprint, Chicago: Univ. of Chicago Press, 1987.

————. *Explaining Epidemics and Other Studies in the History of Medicine*. New York: Cambridge Univ. Press, 1992.

————. "Martin Arrowsmith: The Scientist as Hero." *American Quarterly* 15 (autumn 1963): 447–58. Reprinted in Griffin, *Twentieth-Century Interpretations of "Arrowsmith,"* 47–56.

————. "The Therapeutic Revolution: Medicine, Meaning, and Social Change in Nineteenth-Century America." In Rosenberg and Vogel, *The Therapeutic Revolution*, 3–25.

Rosenberg, Charles E., and Janet Golden, eds. *Framing Disease*. New Brunswick NJ: Rutgers Univ. Press, 1992.

Rosenberg, Charles E., and Morris Vogel, eds. *The Therapeutic Revolution*. Philadelphia: Univ. of Pennsylvania Press, 1979.

Rothfield, Lawrence. *Vital Signs: Medical Realism in Nineteenth-Century Fiction*. Princeton: Princeton Univ. Press, 1992.

Rothstein, William G. *American Physicians in the Nineteenth Century*. Baltimore: Johns Hopkins Press, 1972.

Safire, William. "Health Care Provider, Heal Thyself." *New York Times Magazine*, 11 April 1993, 12.

Scarry, Elaine. *The Body in Pain: The Making and Unmaking of the World*. New York: Oxford Univ. Press, 1985.

Schorer, Mark. Afterword to *Arrowsmith*, by Sinclair Lewis. New York: Penguin, 1961.

Sheridan, Mary S. *Pain in America*. Tuscaloosa: Univ. of Alabama Press, 1992.

Shorter, Edward. *Bedside Manners: The Troubled Relations between Doctors and Patients*. New York: Simon & Schuster, 1985.

Shryock, Richard Harrison. *The Development of Modern Medicine: An Interpretation of the Social and Scientific Factors Involved.* 1936. Reprint, Madison: Univ. of Wisconsin Press, 1979.

Silver, Jonathan M. "Medical Terms—A Two-Way Block?" *Colloquy: The Journal of Physician-Patient Communications* 1 (November 1979): 4–10.

Spiro, Howard M. "Empathy: An Introduction." In Spiro et al., *Empathy and the Practice of Medicine,* 1–6.

———. "What Is Empathy and Can It Be Taught?" In Spiro et al., *Empathy and the Practice of Medicine,* 7–14.

Spiro, Howard M., Mary G. McCrea Curnen, Enid Peschel, and Deborah St. James, eds. *Empathy and the Practice of Medicine: Beyond Pills and Scalpels.* New Haven: Yale Univ. Press, 1994.

Starr, Paul. *The Social Transformation of American Medicine.* New York: Basic, 1982.

Stewart, Moira, and Debra Roter, eds. *Communicating with Medical Patients.* Newbury Park NJ: Sage, 1989.

Trautman, Joanne. "The Image of the Physician in Twentieth-Century Literature." In Carson, Reynolds, and Moss, *Patient Wishes and Physician Obligations,* 38–53.

Uglow, Jenny. *Elizabeth Gaskell: A Habit of Stories.* Boston: Faber & Faber, 1993.

Vogel, Morris. *The Invention of the Modern Hospital.* Chicago: Univ. of Chicago Press, 1980.

Waddington, Ivan. *The Medical Profession in the Industrial Revolution.* Dublin: Gill and Macmillan Humanities Press, 1984.

Walsh, Mary Roth. *"Doctors Wanted: No Women Need Apply": Sexual Barriers in the Medical Profession, 1835-1975.* New Haven: Yale Univ. Press, 1977.

Warner, John Harley. "The Fall and Rise of Professional Mystery: Epistemology, Authority, and the Emergence of Laboratory Medicine in Nineteenth-Century America." In Cunningham and Williams, *Laboratory Revolution in Medicine,* 110–41.

———. "The Idea of Science in English Medicine: The 'Decline of Science' and the Rhetoric of Reform, 1815–45." In French and Wear, *British Medicine in an Age of Reform,* 136–64.

———. *The Therapeutic Perspective: Medical Practice, Knowledge, and Identity in America.* Cambridge: Harvard Univ. Press, 1986.

Weindling, Paul. "Scientific Elites and Laboratory Organisation in *Fin-de-siècle* Paris and Berlin: The Pasteur Institute and Robert Koch's Institute for Infectious Diseases Compared." In Cunningham and Williams, *Laboratory Revolution in Medicine,* 170–88.

West, Candace. *Routine Complications: Troubles with Talk between Doctors and Patients.* Bloomington: Indiana Univ. Press, 1984.

White, Hayden. *Metahistory.* Baltimore: Johns Hopkins Press, 1973.

Williams, Guy R. *The Age of Agony.* London: Constable, 1973.

INDEX

Abel-Smith, Brian, 127
achromatic microscope, 60
affluent classes, rise of doctor's power among, 145–46
Akerknecht, Erwin, 6, 15
Alexander, G. G., 122
American Medical Association, 218–19
anatomy as focus of research, 59–60, 133, 155
Anderson, Elizabeth Garrett, 96
anesthesia, 148–49
Anthropologist on Mars, An (Sacks), 245–48
antisepsis, 148–49
apothecaries, social status of, 21, 27
apprenticeship, as medical education method, 58
Arrowsmith (Lewis), 105, 163–66, 168–69, 171–78, 180, 181
asepsis, 148
Association of American Physicians, 87
Assommoir, L' (Zola), 125–26, 129, 130, 147
auditory resonance diagnostic method, 56. *See also* stethoscope
Auenbrugger, Leopold, 56
auscultation. *See* stethoscope
autobiography, vs. fiction, 195–96
autopsy, 133, 230
Awakenings (Sacks), 244, 245, 246, 247, 249–50

Babbage, Charles, 58
Balint, Michael, 2, 231–32, 238
Balzac, Honoré de: *La Comédie humaine,* 12, 50, 147; *Eugénie Grandet,* 50; *Médecin de campagne,* 33; *Le Père Goriot,* 50

Barbour, Allen, 224
Becoming a Doctor (Konner), 191, 192–96, 199–200, 202, 204, 207–8, 209–10, 213, 215–16
bedside, as patient-focused location, 15–16. *See also* missionary to bedside, doctor as
Beeton, Isabella, 93
Beier, Lucinda, 7
Berger, John, 53
Berger, Stuart, 241
Bernard, Claude, 153–54
Biasin, Gian-Paolo, 83
Bichat, Pierre-Charles-Alexandre, 59
Blackwell, Elizabeth, 96, 99–101, 119
body snatching, and fear of hospitals, 133
Bogdanich, Walt, 240
Bok, Derek, 186
Book on the Physician Himself (Cathell), 3–6, 11, 47, 98, 105, 127–28, 140–41, 165–66
Bostonians, The (James), 89–92, 107, 108, 110, 119, 122
Brave New World (Huxley), 162
Brody, Howard, 222–23, 229
Broussais, François-Joseph-Victor, 59
Buchan, William, 30
Buddenbrooks (Mann), 36, 83
bureaucracy, growth of medical, 169–71, 227–28

Cabanis, Pierre-George, 41
caring: vs. curing, 183, 212, 244; power surrender in exchange for, 199–200, 201. *See also* holistic approach to medicine; missionary to bedside, doctor as
Cassell, Eric, 230

279

Year Long Night, A (Klitzman), 191–93, 195, 196, 197, 198–99, 200–201, 203, 204, 208, 214

Yersin, Alexandre, 175

Zakrzewska, Marie Elizabeth, 96, 104

Zola, Émile: *L'Assommoir,* 125–26, 129, 130; *Le Docteur Pascal,* 33, 50, 148, 158–59; *Nana,* 83; *Le Roman expérimental,* 153; *Le Rougon-Macquart,* 12, 147